Essentials
of Clinical
Neurophysiology

Essentials of Clinical Neurophysiology

Second Edition

Karl E. Misulis, M.D., Ph.D.

Associate Clinical Professor of Neurology,
Vanderbilt University School of Medicine,
Nashville, Tennessee; Neurologist, Semmes-
Murphey Clinic, Jackson, Tennessee

Butterworth–Heinemann
Boston   Oxford   Johannesburg   Melbourne   New Delhi   Singapore

Library of Congress Cataloging-in-Publication Data

Misulis, Karl E.
    Essentials of clinical neurophysiology / Karl E. Misulis. -- 2nd
  ed.
       p. cm.
    Includes bibliographical references and index.
    ISBN 0-7506-9887-X
    1. Electroencephalography. 2. Electromyography. 3. Evoked
potentials (Electrophysiology) 4. Neurophysiology. 5. Neural
conduction. I. Title.
    [DNLM: 1. Electroencephalography--methods. 2. Electromyography-
-methods. 3. Evoked Potentials--physiology. 4. Neural Conduction-
-physiology. 5. Polysomnography--methods. WL 102 M678e 1997]
  RC386.6.E43M57 1997
  616.8'047547--dc21
  DNLM/DLC
  for Library of Congress   96-50458
                                    CIP

British Library Cataloguing-in-Publication Data
A catalogue record for this book is available from the British Library.

The publisher offers special discounts on bulk orders of this book.
For information, please contact:

Manager of Special Sales
Butterworth–Heinemann
313 Washington Street
Newton, MA 02158–1626
Tel: 617-928-2500
Fax: 617-928-2620
For information on all Butterworth–Heinemann medical publications available, contact our World Wide Web home page at: http://www.bh.com/med

10 9 8 7 6 5 4 3 2 1

Printed in the United States of America

For Christa

Contents

Preface   xi

List of Abbreviations and Units of Measurement   xiii

I. **Basic Electronics   1**

Chapter 1 Physics and Biology of Electricity   3

Chapter 2 Circuit Theory   17

Chapter 3 Filters   29

Chapter 4 Amplifiers   37

Chapter 5 Digital Signal Analysis   47

Chapter 6 Displays   55

Chapter 7 Electrodes and Patient-Electrode Interface   63

Chapter 8 Artifacts and Noise   69

Chapter 9 Electrical Safety   73

II. **Electroencephalography   77**

Chapter 10 Physiologic Basis of Electroencephalography   79

Chapter 11 Technical Requirements for Electroencephalography   85

Chapter 12 Electroencephalography Basics   103

Chapter 13 Normal Electroencephalographic Patterns   111

Chapter 14 Activation Methods   129

Chapter 15 Spikes and Sharp Waves   135

Chapter 16 Slow Activity   151

Chapter 17 Brain Death Studies   155

Chapter 18 Neonatal Electroencephalography   159

Chapter 19 Quantitative Electroencephalographic Analysis   169

Chapter 20 Electroencephalogram
Monitoring   173
Chapter 21 Troubleshooting in
Electroencephalography   179

**III.   Nerve Conduction Studies and
Electromyography   183**
Chapter 22   Basic Principles of Nerve Conduction
Studies and Electromyography   185
Chapter 23   Nerve Conduction Studies   195
Chapter 24 Electromyography   215
Chapter 25 Special Tests of Neuromuscular
Transmission   229
Chapter 26 Quantitative Electromyogram
Analysis   239
Chapter 27 Evaluation of Common Neuromuscular
Problems   243
Chapter 28 Disorders of Peripheral Nerve   251
Chapter 29 Disorders of Muscle   263
Chapter 30 Disorders of Neuromuscular
Transmission   271
Chapter 31 Troubleshooting in Nerve Conduction
Studies and Electromyography   275

IV.   Evoked Potentials   283
Chapter 32 Evoked Potential Basics   285
Chapter 33 Brain Stem Auditory-Evoked
Potentials   293
Chapter 34 Visual-Evoked Potentials   305
Chapter 35 Somatosensory-Evoked Potentials   317
Chapter 36 Evoked Potential Monitoring   327
Chapter 37 Troubleshooting in Evoked
Potentials   331

V.   Polysomnography   333
Chapter 38 Physiologic Basis of Sleep and
Sleep Disorders   335
Chapter 39 Technical Aspects of
Polysomnography   341

Chapter 40 Interpretation of Polysomnographic
    Recordings   347

Glossary   353
Annotated Bibliography   359
Index   361

Preface

It has been 4 years since the first edition of this book was published. I have incorporated new advances in clinical neurophysiology into this edition, along with suggestions from friends, colleagues, and reviewers. The purpose of this text remains to provide information essential for the performance of neurophysiologic studies. Information in this text should be supplemented by comprehensive texts; an annotated bibliography is included in this text.

I would like to acknowledge the work of all of the people cited in the first edition, plus express my sincere appreciation to my partners at the Semmes-Murphey Clinic for their input and patience during completion of this task.

K.E.M.

List of Abbreviations and Units of Measurement

Neurodiagnostic Terminology

BAEP	Brain stem auditory-evoked potential
BSAP	Brief small-amplitude polyphasic
CMAP	Compound motor action potential
EEG	Electroencephalography
EMG	Electromyography
EP	Evoked potential
MUP	Motor unit potential
NCV	Nerve conduction velocity
SNAP	Sensory nerve action potential
SEP	Somatosensory-evoked potential
VEP	Visual-evoked potential

Muscles

The following abbreviations are routinely used by many electromyographers in annotating studies.

ADM	Abductor digiti minimi (or ADQ, abductor digiti-quinti)
APB	Abductor pollicis brevis
EDB	Extensor digitorum brevis
FDP	Flexor digitorum profundus (suffix is 1&2 or 3&4, indicating median or ulnar innervated portions, respectively)
FDS	Flexor digitorum superficialis

1stDI	First dorsal interosseus
LG	Lateral gastrocnemius
MG	Medial gastrocnemius
RF	Rectus femoris
TA	Tibialis anterior
VM	Vastus medialis

Disorders

ALS	Amyotrophic lateral sclerosis
DMD	Duchenne muscular dystrophy
FSH	Facioscapulohumeral dystrophy
MG	Myasthenia gravis
MS	Multiple sclerosis
SMA	Spinal muscular atrophy

Units of Measurement

amp	Ampere
cm	Centimeter
dB	Decibel
Hz	Hertz
kHz	Kilohertz
kohm	Kilo-ohm (1,000 ohms)
mm	Millimeter
ms	Millisecond (0.001 second)
µs	Microsecond (0.000001 second)
mV	Millivolt (0.001 volt)
µV	Microvolt (0.000001 volt)
sec	Second
V	Volt

I

Basic Electronics

1

Physics and Biology of Electricity

Atomic Structure and Charge

Every atom has a nucleus composed of positively charged protons and uncharged neutrons. Negatively charged electrons orbit the nucleus. In most atoms, the number of electrons is equal to the number of protons in the nucleus, and there is no net charge. If the number of electrons is less than the number of protons, then the atom has a net positive charge. If the number of electrons is greater than the number of protons, then the atom has a net negative charge. This is illustrated in Figure 1.1. The atom in Figure 1.1A has a full outer orbital and no net charge. The atom in Figure 1.1B has one empty electron position but still no charge. This atom could donate or accept an electron. Figure 1.1C shows the same atom as Figure 1.1A, but the atom has lost an electron. The atom has a charge of +1, because there are now more protons in the nucleus than electrons in orbitals. Figure 1.1D shows the same atom as Figure 1.1B, but the atom has filled its empty orbital with an electron. The atom has a charge of −1. This is a fairly stable system, in that the orbitals are completely filled.

In the universe, there is electrical neutrality; however, there are local concentrations of charge throughout biological and physical systems. These local concentrations are responsible for all electrical activity from cellular membrane potentials to the power behind neurodiagnostic equipment.

Conductors, Semiconductors, and Nonconductors

Every atom can be induced to give up an electron, but the energy required differs greatly between atoms. Atoms that give up electrons easily can be *conductors*. Conductors allow electrons to pass from

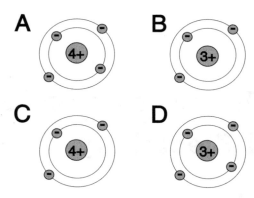

Figure 1.1 Diagram of atomic structure. The rings signify the outer orbitals. A. Atom has a full outer orbital and no net charge. B. Atom has one empty electron position but maintains electrical neutrality. This atom could easily accept an extra electron. Although it would give the atom a negative charge, the orbital would be filled. C. Atom has lost an electron and has a +1 charge. This is a stable state since there are no partially filled orbitals. D. Atom has accepted an electron and has a −1 charge. This is essentially the atom shown in B with the extra electron.

atom to atom, thereby conducting electron flow. Elements such as helium and silicon require so much energy to give up an electron that this action almost never occurs in nature. Such elements are *nonconductors*. Iron easily donates electrons and is stable at two different charge states (+2 and +3). Therefore, iron is an excellent conductor. Iron atoms have a loosely held electron and an empty electron orbital. With charge movement, iron accepts an electron and then releases it. *Semiconductors* are materials that can donate and accept electrons more easily than nonconductors but not as well as conductors. They are discussed in detail in Chapter 4.

Figure 1.2 shows three views of a conductor. Figure 1.2A is the atomic structure of the wire. The 3+ in the circle indicates the valence of the nucleus. The area encompassed by the arcs signifies the orbitals shared by adjacent atoms. A stable situation occurs, even without electric neutrality, when two electrons share an orbital. The *e*s in the circles represent electrons filling some, but not all, orbital positions. The conductor is electrically neutral, which means that there is one electron for each nucleus valence. Figure 1.2B is a less enlarged view of a conductor. It could be considered a magnified view of a wire, which is essentially a cylinder. A potential difference is applied across the conductor, causing electrons to move in the direction indicated by the arrow. Figure 1.2C is a schematic diagram of a conductor

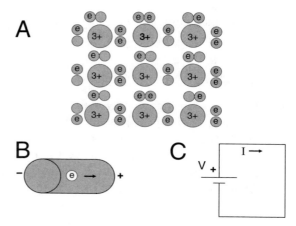

Figure 1.2 Diagram of a conductor. A. Diagram of the atomic structure of a conductor with shared orbitals. The central circle with the number indicates the valence of the nucleus. The circles with *e*s indicate electrons in the outer orbitals. Not all of the protons and electrons are shown. B. A somewhat less enlarged view. C. A schematic diagram of a conductor connected to the terminals of a battery. The plus symbol indicates the positive terminal of the battery. Electrons flow from the negative terminal, through the conductor, to the positive terminal.

attached to a battery. (From this figure on, all electronic equipment is drawn in standard electronic schematic format.) Energy is imparted to the system to make electrons move from one atom to another. The energy required to make the electrons move may be obtained from a variety of sources (e.g., alternating current line voltage, a direct current battery, the electrochemical fluxes of a neuron, or a magnetic field). The driving force for electrons is a potential difference, which is measured in volts. The voltage causes electrons to flow through the wire from the negative terminal and into the positive terminal.

When no energy is applied to the conductor, electrons move randomly, with no net flow in any direction. When a potential difference is created through the wire by a power source, the electrons will have a net movement away from the negative side and toward the positive side. The net movement of electrons through a conductor is *current*. Current is the amount of charge moving through a conductor per unit time. The unit of measurement of current is the ampere, or amp. The unit of measurement of charge is the coulomb. One coulomb is equivalent to 6.24×10^{18} positive or negative charges. One amp of current is equivalent to the movement of one coulomb of charge per second through a conductor; or

$$I = \frac{Q}{t} \quad \text{or} \quad \text{Current} = \frac{\text{Charge}}{\text{time}}$$

We envision that electrons with high energy content flow out of the negative pole, through the wire, and into the positive pole. More accurately, the battery imparts energy to the electrons of the conductor in proximity to the negative pole. Thus, electrons are coaxed to leave their orbitals and flow toward the region of less negative charge—that is, the positive pole. There is a cascading action, with successive electrons in the conductor traveling toward the positive pole. The flow of current was described earlier as the movement of negative charge. However, conventional terminology speaks of the flow of positive charge, which was designated before subatomic structure was understood. One can envision that if electrons are moving from left to right in a conductor, they are essentially skipping from atom to atom, temporarily filling empty orbitals. This is conceptually equivalent to having empty orbitals of atoms moving from right to left. Of course, this does not actually happen. The flow of positive charge is referred to as the flow of holes, which travel in the opposite direction of electron flow. For most of the rest of this discussion, we use the convention of considering current as the flow of positive charge.

Electronic equipment is composed of complex circuitry that can be broken down into functional modules. The basic modules are amplifiers, filters, stimulators, and displays. Each of these is discussed in subsequent chapters after a discussion of circuit theory in Chapter 2.

Electrical Properties of Biological Tissues

Ion Fluxes and Membrane Potentials

Nerve and muscle membranes conduct electricity in a fashion similar to that of wires. When recording electrical activity from a patient, the tissues become an integral part of the circuit. Most of the charge movement in biological tissues can be attributed to passive properties of the membrane or to changes in ion conductance. The important positively charged ions are potassium (K^+), sodium (Na^+), and calcium (Ca^{2+}). The important negatively charged ions are chloride (Cl^-) and proteins ($Prot^-$). Positive ions are *cations*, while negative ions are *anions*. Neuronal membrane has a resting potential of approximately –75 mV due to differential permeability to ions. The sodium-potassium pump forces K^+ into the cell and Na^+ out of the cell.

At rest, the permeability of neuronal membrane to K^+ is greater than to any other ion. Therefore, K^+ diffuses out of the cell and down its chemical gradient. Anionic proteins cannot accompany the K^+ through the membrane, so the interior of the cell becomes negative compared with the exterior. The buildup of charge opposes the further efflux of K^+. When the potential difference is approximately –75 mV, the efflux of K^+ stops. This potential is the equilibrium potential, which is the electrical gradient sufficient to prevent K^+ from flowing down its chemical gradient. The combination of electrical and chemical influences on an ion is its *electrochemical gradient*. This discussion describes the equilibrium potential for K^+ (which is termed E_{K^+}), but the same principle can be applied to every ion. Permeability of the membrane to each ion is termed *conductance* (G). The contribution of each ion to the membrane potential is determined by its conductance. The resting membrane potential approximates E_{K^+} because G_K is so much larger than G_{Na}, G_{Cl}, and so on. The Nernst equation describes the equilibrium potential of ions as a function of their concentrations:

$$E_{Na} = -58 \log \frac{[Na]_i}{[Na]_o} \quad \text{for sodium}$$

$$E_K = -58 \log \frac{[K]_i}{[K]_o} \quad \text{for potassium}$$

$$E_{Cl} = -58 \log \frac{[Cl]_o}{[Cl]_i} \quad \text{for chloride}$$

where E_{Na}, E_K, and E_{Cl} are the equilibrium potentials for sodium, potassium, and chloride, respectively, and the bracketed letters signify the concentrations of the respective ions. The i and o after the bracket indicate that the concentration is *inside* or *outside* of the cell. The formula for E_{Cl} shows outside-inside concentration reversed in comparison with E_{Na} and E_K, because chloride is negatively charged. An equilibrium potential can be described for each ion. However, these ions are the most integrally involved in the resting membrane potential. In addition to these ions, calcium (Ca^{2+}) is important for action potentials.

The membrane potential depends on which ions have the greatest conductance. Since potassium has the greatest conductance at rest, then the resting membrane potential is closest to E_K or –75 mV. When an excitatory neurotransmitter activates the postsynaptic receptors, the conductance to sodium is increased. Therefore, the membrane potential approaches E_{Na}

(which is approximately +45 mV) and can be described as a function of the equilibrium potentials of individual ions weighted by the conductance to each ion. This relationship is described in the Goldman constant field equation.

$$V = -58 \log \frac{G_K[K]i + G_{Na}[Na]i + G_{Cl}[Cl]o + \ldots}{G_K[K]o + G_{Na}[Na]o + G_{Cl}[Cl]i + \ldots}$$

The ellipses at the end of the numerator and denominator indicate that additional ions will contribute to the equation, but at rest they are such minor contributors that they are not shown here. This equation appears complex but is simplified when one considers which ions are of predominant importance. At rest, the conductance to sodium and chloride is relatively low compared to that of potassium, so the factors for Na$^+$ and Cl$^-$ become insignificant compared to that for K$^+$. Therefore, the equation can be reduced to essentially to:

$$V = -58 \log \frac{G_K[K]i}{G_K[K]o}$$

Since the G_K drops out:

$$V = -58 \log \frac{[K]i}{[K]o}$$

This is essentially the same as the equilibrium potential for K$^+$. Therefore, the resting potential approaches –75 mV but is not exactly that value because of a small contribution from Cl$^-$ and Na$^+$.

Action Potential

Action potentials develop in nerve and muscle fiber in response to depolarization. Neurotransmitter molecules bind to the post-synaptic membrane receptors. These receptors open channels for the influx of sodium, thereby depolarizing the cell. An action potential only develops if the depolarization reaches the threshold that is determined by the voltage-dependent property of sodium channels. Depolarization causes the opening of additional sodium channels. With faster and greater depolarization, more and more channels open. Of course, each open channel further increases the conductance to sodium, producing further depolarization. Eventually, the depolarization is sufficient to be regenerative. That is, a vicious cycle is established whereby depolarization produces more depolarization. This is *threshold*. The sodium conductance is so great that the membrane potential overshoots zero and becomes positive. The sodium channels are not only voltage dependent but also time dependent. Time

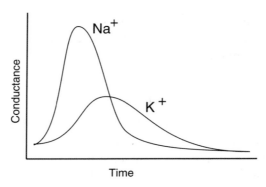

Figure 1.3 Sequence of ion conductance changes during an action potential. The initial phase of sodium (Na) conductance causes the depolarization. Potassium (K) conductance subsequently increases, resulting in repolarization. Since the potassium conductance outlasts the drop in sodium conductance, there is some hyperpolarization of the membrane following the action potential.

dependent means that the channels can stay open only for a specified period of time. After that time they close, even though the cell is depolarized. With closure of the sodium channels, conductance to sodium declines, and the membrane potential once again approaches the equilibrium potential of potassium.

Figure 1.3 shows changes in membrane potential and ion conductances with an action potential. The upper curve shows the changes in sodium conductance discussed in the previous section. The lower curve is potassium conductance. Since the chemical gradient for potassium favors efflux, the late increase in potassium conductance causes repolarization of the cell and even some hyperpolarization as the membrane potential approaches the equilibrium potential for potassium.

It should be evident from this discussion that incremental depolarization can add together to bring an area of membrane to threshold for action potential generation. This summation must occur within a short time, however, because the sodium channels are not only voltage-dependent but time-dependent. If a membrane is gradually depolarized, sodium channels will open at specified voltage levels and close a short time later. The recently open channels will be closed by the time there is opening of additional channels. The recently open channels cannot open again until the membrane repolarizes. This is similar to a gun's trigger mechanism;

after the trigger is pressed, it cannot be pressed again until the weapon is cocked. For a neuronal membrane, this is accomplished only by repolarization of the membrane.

Nerve Conduction

Nerve cells conduct their impulses to subsequent neurons by two methods, *electrotonic conduction* and *action potential propagation*. When the electrical impulse is conducted to the nerve terminal, the depolarization promotes release of vesicles of the neurotransmitter that act on the postsynaptic cells.

Electrotonic conduction is only effective over relatively short distances. Depolarization of a point of membrane results in the spread of the depolarization to adjacent membrane. The magnitude of the depolarization falls off with increasing distance. If the depolarization is not sufficient, there may be no change in the amount of transmitter released from the nerve terminal.

Action potential propagation occurs when electrotonically conducted depolarization is sufficient to create an action potential in an adjacent membrane. This depolarization then excites the membrane adjacent to it, and so on. Therefore, the action potential is propagated down the axon, with no loss of depolarization throughout the course. Therefore, action potential propagation allows the signal to be conducted along much longer distances than electrotonic conduction. Action potentials are generated in the axon hillock, which is at the origin of the axon from the cell body (soma). The axon hillock is depolarized by stimulation of receptors, on primarily dendrites, that produce depolarization that is conducted toward the soma.

Saltatory conduction relies on electrotonic conduction and action potential propagation, but the velocity of conduction is much faster. Myelin sheaths separate nodes of excitable membrane, so that an action potential at one node can be conducted electrotonically to the next node. At that node, an action potential is produced that then activates the next node and so on. Electrotonic conduction between nodes is much faster than action potential propagation, so that conduction is faster than in unmyelinated fibers. Normally, electrotonic spread of potential difference would not be sufficient to bring an area of membrane to threshold so far from the starting node, but the myelin sheath greatly increases the membrane impedance, so that the *length constant* is increased (i.e., the length over which the potential decays is decreased because it is more difficult for ions to move between the axoplasm and interstitial fluid with the myelin sheath).

Synaptic Transmission

Depolarization of the nerve terminal results in opening of ionic channels, including those that admit calcium. Calcium entry promotes the release of transmitter from the presynaptic terminal; the transmitter molecules then cross the junction to bind to receptors on the postsynaptic membrane. Chemical transmission is the predominant mode of neuronal communication, although there are also electrical junctions through which electrical potentials can be conducted directly from one cell to another. Figure 1.4A shows release of transmitter from the presynaptic terminal onto the postsynaptic membrane. Changes in potential are conducted electrotonically across the membrane, as shown in Figure 1.4B. Figure 1.4C shows the postsynaptic potentials recorded, with one potential not reaching threshold but the second reaching threshold for action potential generation.

Chemical transmission can be excitatory or inhibitory; the action is dependent on the postsynaptic receptor rather than the particular chemical. If the chemical binding elicits influx of sodium and depolarization of the postsynaptic membrane, the response is excitatory; this is an excitatory postsynaptic potential (EPSP). On the other hand, if binding of the chemical to the receptor produces an increased conductance to potassium, chloride, or both, the effect is inhibitory. The movement of these ions will prevent the postsynaptic membrane from reaching threshold; this is an inhibitory postsynaptic potential (IPSP). The most common excitatory transmitter in the brain is glutamate. Gamma-aminobutyric acid and glycine are inhibitory transmitters. There are many other transmitters, and the list of identified agents continues to grow.

EPSPs usually occur due to increased conductance to sodium, calcium, or both. As the conductance to sodium increases, the influx diminishes the resting membrane potential so that the cell approaches zero potential. Because the conductance to sodium is greater than that to any other ion, the membrane potential approaches the equilibrium potential for sodium, which is positive (approximately +45 mV).

Several EPSPs may be needed to generate sufficient depolarization to produce a regenerative action potential. Therefore, the release of transmitter is dependent on action potential generation and is, therefore, all or none. Some interneurons do not generate action potentials. Instead, depolarization of the postsynaptic membrane is electrotonically conducted to the cell's terminal. This depolarization, in turn, produces release of transmitter. Since the release of transmitter is directly related to the degree of depolarization, the transmission is graded, as compared with the all-or-none transmission of action potential generating neurons.

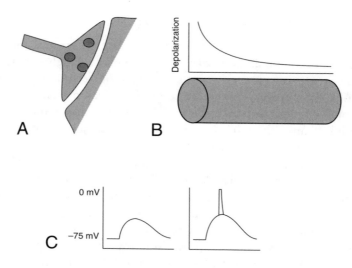

Figure 1.4 Synaptic transmission and action potentials. A. Basic mechanisms of synaptic transmission. Depolarization of the terminal on the left causes release of transmitter vesicles into the cleft. The transmitter binds to the postsynaptic receptor on the postsynaptic membrane across the synaptic cleft. B. Electrotonic depolarization of adjacent membrane. The inward current on the left results in depolarization of membrane further to the right. C. Effect of depolarization on membrane potential. On the left is a potential that does not reach threshold. On the right is a potential that reaches threshold and results in an action potential.

IPSPs are typically due to increased conductance to potassium, chloride, or both. The equilibrium potential for potassium is more negative than the resting membrane potential, so increased potassium conductance hyperpolarizes the cell. The equilibrium potential for chloride is more positive than the resting membrane potential but is still negative at approximately −55 mV. Therefore, increased conductance to chloride depolarizes the membrane but effectively prevents the membrane potential from becoming much less than −55 mV.

Generation of Electrical Activity by Nerve and Muscle

The generators of EEG and EMG activity are discussed in greater detail in Chapters 10 and 22, respectively. In general, the potentials recorded in clinical neurophysiologic studies have as origins (1) action potentials in nerve fiber bundles, whether they be peripheral nerves or central nerve tracts, and (2) extracellular potentials generated by movement of ions into and out of cells during depolarization and repolarization. Since most electrophysiologic recordings are extracellular and at some distance from the origin of the potential, detecting most responses depends on simultaneous activation of many nerve or muscle fibers, because their electrical activity combines to produce a compound potential. These potentials are conducted through the tissue of the body and detected by the electrodes. This introduces the concepts of *volume conduction* and *field potentials*.

Field Potentials and Volume Conduction

The influx of sodium during an action potential is effectively an inward current. An intracellular electrode would see this as a positive potential, because the interior is becoming more positive than it was at rest. An extracellular electrode would see this as a negative potential because of the shift of positive charge from the extracellular space into the cell. The extracellular potential can be recorded at a considerable distance from the cell and is known as a *field potential*. The movement of charge from excitable tissue through surrounding tissues is called *volume conduction*. Field potentials are often described as near-field and far-field potentials. Near-field potentials are recorded by electrodes close to the membrane, whereas far-field potentials are recorded at a distance. To illustrate, consider a peripheral nerve conducting a volley of action potentials. Refer to Figures 1.5, 1.6, and 1.7. The near-field potential can be recorded by a unipolar or bipolar recording arrangement. For a unipolar recording, the active electrode (G1, for Grid 1 from tube terminology) is directly overlying the nerve, and the reference (G2) is on the same limb but not overlying the nerve (see Figure 1.5). As the wave of depolarization passes under G1, the inward current causes a prominent negative wave. As the wave passes, the potential returns to baseline.

Bipolar recording is similar to a unipolar recording except that G2 is over a distal segment of the nerve (see Figure 1.6). The initial negative component is as previously described. As the depolarization passes under G2, however, a positive phase occurs because the amplifier is measuring the difference in potential between G1 and G2. Depolarization at G1 makes G1 negative relative to G2. Depolarization at G2 makes G2 negative relative to G1, but this means that G1 is positive relative to G2. Therefore, the recording is biphasic. The far-field potential is recorded with G1 at a distance from the current

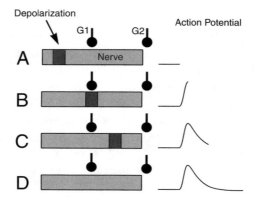

Figure 1.5 Unipolar near-field potential. This diagram should be compared with the two that follow. For each figure, the cascading figures show the effect of propagation of an action potential on the recording. The wave of depolarization travels from left to right. G1 is the active electrode. G2 is the reference and is not overlying the excitable membrane. A. Wave of depolarization has not yet reached the membrane under the electrode. B. Maximal negativity occurs when the wave of depolarization is directly under the recording electrode. C. The potential decays as it passes away from the active recording electrode. D. The depolarization is long gone and the potential is back to baseline.

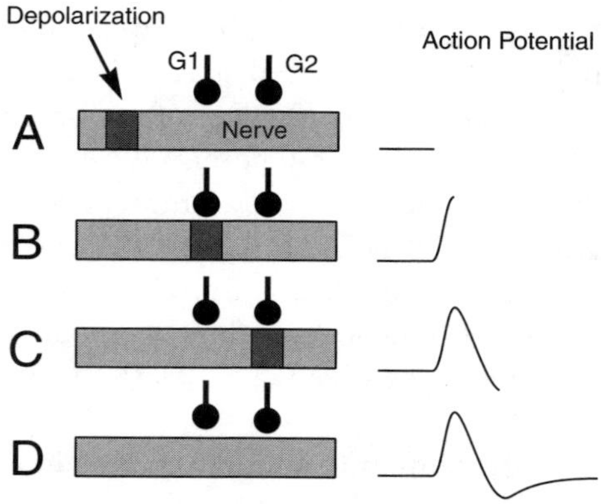

Figure 1.6 Bipolar near-field potential (compare with Figures 1.5 and 1.7). The recording setup is similar to that of Figure 1.3 except that G2 is located over a distal nerve segment. A. The wave of depolarization has not yet reached the electrodes. B. Maximal negativity occurs as the wave of depolarization passes under G1. C. Maximal positivity ensues as the wave of depolarization passes under G2. D. The depolarization is passed and the potential returns to baseline.

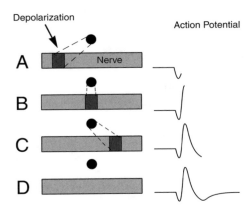

Figure 1.7 Far-field potential (compare with Figures 1.5 and 1.6). G1 is distant from the nerve. G2 is not shown and is located distant from G1. A. The advancing front of depolarization produces a positive far-field potential. B. As the depolarization travels beneath the electrode, a negative potential is seen. C. The receding phase of repolarization produces a following positive phase. D. The potential has passed and the potential has returned to baseline.

generator and G2 at a greater distance, typically in a different tissue compartment (see Figure 1.7). The far-field potential is a stationary wave that is due to the moving front of depolarization in the axons. Since the far-field potential is recorded at a distance, it is not governed by exact electrode position. If the nerve volley comes close to the active or reference electrode, a component of near-field potential can be seen. Most of the potentials recorded in clinical neurophysiology are far-field potentials. The notable exception is the compound action potentials of nerve conduction studies, which are largely near-field potentials.

2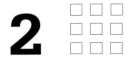

Circuit Theory

A circuit is a closed loop or series of loops composed of circuit elements. Current requires a closed loop in order to flow; it will not flow into the blind end of a conductor. Circuit elements include power supplies, resistors, capacitors, inductors, and transistors. This chapter first discusses circuit elements and then presents the laws governing the function of electric circuits.

Circuit Elements

Power Supply

The power supply provides the energy to drive electrons (or holes) around the circuit. It produces a potential difference that the electrons flow down. Power can come from many sources, including alternating current line voltage, direct current batteries, or the voltage change across neuronal membranes. The potential difference is measured in volts (V).

Resistors

A resistor opposes the flow of electrons by converting the energy imparted to the electrons into heat. Thus, the electrons leaving a resistor have lost a considerable amount of energy. Resistance (R) is measured in ohms, which are named after the nineteenth-century German physicist Georg Ohm. If a volt meter is placed across the terminals of a resistor, a recordable voltage difference is produced when current is flowing. This is termed the *voltage drop* across the resistor and is indicative of the amount of energy dissipated by the resistor. If no current is flowing, there is no energy to dissipate, and the volt meter would report no voltage drop.

Capacitors

Capacitors store energy in the form of separation of charge. Briefly, a capacitor is made up of two plates of conducting material separated by a thin layer of a nonconducting material. Current flowing through the circuit results in the buildup of excess electrons on one plate and excess holes on the other plate. The dynamic of the charging and discharging of these plates is responsible for the frequency dependence of many electronic circuits. A more in-depth discussion of capacitors appears later in this chapter in the section on Theory of Capacitors. Frequency dependence makes the capacitors crucial to filters, which are discussed again in Chapter 3 in the section on Filters.

Inductors

Inductors store energy in the form of a magnetic field. Briefly, an inductor is a length of conducting wire that is wound into a very tight coil. The passage of current through the coil creates a strong magnetic field. This magnetic field can, in turn, influence the flow of current. The result is a complex relationship between the applied voltage and subsequent current. Inductors are included in most electronic equipment. The process of induction is especially important in the generation of noise, though this type of induction is not intended. Inductors are discussed in more detail later in this chapter in the section on Theory of Inductors.

Semiconductors

Semiconductors are key elements of modern amplifiers and filters and are discussed in Chapter 4. They conduct electricity better than nonconductors but not as well as conventional conductors, that is, they semiconduct.

Laws Governing Circuit Theory

Ohm's Law

Ohm's law describes the relationship between current (I), resistance (R), and voltage (V) in a circuit or a circuit element.

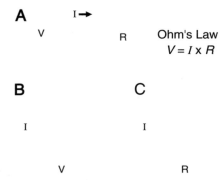

Figure 2.1 Ohm's law. A. A simple circuit diagram of a resistor in series with a battery. By Ohm's law, the voltage of the battery (*V*) is equal to the current (*I*) times the resistance of the resistor (*R*) (*V* = *I* × *R*). Although Ohm's law applies to this simple circuit, it is defined to apply to the voltage dissipated by individual resistors within more complex circuits. B. A graph showing the relationship between voltage and current. C. A graph showing the relationship between resistance and current.

$$V = I \times R$$

Ohm's law: The applied voltage is equal to the current multiplied by the resistance of the circuit.

This formula is used mainly to describe resistive circuits. Figure 2.1 shows a simple circuit that illustrates Ohm's law. The schematic in Figure 2.1A shows a resistor in series with a battery. The voltage of the battery (*V*) is equal to the induced current (*I*) times the resistance of the resistor (*R*). The same general principle is operative with capacitors, although the resistance of capacitors is dependent on the frequency of the applied voltage. The formula *V* = *I* × *R* may not seem intuitively obvious, but the relationship becomes clearer when permutations of the formula are considered (see Figure 2.1).

- When resistance is fixed, the applied voltage and resulting current have a direct relationship. Therefore, an increase in applied voltage produces a proportionately greater current flow.
- When voltage is constant, resistance and current have an inverse relationship. Therefore, an increase in resistance produces a reduction in current.

Ohm's law is the basis by which other circuit laws are derived.

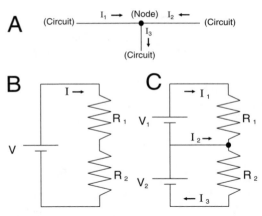

Figure 2.2 Kirchhoff's laws. A. Kirchhoff's current law. This is a schematic diagram of the junction point of three conductors. I_1, I_2, and I_3 are the currents in each conductor. The current flowing into the node must equal the current flowing out. B. Kirchhoff's voltage law. A battery is in series with two resistors, R_1 and R. The voltage applied must be equal to the sum of the voltage drops across the two resistors. C. Kirchhoff's voltage law applies to each of the three potential loops in this schematic diagram: (1) the upper loop with battery V_1 and resistor R_1, (2) the lower loop with battery V_2 and resistor R_2, and (3) the large loop encompassing both batteries and both resistors.

Kirchhoff's Current Law

Kirchhoff's current law states that for any node, the sum of the currents flowing into and out of the node is zero. A *node* is a junction point of two or more conductors. Figure 2.2A shows one node in a circuit. The loops of the circuit are all complete, but the remainder of the elements making up the circuit are not shown. I_1, I_2, and I_3 are the currents flowing through the three wires into and out of the node. The node has no capacity to store or produce energy and has no ability to alter energy imparted to it. Therefore, the sum of all the current flowing into a node equals the current flowing out.

Expressed mathematically:
$$I_3 = I_1 + I_2$$
or, rearranging:
$$I_1 - I_2 - I_3 = 0$$
Since currents flowing out of the node are actually negative:
$$I_1 + I_2 - I_3 = 0$$
Or, for any node:
$$\Sigma I_i = 0$$

Kirchhoff's Voltage Law

Kirchhoff's voltage law states that for any circuit loop, the sum of the voltage sources is equal to the sum of the voltage drops. In other words, for any loop of a circuit, the energy imparted to the loop must equal the energy dissipated. This makes sense, because the circuit elements use all available power coming from the power source. Figure 2.2B shows a battery forming a circuit loop with two resistors in series. The energy is imparted by the battery (V), and the voltage is dissipated by resistors R_1 and R_2. Current (I) flows from the battery through the two resistors. Since there is only one path, the current is equal through all portions of the loop. If the current is multiplied by the resistance of one of the resistors (R_1), the product is called the *voltage drop* across the resistor (V_1). This is an adaptation of Ohm's law $(V = I \times R)$, where the voltage drop across a resistor is equal to the resistance of the resistor (in ohms) multiplied by the current flowing through the resistor (in amps). Kirchhoff's voltage law can be reworded to read for any circuit loop, the sum of the voltage sources is equal to the sum of the voltage drops.

Expressed mathematically:
$$V_T + V_1 + V_2 = 0$$
or, for any loop:
$$\sum V_i = 0$$

Kirchhoff's voltage law applies to any loop, even though it may be part of a larger circuit. In Figure 2.2C, Kirchhoff's voltage law applies to both the top and bottom loops. In fact, it also applies to the large loop that encompasses both batteries and both resistors.

Theory of Resistors

Resistors impede the flow of electrons through a circuit. Energy is dissipated because resistors convert the energy imparted to the electrons by the power supply into heat. Since the electrons have less associated energy, they flow less forcefully down their electrical gradient toward the ground. Therefore, resistors decrease the effective voltage of the electrons— that is, a voltage drop occurs. If the two terminals of a battery are connected by a wire (Figure 2.3A), a massive flow of current between the terminals would quickly destroy the battery. However, if a resistor is placed in the wire (Figure 2.3B), some of the energy imparted to the electrons would be converted to heat and fewer electrons would flow to the positive terminal. The current would be reduced.

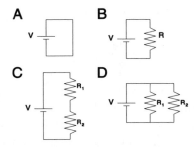

Figure 2.3 Theory of resistors. A. The terminals of a battery are connected by a wire, resulting in a massive but brief flow of current. The current stops as the battery is discharged. B. The leads of a resistor are connected to the terminals of the battery. Current flows from the positive terminal through the resistor and into the negative terminal. Energy is dissipated at the resistor as heat. C. Two resistors are connected in series. The total resistance of the circuit in C can be represented as an equivalent resistance (R_{eq}). This would look similar to diagram B, with R being R_{eq}. D. Two resistors are connected in parallel. The total resistance can be represented as R_{eq} as for C.

Series Resistance

If current runs through two or more resistors connected serially, energy will be dissipated by both resistors. In Figure 2.3C, V is the total voltage delivered to the battery, I is the current through the entire circuit, R_1 and R_2 are the resistances of the two resistors, and V_1 and V_2 are the voltage drops across the two resistors. Figure 2.3B can represent the same circuit with the serial resistors represented as a single equivalent resistance. The purpose of these equations is to determine the equivalent resistance of the two resistors connected in series.

From Ohm's Law:
$$V_1 = I \times R_1 \text{ and } V_2 = I \times R_2$$
And from Kirchhoff's voltage law:
$$V = V_1 + V_2$$
and the equivalent resistance of the system is
$$R_{eq} = \frac{V}{I}$$
then:
$$R_{eq} = \frac{(I \times R_1) + (I \times R_2)}{I} = R_1 + R_2$$
Thus for series resistances:
$$R_{eq} = \Sigma R_i$$

For resistors in series, the total resistance is equal to the sum of the individual resistances.

Parallel Resistance

In a circuit with branch points, the laws for circuit loops still apply for each loop. In Figure 2.3D, the total current (I_T) traveling from the positive and negative terminals of the battery splits into the two parallel resistor arms. The amount of current down each path depends on the relative resistances. From Kirchhoff's voltage law, the voltage drop across R_1 equals that across R_2, which equals the imparted voltage of the battery (V), since there are three circuit loops that can be examined. The parallel resistances can be represented by an equivalent resistance (termed R_{eq}) as in Figure 2.3B. Thus:

From Ohm's law:
$$V_1 = I_1 \times R_1 \text{ and } V_2 = I_2 \times R_2$$
rearranging:
$$I_1 = \frac{V_1}{R_1} \text{ and } I_2 = \frac{V_2}{R_2}$$

Since from Kirchhoff's current law:
$$I_T = I_1 + I_2$$
Substituting from the equations above:
$$\frac{V}{R_T} = \frac{V_1}{R_1} + \frac{V_2}{R_2}$$

But we know from Kirchhoff's voltage law that:
$$V_1 = V \text{ and } V_2 = V$$
So, substituting the last equations:
$$\frac{V}{R_T} = \frac{V}{R_1} + \frac{V}{R_2}$$

V drops out of both sides of the equation:
$$\frac{1}{R_T} = \frac{1}{R_1} + \frac{1}{R_2}$$

or:
$$\frac{1}{R_T} = \Sigma \frac{1}{R_i}$$

For resistors in parallel, the total resistance is equal to the reciprocal of the sum of the reciprocals of the individual resistances.

One corollary of this formula is that total resistance is always less than any of the individual resistances. This makes sense because, for any resistor, if you provide an additional pathway, electrons will find the path easier. To illustrate, consider the analogy of a bucket of water. If a small hole is placed in the bottom of the bucket, a small stream of water will flow out because of the high resistance. If there are two small holes, the flow will be substantially faster, even though each hole has relatively high resistance. This is because the resistance of each resistor is a lot less than the resistance of the bucket walls to the flow of water, and conduit for flow, no matter how high the resistance, will reduce the total resistance to water flow.

Conductance (G) is the reciprocal of resistance. In the analogy, the ability of each hole to allow water flow is the conductance of that hole. The greater the resistance, the less the conductance, and vice versa. If there are several resistors in parallel (or several holes in the bucket), then the total conductance is equal to the sum of the individual conductances.

Expressed mathematically:
$$G_T = G_1 + G_2 + G_3 + ...$$
Where G_T is the total conductance and G_1, G_2, and G_3
are the conductances of the individual resistors.
Since conductance is the reciprocal of resistance:
$$\frac{1}{R_T} = \frac{1}{R_1} + \frac{1}{R_2} + \frac{1}{R_3} + ...$$

This last formula arrives at the same conclusion as the previous calculations for parallel resistances.

Theory of Capacitors

Capacitors store energy by separating electrons from holes. They are composed of two thin plates of conducting material separated by a thin layer of nonconducting material. Figure 2.4A shows an electrical diagram of a capacitor. Wires are attached to the two plates for connection with the rest of the circuit, which in this case consists only of a battery. Figure 2.4B is a close-up of the same capacitor showing electrons flowing onto one side of the plate from the negative terminal of the battery, while holes flow onto the other side from the positive terminal. Actually, on the positive side, electrons flow from the plate and into the positive terminal, leaving holes. Considering this structure, it is evident that electrons cannot flow through the capacitor, since they cannot jump the thin gap between the plates. Because the plates

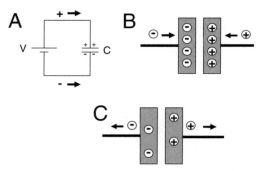

Figure 2.4 Theory of capacitors. A. A capacitor is connected to the terminals of a battery. Charge flows from the battery to the plates of the capacitor. Current (I) flow stops when the charge on the capacitor is equal to and opposite the charge of the battery. B. Close-up of the plates of the capacitor with the leads to the battery on the right and left sides. Circles with (+) symbols indicate movement of "holes," while circles with (–) symbols indicate movement of electrons. C. When the potential difference is abolished, the holes and electrons stream off of the plates. This requires an intact circuit (not shown).

are so close, electrons sent to one plate repel electrons on the other plate, making them travel out the other wire. Thus, electrons can flow onto one plate, which in turn causes electrons to flow from the next, producing an apparent current flow through the capacitor, although the current is not being carried by the same electrons. This current is a capacitative current, since no electrons actually complete the journey through the capacitor.

Capacitative current results in a buildup of voltage difference across the capacitor. Subsequently, the negative charge on one plate counterbalances the potential difference of the power supply. When the voltage across the capacitor plates is equal to but opposite from the voltage of the power supply, the flow of electrons stops. Figure 2.4C shows the capacitor after the potential difference is turned off. (The complete circuit is not shown.) The potential difference across the capacitor forces electrons off one side of the plates and holes off the other. In other words, electrons flow off the plate that has an excess of electrons, through the circuit, and onto the plate with a deficit of electrons (excess holes), thereby filling the holes and discharging the voltage across the capacitor. Thus, following cessation of applied voltage, there is reversal of flow of current due to the voltage difference developed across the plates of the capacitor.

The characteristics of a capacitor depend on its capacitance (*C*), which is measured in farads (named after Michael Faraday, an eighteenth-century

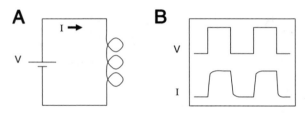

Figure 2.5 Theory of inductors. A. A diagram of an inductor. A coil of wire is connected to the circuit by the two ends of the wire. A magnetic field is oriented along the axis indicated by the arrow. B. A graph of the effects of changing applied voltage on current through an inductor. An inductor resists changes in current.

English chemist and physicist). This property reflects how much charge can be built-up on a capacitor for a given voltage. If the capacity (capacitance) is low because the plates are small, then a relatively high voltage will be built-up after very little current flow. In contrast, if the capacitance is large, then much more current must flow onto the plates in order to develop a comparable voltage. Expressed mathematically:

$$I = k \frac{dV}{dt}$$

where k is a proportionality constant that represents the capacitance of the capacitor. The value k can be used to represent the capacitance of the capacitor, therefore, becoming C. Thus:

$$I = C \frac{dV}{dt}$$

In other words, the capacitative current is proportional to the rate of change of voltage. This is an important concept. The implication of this relationship is that capacitative current is frequency dependent. Frequency dependence is an important factor used in designing high- and low-frequency filters (see Chapter 3). Capacitance is also important in generation of noise in neurodiagnostic recordings and is further discussed in Chapter 8.

Theory of Inductors

Inductors store energy in the form of a magnetic field created by the movement of charge. When current flows through a wire, it produces a weak magnetic field that is oriented circumferentially to the wire (Figure 2.5). An inductor consists of a coil of conducting wire with two leads incorporated into a circuit. When current flows through the wire, the coiling makes the magnetic fields orient in the same direction, along the axis of the coil. The influence of the magnetic field on the flow of electrons is to oppose a change in current. Current through an inductor cannot change instantaneously. If the voltage is increased, some of the additional energy will also increase the magnetic field. Therefore, current does not build up as much as would be expected without an inductor in the circuit. If current is decreased (by reducing the voltage), some of the energy in the magnetic field will be imparted to electrons in the conducting coil, thereby transiently maintaining current. This exchange of energy occurs because the greatest effect on the flow of electrons is not the presence of a magnetic field, but the change in a magnetic field. The process of induction, which is an important cause of noise in neurodiagnostic recordings, is discussed in Chapter 8.

3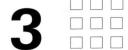

Filters

All biological signals can be broken down into fundamental frequencies, with each frequency having its own intensity. Display of the intensities of all frequencies is called a power spectrum. In clinical neurophysiology, we are usually interested in signals of a particular frequency range or *band width*. The band width differs for individual studies. Certain frequencies are less clinically useful and may actually obscure important information. Therefore, unwanted frequencies are filtered out of the displayed signal. Figure 3.1 shows how a biological signal is composed of its fundamental frequencies. The diagram in Figure 3.1A shows how a high-frequency signal, such as spikes, can be added to a low-frequency signal, such as a sine wave, to produce a complex waveform. The diagram in Figure 3.1B shows power spectra for the corresponding signals. The complex signal is composed of both high- and low-frequency components. Filters can be active or passive. Active filters use exogenous energy to alter the waveform, while passive filters do not. This chapter discusses passive filters first. Fundamental to the passive filter is the resistor-capacitor (RC) circuit.

Resistor-Capacitor Circuits and Passive Filters

The key to filter theory is the RC circuit, which is illustrated in Figure 3.2A. A resistor (R) and capacitor (C) are in series with a power source that is the signal voltage (V_S). The effects of a sudden change in voltage (*step voltage*) on current and voltage drops across the resistor and capacitor are illustrated in 3.2B. Immediately after the voltage is turned on, current (I) begins to flow through the circuit. As current flows, a voltage difference develops between the two terminals of the resistor (since $V_R = I \times R$). This current also results in a build-up of charge on the capacitor as capaci-

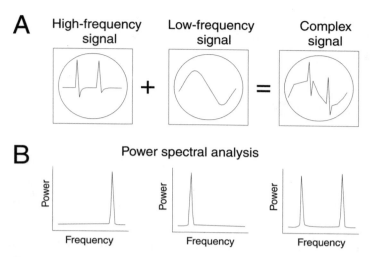

Figure 3.1 Frequency components of biological signals. A. Diagram of oscilloscope traces of a complex signal. The left diagram shows a signal composed mainly of fast frequencies. The middle shows a signal composed of a slow wave. The right trace is the summation of the two. B. Power spectral analysis of the signals shown in A. Summed signal can be represented as a sum of the power spectral analysis; a complex signal can be broken down into fundamental frequencies.

tative current flows. The charge on the capacitor opposes the flow of further current, ultimately stopping flow when the voltage on the charged capacitor is equal and opposite to the applied signal voltage. When no current is flowing, there is no voltage across the resistor ($V_R = I \times R$ with $I = 0$).

When the voltage is suddenly decreased to baseline, the only source of current is the charged capacitor. Electrons flow off the lower plate toward the battery. Likewise, electrons from the battery flow through the conductor and through the resistor to occupy the holes on the upper plate of the capacitor. Current is flowing opposite to the direction it was flowing when the voltage was applied. In summary, when there is a sudden change in voltage, the voltage is high across the resistor and low across the capacitor. As voltage increases on the capacitor, the voltage across the resistor decreases exponentially and eventually falls to zero as the current stops.

For the capacitor:

$$I = C \times \frac{dV}{dt}$$

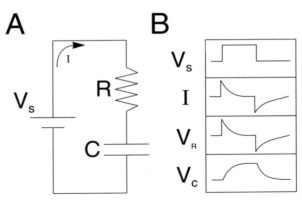

Figure 3.2 Resistor-capacitor circuit. A. A schematic diagram of the resistor (R) and capacitor (C) connected in series to a battery. B. The effects of a step voltage on current and voltage drops across the resistor and capacitor. The resistor has a voltage across it only when current is flowing. The capacitor develops a potential between the plates that is proportional to the total charge flowing onto the plates. The formula for V_R is Ohm's law. The formula for V_C is the formula for voltage across a capacitor. (V_S = signal voltage; I = current; V_R = voltage difference across the resistor; V_C = voltage difference across the capacitor.)

Where C is the capacitance and dV/dt is the change in voltage with time. Since, in Figure 3.2A, the voltage across the capacitor (V_C) represents the cumulative flow of charge onto the plates, V_C is inversely proportional to the capacitance and directly proportional to the total amount of charge that has gone onto the plate (i.e., the integral of current with respect to time).

Or:

$$V_C = \frac{1}{C} \times \int I \, dt$$

For the resistor, from Ohm's law:

$$V_R = I \times R$$

Since from laws of capacitors:

$$I = C \times \frac{dV}{dt}$$

then:

$$V_R = R \times C \times \frac{dV}{dt}$$

This means the following:

- The voltage drop across the resistor (V_R) is greatest when the signal voltage (V_S) is changing, and
- The voltage across the capacitor (V_C) is greatest when the signal voltage is not changing (at steady state).

In other words, if the voltage across the two elements of the circuit is measured, the voltage differences across the resistor responds to changes in signal voltage and cuts out low frequencies, whereas the voltage difference across the capacitor responds to steady-state signal voltages and cuts out high frequencies. This is the basis for high- and low-frequency filters. The signal is applied across an RC circuit with an amplifier looking at the voltage across either the resistor or the capacitor. If the amplifier is measuring the voltage across the capacitor, the device is a high-frequency filter. If the amplifier is measuring the voltage across the resistor the device is a low-frequency filter. Electrical devices use high-frequency filters and low-frequency filters in tandem to eliminate the high and low ends of the frequency spectrum. The voltage of a battery that is being turned on and off is essentially a square-wave pulse that has both high- and low-frequency components, a slow-frequency step component and a fast-frequency phasic component, representing the rise and fall of the step (as the switch is turned on and off). In reality, biological signals are complex and are made up of a mixture of fast and slow frequencies. The exponential rate at which current and voltage rise and fall in an RC circuit is described by the time constant (TC). The TC, measured in seconds, is the time required for a step voltage to charge the capacitor to within 37% of the signal voltage. Thirty-seven percent is derived from the reciprocal of the natural logarithm, e, which is approximately 2.7 ($1/e = 0.37$, or 37%). The TC is dependent on the resistance and capacitance of the RC circuit. The larger the capacitance, the longer the current will have to flow to charge the capacitor. The larger the resistance, the less current will flow, again requiring a longer time to charge the capacitor. In other words, the TC is directly proportional to both capacitance (C) and resistance (R). Thus:

$$TC = k \times R \times C$$

Where TC is the time constant and k is a proportionality constant. Since this is an exponential function, and TC is defined as the time to $1/e$ of maximum, then the proportionality constant drops out, leaving:

$$TC = R \times C$$

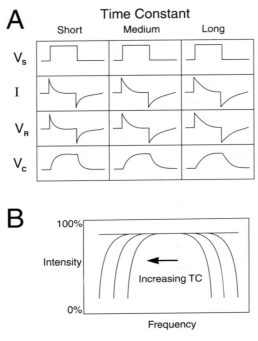

Figure 3.3 Effect of time constant (TC) on frequency response. A. Changes in response to a step voltage with different time constants. B. Frequency response curves with differing time constants. While the term *time constant* is usually used to indicate the response of the low-frequency filter, change in time constant governs response of the high-frequency filter. (V_S = signal voltage; I = current; V_R = voltage difference across the resistor; and V_C = voltage difference across the capacitor.)

Using this relationship, filters of the desired time constants are selected, allowing passage of the appropriate frequency band to the amplifier while rejecting the others. Separate TCs are selected for both the high- and low-frequency filters so that the appropriate band width is selected. Figure 3.3A illustrates the effect of varying TC on the voltage profiles developed across a resistor (V_R) and capacitor (V_C). High-frequency filters look at V_C, and low-frequency filters look at V_R. The limitation of the voltage profiles imposed by the selected filters is the frequency response curve. Figure 3.3B shows the effect of changing the TC on the power spectrum allowed by the filters. Effects on both high- and low-frequency filters are shown. The half-amplitude frequency is the frequency for either high- or low-frequency filters in which the ratio of output to input voltage has fallen by one-half (6 decibels [dB]). The term *turnover frequency* refers to the frequency at which the decrease in frequency response has fallen to approximately 70% (3 dB) of the maximum. Below the turnover frequency, the rate of decrease is accelerated. The speed of this decline is termed the *roll-off* and is expressed as dB/octave. For example, the roll-off may be 6 dB/octave—that is, the response is cut in half (6 dB) for each octave change in frequency. For both high- and low-frequency filters, this frequency can be calculated from the resistance and capacitance of the circuit by the following formula:

$$70\% \text{ frequency} = \frac{1}{2\pi RC}$$

An example of the use of this formula is the determination of turnover frequency of machines in which the low-frequency filter specification is given as time constant rather than frequency. Some EEG machines represent the low-frequency filter settings by the TC, since this is easy to measure on the calibration pulses. Most EEG machines represent the high-frequency filter by the 3-dB (70%) frequency.

Active Filters

Active filters require energy to modify the input waveform. They are composed of an amplifier and other circuit elements. Feedback loops reduce the amplification of signals that are above or below a specified frequency. A power supply, such as a battery or transformer, drives the amplifier. The principles of frequency-dependent response are the same as that described for passive filters, but the circuitry is much more complex. Most equipment used in clinical neurophysiology uses active filters. It is not important to understand circuit schematics of active filters. Rather, it is more important to grasp the concepts of frequency response and the fundamentals of filter theory.

Digital Filters

Analog-to-digital conversion is discussed in Chapter 5; however, digital filtering will be considered briefly here. The computer converts the analog signal into digital format after some preamplification and filtering. Digital filters do not compensate for the distortions in the signal made by previous analog filters. Digital filters allow for further modification of the signal, however. Digital filters are essentially calculations performed on the digitized data. A common method of digitally filtering is to perform a Fourier transformation of a segment of data, reduce the value of selected frequencies, and then compute the inverse Fourier transformation. Other methods use interrelationships between data points in complex calculations that will not be discussed here. The effects of digital filtering are difficult to represent graphically and even more difficult to understand conceptually. Digital filtering does not result in a smooth frequency-response curve, as does analog filtering. One specific type of digital filter does not produce the phase distortions characteristic of analog filters; however, a frequently employed digital filter does. The commonly held belief that all digital filters prevent phase distortions is incorrect.

60-Hertz Filters

EEG machines have a 60-Hz filter, which is sometimes referred to as a *notch filter*. This filter subtracts out activity in the 60-Hz range (the frequency of line power), thus removing artifact from line voltage that affects the physiologic recording. The 60-Hz filter also cuts some frequency response slightly above and below 60 Hz, however. Using the 60-Hz filter during recording of EEG activity can distort the recording of muscle activity by making it resemble beta activity. Therefore, this filter should not be used to compensate for 60-Hz noise caused by high-electrode impedances.

4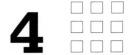

Amplifiers

Amplifiers are integral to all equipment used in clinical electrophysiology. Transistors are the critical component of modern amplifiers. They replaced vacuum tubes, which had a limited life span and were much more expensive to make. Most amplification is performed by integrated circuits or chips, which are wafers that contain many components in complex circuits.

Transistors are a class of semiconductors. Understanding semiconductors is essential to understanding transistors and amplifiers.

Semiconductor Theory

Semiconductors are poorer conductors than some materials but are better than others—that is, they semiconduct. The solid materials that make up semiconductors do not conduct as well as most metals having fewer loosely held electrons or fewer holes. Silicon and germanium, which normally have very low conductance, are doped with impurities to increase the numbers of holes and electrons available for movement in an electric field. The doping process controls the degree of conductance. Doping the tetravalent base material (e.g., silicon or germanium, Figure 4.1A) with a pentavalent element (e.g., arsenic) causes one electron to be held less tightly than the others, so that it is available for conduction of charge (Figure 4.1B). Since the loosely held charge is negative, the material is referred to as an *N-doped material*. If, on the other hand, the material is doped with a trivalent element (e.g., gallium), the absence of sufficient electrons to fill all of the orbitals will leave a hole or place of deficiency of an electron, even though there is electrical neutrality (Figure 4.1C). This is *P-doped material*. Thus, N-doped materials have electrons available for movement, whereas P-doped materials have areas that have a potential space for electrons.

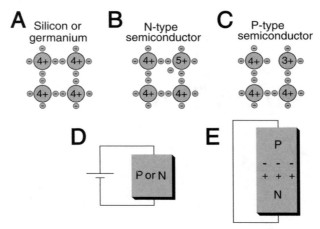

Figure 4.1 Semiconductors. A. Parent structure of semiconductors. This matrix of tetravalent atoms is essentially a nonconductor. B. N-doped semiconductor. The pentavalent atom has an "extra" electron that is available to conduct current. C. P-type semiconductor. The trivalent atom causes a hole in the electron orbitals that can accept electrons moving in transit as current. D. Semiconductor connected to a battery. Current will flow regardless of whether the semiconductor is N-type or P-type. E. An N-P junction. Some electrons from the N-doped side will cross into the P-doped side and fill the empty orbitals. This migration progresses until the charge built up across the junction is sufficient to inhibit further movement of electrons.

Current can flow either way through N- or P-type semiconductor material. If a battery is connected to two ends of one of these materials, electrons will flow in and a corresponding number of electrons will flow out (Figure 4.1D). The useful properties of semiconductors appear when two or more dissimilar semiconductors are adjacent (Figure 4.1E). This figure shows adjacent N and P semiconductor materials, termed an *NP junction*. When these materials are placed together, electrons diffuse from the N region to the P region, filling some of the empty orbitals of the P region. This diffusion occurs until the relative attraction of the empty orbitals of the P material for electrons is counterbalanced by a charge differential built up across the junction. This is similar to the physiologic basis for the resting membrane potential in neural tissue. In NP junctions as well as neural membranes, an electrical field is built up at the junction that establishes an equilibrium with the driving force for flow of electrons. If voltage is applied so that positive current flows into the P region and negative current into the N region, then the electrical field built up at the junction of the semi-

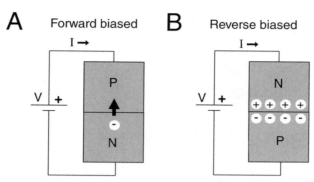

A   Forward biased   **B**   Reverse biased

Figure 4.2 Diode function. A. Forward-biased junction. Current can flow because the applied potential dissipates the junction potential, allowing more electrons to cross the junction. Electrons flow from N to P. The arrow indicates the flow of positive current. B. Reverse-biased junction. The applied potential only accentuates the junction potential, preventing flow of current. In the region of the junction, the N-doped material is depleted of electrons, whereas the P-doped material has the orbitals filled. (I = current; V = volts; N = N-doped semiconductor material; P = P-doped semiconductor material.)

conductors is reduced and current can flow (Figure 4.2A). If, on the other hand, positive voltage is applied at the N region, the diffusion potential is augmented and the flow of current is blocked (Figure 4.2B), because the electrons from the N material have crossed to the other side of the junction to fill the empty orbitals of the P material and are unavailable for conduction of current. Similarly, the holes of the P material near the junction are filled. Thus, this junction allows for conduction only in one direction, and the junction is functioning as a diode. If the voltage applied across the semiconductor junction results in flow of current, it is forward biased. If the voltage is applied in the opposite direction, so that no current flows, it is reverse biased.

Transistors

The term *transistor* is derived from the words *transfer* and *resistor*, since the transistor controls the transference of energy across a resistance. Transistors work like vacuum tubes in older electrophysiologic equipment. In both tubes and transistors, a small gating current controls the flow of a much greater current along another pathway. This is analogous to an automobile, in which the relatively small amount of force applied to the gas

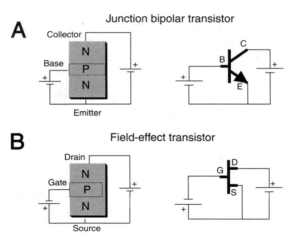

Figure 4.3 Transistor construction. For both sections of this figure, a diagram illustrating composition is on the left, and a schematic diagram is on the right. A. Junction bipolar transistor. Potential applied across the base and emitter controls current flow from the collector to emitter. The upper junction is reverse biased and will not conduct, but with applied potential, the "excess" electrons are removed, allowing current to flow. B. Field-effect transistor. Potential applied across the gate and source controls current flow between the drain and source. An applied potential blocks conduction through the thin N segment. No free electrons are available for conduction. (G = gate; D = drain; S = source; C = collector; B = base; E = emitter.)

pedal by the driver's foot proportionately controls the much greater force of the engine.

There are several types of transistors, but they essentially operate on the same principle. Schematic diagrams of a field-effect transistor and a junction bipolar transistor are shown in Figure 4.3. Both have three connections to the transistor. Conductance between two of the terminals (*drain* and *source* or *emitter* and *collector*) is influenced by the voltage bias delivered across the third (*gate* or *base*). In transistors, a small controlling voltage can gate the flow of electrons through a circuit with larger voltage by changing the resistance of the transistor. Therefore, amplification is one of the most common uses for transistors. The junction bipolar transistors are of two types, NPN and PNP. The letters refer to the configuration of the three layers that make up the transistor. N stands for negative and P stands for positive, as is detailed in the preceding section on semiconductors. Thus, the NPN has positively doped material in the middle layer, whereas PNP has negatively doped material in the middle layer. For either type of junction bipolar transistor, the controlling terminal is the base, and the controlled current flows between the emitter and collector.

For an NPN bipolar junction transistor (Figure 4.3A), the base-emitter junction (between P and lower N wafers) is forward biased, so that current can flow. In contrast, the pathway through the transistor from emitter to collector includes the reverse-biased upper N-P junction, as well as the forward-biased P–lower N junction. Therefore, little current will flow in the collector-emitter circuit. When voltage is applied across the base and emitter and the electrical barrier between P and lower N is reduced, however, the barrier between P and upper N is reduced as well. This is because the equilibrium potential at upper N-P, which normally prevents current flow, is reduced by electrons on the P side of the junction that are being sucked off into the base, leaving available holes. As a result, conduction between the collector and emitter is facilitated. The way the transistor is designed, the base P material is very thin, so only a very small base-emitter voltage must be applied to facilitate large conductances between collector and emitter. Thus, controlling voltage across base and emitter governs conductance of a much greater voltage applied across the collector and emitter. This is the basis of amplification using the junction bipolar transistor. Field-effect transistors function similarly to bipolar junction transistors, but the movement of charge is somewhat different. Field-effect transistors transform a small increase in controlling voltage to a large decrease in controlled current (Figure 4.3B). In this case, the gate-source junction (controlling circuit) is reverse biased, so that virtually no current flows through the junction when voltage is applied. In contrast to the junction bipolar transistor, the field-effect transistor has a drain and source of contiguous N-type materials that allow unobstructed current flow. However, as voltage is applied across the gate-source circuit, the region of depletion of electrons and holes (at the junction of the N and P regions) is enhanced. This effect is most pronounced at the thin connecting segment between the drain and source. Carriers of charge are removed from this segment. Within a certain range this effect is proportional. Therefore, whereas this action is similar to that of the junction bipolar transistor, the effect is actually opposite in sign, (i.e., increasing gate-source voltage decreases drain-source conductance).

Amplifiers

Amplifiers are quite complex compared to RC circuits and transistors. Their function is conceptually easy to understand, however. They magnify the signal so that it can be displayed. Figure 4.4A shows a

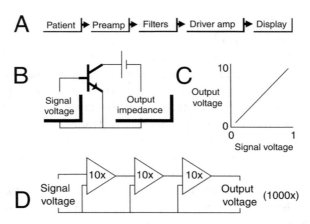

Figure 4.4 Amplifiers. A. Pathway of signal movement from patient ultimately to the display of the apparatus. B. Schematic of a single-stage amplifier. The signal voltage controls the impedance to flow through the resistor. This controls current through the right side of the circuit. The voltage drop across the output impedance is greater than the input voltage. C. Input-output relationship of the amplifier shown in B. D. Three-stage amplifier. Each stage represents approximately 10× gain, for a net gain of 10^3 or 1,000×.

schematic diagram of the pathway of electrical information from the patient to display. Shortly after the biological signal enters the electrophysiologic device, and before any signal processing takes place, a preamplifier boosts the signal.

There are two reasons for preamplification: (1) so that the filters have sufficient signal voltage to deal with and (2) so that the level of signal voltage is much higher than that of system noise. The filters are positioned after the preamplifier to exclude unwanted information before the signal is sent to the driver amplifier. The function of the driver amplifier is to increase the signal intensity sufficiently to drive a chart pen or oscilloscope beam. Both amplifiers require an exogenous power source whose output is controlled by the signal voltage. Figure 4.4B shows a transistor circuit with a signal voltage that varies between 0V and 1V. The signal voltage controls conductance through the right side of the circuit, so that the output impedance sees proportionately between 0V and 10V of a 20V output power supply (Figure 4.4C). The gain of this simple amplifier is 10×. Depending on the size of the output power supply, the potential gain could potentially be much larger. However, semiconductors break down at high differential voltages so the amplification of each amplifier stage is fixed at 9×. For example, to get a gain of 1000×, at least three stages must be used. Thus, the amplifier stages are placed in series, as in Figure 4.4D. Ideally, each amplifier stage should draw minimal current from the preceding stage. Otherwise, amplification is decreased, and the signal may be distorted. The distortion is due to frequency-dependent effects of the amplifier-to-amplifier connection, by virtue of capacitance in the transistors and in other components of the amplifiers. In conventional neurodiagnostic equipment, the draw of current from the signal voltage source and from the preceding amplifier stage is many orders of magnitude less than the output current and is therefore negligible.

Differential Amplifiers

The differential amplifier, sometimes called a *balanced amplifier*, is used extensively in neurophysiologic equipment. Its major advantage is the property of common mode rejection. A standard amplifier compares a signal voltage in the active input to a common reference (Figure 4.5A). Unwanted signals are amplified to the same degree as biological signals. The main unwanted signal in clinical situations is 60-Hz activity, which is caused by line voltage passing through nearby electrical circuits. The differential amplifier is designed to reject unwanted signals through the use of an inverting circuit. The power supply voltage is inverted, so that a positive input voltage results in a proportional negative output voltage. In all other respects it functions as a standard amplifier. In Figure 4.5B, the signal voltages V1 and V2 are compared. The standard amplifier is labeled +10×, whereas the inverting amplifier is –10×. The output voltage is the sum of the two amplifiers. The effect of this arrangement is that any signal applied in common to the two electrodes (V1 and V2) cancel each other out and are not seen in the output (i.e., the modes in common to the two electrodes are rejected, which is called *common mode rejection*). The 60-Hz activity affects both inputs equally and is canceled out. This results in an improved output signal (Figure 4.5C). The common mode rejection does not work as well on high-amplitude signals because the input impedance and the amplifying characteristics of the two amplifiers are not exactly the same. The common mode rejection ratio (CMRR) is equal to applied common input voltage divided by the output voltage.

$$\text{CMRR} = \frac{\text{Common signal voltage}}{\text{Nonamplified output voltage}}$$

For modem amplifiers the CMRR is about 10,000 to 1. However, the CMRR can be degraded by very high or very different electrode impedances that serve to change the signal voltage perceived by the inputs of the

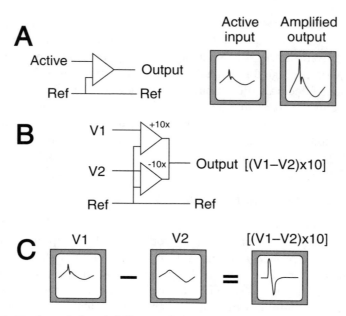

Figure 4.5 Single-ended and differential amplifiers. A. Single-ended amplifier. The output is a magnified representation of the input. B. Differential amplifier. The output is a magnified representation of the difference between signals V1 and V2. C. Simulated oscilloscope traces of the inputs and output of the differential amplifier shown in B. The slow activity in common to both inputs is magnified equally but cancels out because the second channel output is inverted. The spike, which is only seen in V1, is amplified in the output.

amplifiers. The differential amplifier is used for EEGs in montages that compare two electrodes. In Figure 4.6, the preamplifiers first boost the signal for ease of filtering and noise reduction and then feed the amplified signals to the amplifiers. In this diagram, the standard and the inverting amplifiers are included in one amplifier symbol (i.e., the V2 for one channel is the V1 for the next). This is an example of the left parasagittal portion of the longitudinal bipolar montage. This serial bipolar arrangement is responsible for the reversal of localized cortical potentials. Using Figure 4.6 as an example, consider the display of a surface negative spike focus at C3. The amplifier arrangement would deliver a negative potential to the top input of a differential amplifier, causing an upward pen deflection, and a negative potential to the bottom input, causing a downward pen deflection. The signal produced by a negative potential at C3 is seen predomi-

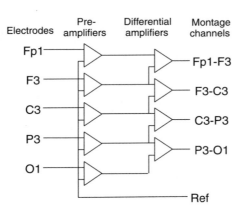

Figure 4.6 EEG amplifier. Preamplifiers boost signal intensity and feed their output to the differential amplifiers. In this figure, the differential amplifiers are represented as a single symbol. The electrodes and connections comprise the left parasaggital portion of the longitudinal bipolar montage. Note that in this bipolar montage, the secondary (inverted) input for one channel is the primary (noninverted) signal for the next.

nantly in two channels, F3-C3 and C3-P3. In the F3-C3 channel, the negative spike in the bottom input to the differential amplifier causes a downward pen deflection and the negative potential in the top input of the C3-P3 channel of the differential amplifier causes an upward pen deflection. Therefore, the two spikes point toward one another (toward the focus) when the two channels are displayed serially on paper.

5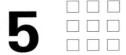

Digital Signal Analysis

Visual inspection is the first and often most important type of signal analysis. A neurophysiologist or technician looks at the signal, whether it be EEG, EMG, or evoked potential (EP), and answers several questions.

- Is the recording equipment functioning properly?
- Is there a biological signal from the patient?
- Is there an artifact that interferes with the assessment of the recording?

Only after satisfactorily answering these questions does the individual attempt to characterize the recording. Visual analysis usually suffices for EEG, but for EMG and EP, quantitation of the response improves diagnostic accuracy. Measurements of latency and amplitude can be compared with the results obtained from the same nerves of patients of similar ages and temperatures. These measurements add diagnostic sensitivity to the interpretation, since there is usually general agreement as to what constitutes a normal or abnormal response. Measurements of latency and amplitude do not require digital signal analysis, but in practice, modern neurophysiologic equipment uses digital analysis not only to facilitate measurements but also for routine display.

Digital analysis for EMG and EP has not only aided making measurements but also has allowed for averaging of responses. In fact, without averaging multiple responses, most EPs could not be identified. Although digital analysis of EMG and EP responses is important, it is crucial that the technician, the neurophysiologist, or both look at the raw signal. Data that are averaged, filtered, retouched, and measured may look plausible, but the old adage, "garbage in, garbage out," still holds true.

Digital analysis has been more problematic for EEG than for EMG and EP. The spectrum of normal and abnormal waveforms is huge, and waves must be interpreted in the context of wake-sleep state and coexisting EEG patterns. Therefore, digital analysis of EEG has focused on selected pieces of data, such as frequency content, without attempting to make correlations between waves and patterns. *Power spectral analysis* and *brain mapping* (Chapter 19) are two applications of this technique. A larger use of a digitized EEG signal is not for analysis, per se, but for display on computer screens. Digital EEG display has several advantages, two of which are (1) the ability to reformat the stored display so that a single epoch can be viewed in different montages, and (2) the ability to change gain and filter settings after the recording has been made at the convenience of the neurophysiologist. Digital EEG analysis is used as a tool to display EEG data and to add a bit of quantified information, but it is still secondary to visual analysis.

Analog-to-Digital Conversion

An *analog signal* is a wave that fluctuates continuously in voltage. Digital conversion consists of measuring the voltage at regular intervals and recording the voltage in a region of computer memory (Figure 5.1). Computers store information in digital format, so the analog voltage at each specified time is converted into a binary format by dividing the voltage range into several levels, which are coded in binary format. For example, with a two-bit analog-to-digital (A/D) converter, the possible combinations of the two bits are shown in Table 5.1.

The number of possible voltage levels is equal to 2 raised to the power of the number of bits. For example, $2^2 = 4$ and $2^3 = 8$. Most neurodiagnostic equipment uses A/D converters of at least twelve bits, and $2^{12} = 4,096$. Four thousand voltage levels are more than sufficient to accurately represent any physiologic analog signal. Time resolution of the A/D converter depends on capabilities of the converter, duration of the recording epoch, and the number of channels to be sampled. Speed of conversion can be described by at least three terms: sampling rate, intersample interval (ISI), and dwell time. *Sampling rate* is the preferred term. It simply indicates the number of conversions per second. *ISI* is the inverse of sampling rate, and is expressed as either ms or μs. *Dwell time* is similar to ISI, but should probably not be used. It is a misleading term in that one might conceive of the A/D converter "dwelling" on the sample for the entire time, perhaps continuously sampling during that interval. In reality, the converter takes its sample then waits until the internal clock indicates that it is time to take the next sample.

Virtually all A/D converters can convert at least 40,000 samples per second. Most are much quicker. An A/D converter can sample several channels; however, it must do so sequentially. For example, a measurement is made

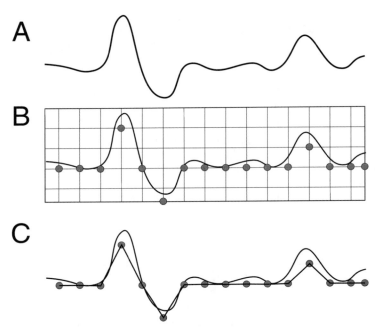

Figure 5.1 Analog-to-digital conversion. A. Analog biological signal that is to be digitized. B. Grid placed over the signal. Each vertical line is the time of sampling. Each horizontal line is a voltage level that can be discerned by the digital converter. At each sampling time, the highest voltage level crossed is the digital voltage recorded. A dot at the intersection of the time and voltage line indicates the digitally measured data point. C. Waveform reconstructed from the digitized data. The wave is essentially lines connecting the digitized data points.

from channel 1, then channel 2, then channel 3, then channel 4, then back to channel 1. In this example, the maximum conversion rate per channel would be 40,000/4, or 10,000, samples per second. Clearly, the more channels sampled, the poorer the time resolution of the averaged signal. Epoch duration determines how many samples will be needed. The sampling rate must be set to be appropriate to the epoch duration. For example, if one wants to sample an epoch of 10 seconds for a sympathetic skin response, a sampling rate of 100,000 per second would be excessive. Not only is that degree of resolution not necessary, but the computer memory would also be monopolized by the 1,000,000 data points required. On the other hand, sampling at too slow a rate degrades the recording.

Table 5.1   Binary-to-Decimal Conversions

Bit 1	Bit 2	Bit 3	Decimal Value
	Two-bit format		
0	0	—	0
0	1	—	1
1	0	—	2
1	1	—	3
	Three-bit format		
0	0	0	0
0	0	1	1
0	1	0	2
0	1	1	3
1	0	0	4
1	0	1	5
1	1	0	6
1	1	1	7

Aliasing refers to an error that occurs when the sampling rate is too slow for the frequency components of the signal (Figure 5.2). Figure 5.2A shows a sine wave, which is simpler than virtually all biological signals. The vertical lines are the sampling times, and the dots are the voltages measured at each sampling time. Figure 5.2B is the waveform reconstructed from the data points measured in Figure 5.2A. The wave has a sine-like appearance; however, the frequency of the wave is much lower than that of the original signal. In order to adequately represent a digitized signal, the sampling rate must be at least twice the frequency of the fastest component.

Quantitative Analysis

The spectrum of quantitative analysis is huge, but commonly used applications include scalar measurements made on the digital signal, averaging, frequency analysis, digital filtering, artifact rejection, and spike detection. Digital filters are discussed in Chapter 3. Spike detection frequency analysis and brain mapping are discussed in Chapter 19. Artifact rejection is discussed in more detail in Chapter 32.

The most common measurements made from digitized signals are for nerve conduction studies where latency and amplitude are of prime importance. The digitized signal also allows measurement of the integrated amplitude of the waveforms, since integrated amplitude is a better estimate of the number of axons or muscle fibers activated than absolute amplitude.

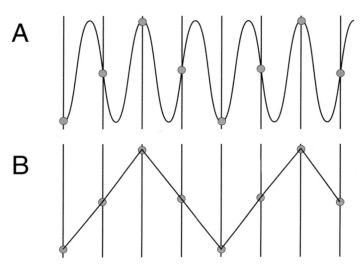

Figure 5.2 Aliasing. A. Sine-wave signal. Vertical lines are sampling times of the analog-to-digital converter. Dots are measured voltages at each sampling time. B. Waveform reconstructed using the data points measured in A. The frequency of this wave is much less than that of the original signal.

Averaging

Averaging is needed for neurodiagnostic studies that require the identification of small amplitude potentials (i.e., EPs and sensory nerve action potentials). The steps to averaging are as follows:

1. Recording of analog signals
2. Digitization of the signal
3. Storage of the data points into memory
4. Acquisition and digitization of additional trials with addition of data to corresponding data points already in memory
5. Division of data registers by the number of trials
6. Display of the averaged waveform.

Signal averaging consists of acquisition of multiple trials, digitization of each trial, and averaging of the digital data in the computer's memory. The first trial is stored directly in the computer's memory. Subsequently, each additional trial is recorded in memory and the total divided by the number of acquired trials. In this way, the computer memory holds a running average of the trials.

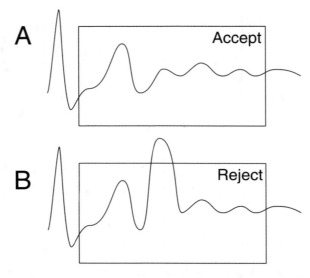

Figure 5.3 Artifact rejection. An electronic window is represented by vertical lines. A. The potential falls completely within the window. Therefore, this trace will be accepted into the average. The stimulus artifact at the beginning of the trace occurs before the sampling begins; therefore, this does not prevent acceptance of the trial. B. A high-voltage transient falls outside of the window. The entire trace will be rejected. The display will usually indicate *Accept* or *Reject* on the display.

Averaging allows detection of a response time-locked to the stimulus, since electrical activity not related to the stimulus is averaged out. However, artifact that is time-locked to the stimulus will also be averaged and can be misinterpreted as a viable response. The improvement in ability to detect the desired signal over unrelated electrical activity, or *noise*, is quantified in the signal-to-noise ratio, which is discussed in detail in Chapter 8.

Artifact Rejection

Artifact rejection is an essential part of every signal averaging program (Figure 5.3). The averager rejects from the average any trial that appears contaminated by artifact. An electronic window is preset so that the averager can distinguish artifact from physiologic signals. The entire trial is rejected if it contains any potentials whose amplitude is outside the window, because high-voltage inputs to an amplifier may produce a temporary block of the amplifier response, which would cause instability of amplification and unpredictable frequency response for several seconds.

Power Spectral Analysis

Power spectral analysis consists of separating the waveforms into fundamental frequencies, determining the relative amplitudes of each frequency in the signal for a specified epoch. Power spectra were introduced in Chapter 3.

Calculation of power spectra involves complex formulae. A common approach is to determine the variance in voltage for the selected epoch. Then, discrete frequencies are tested against the signal to determine how much of the variance can be accounted for by the specified frequency. The greater the amount of signal that can be accounted for by the frequency, the greater the frequency in the signal.

Power spectra are displayed in various formats. Common methods are graphical and colorimetric. Graphic methods display frequency on the X axis and power on the Y axis. For each epoch and channel of information, a separate graph can be displayed, or the graph can be a sum or average of activity across multiple channels. Color displays can be expressed by showing a color that roughly indicates power. For example, a channel that shows mainly slow activity could be represented by blue, while a channel that has predominantly fast activity can be represented by red or yellow. The possible variations are endless. Formatting the data for display is easy when the calculations are done.

6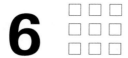

Displays

Displays are generally either video screen or paper. Both are mainly used to show changes in signal over time, but other types of information can also be shown. Printed reports will include sample traces as well as measurements.

Screen Displays

Cathode Ray Tube

Evoked potential and EMG equipment use cathode ray tubes (CRT), which have the ability to display much faster signal changes than the pen display of EEG. This is because the projected electrons have little mass or inertia. The pen, on the other hand, has substantial inertia by virtue of the coil, pivot, and mass of the pen mechanism.

The CRT uses a controlled beam of electrons (the cathode ray) to excite phosphors on the screen for visible display (Figure 6.1). The source of the electrons is a hot cathode. A large amount of energy is imparted to the electrons so that they can escape the parent metal. The electrons are accelerated and focused into a beam by a series of plate electrodes, chiefly anodes, that attract electrons. After the beam is focused, it passes between two sets of deflecting plates oriented at right angles to each other. The deflecting plates control the horizontal and vertical movement of the beam. For EMG and evoked potential, the amplified signal voltage is applied across the plates that control vertical movements.

Time base signal controls the horizontal movements. The *time base* is a voltage delivered to the horizontal deflecting plates that causes the beam to move gradually from left to right with time. At the completion of the sweep the horizontal plate voltage quickly changes so that the beam is ready to make another sweep. The time base refers to the speed of the horizontal

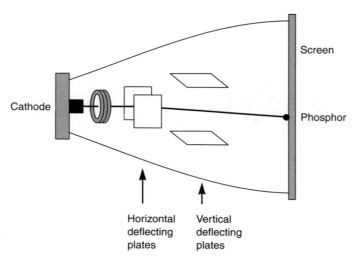

Figure 6.1 Cathode ray tube. A hot cathode creates an electron source that is accelerated and focused by the anode. Output from the time base is delivered to the plates governing horizontal deflection of the electron beam. Output from the driver amplifier is delivered to the plates governing vertical deflection of the electron beam. Impact of the electron beam onto the screen causes phosphorescence and emission of photons.

ramp voltage and therefore to the speed of movement of the beam across the screen. Figure 6.2A illustrates the actions of different time base settings on the voltage applied to the horizontal deflecting plates of the CRT.

The sweep can be triggered in several ways, as is shown in Figure 6.2B. In EMG needle studies, the sweep begins as soon as the previous sweep is completed. In stimulus-triggered sweeps, the time base begins the horizontal ramp when it receives a pulse from the stimulator. Line triggering is more complicated. In line triggering, the sweep is triggered when a signal of sufficient amplitude and rise time is received along the biological signal channel. This type of triggering is used to examine jitter on EMG.

On the CRT, electrons transfer energy into the phosphor on impact. As energy is lost, photons of light are emitted from the phosphor for visual display.

When studying nerve conduction velocity, the amplification is chosen so that the beginning deflection, or *takeoff*, and peak of the signal are easily measured. The time base is selected so that the waves of interest are displayed farthest apart while still at the same sweep speed. Error is intro-

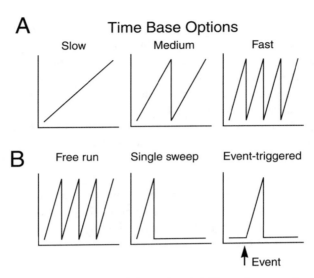

Figure 6.2 Time base. Diagram of the voltage delivered across the horizontal deflecting plates in response to the time base signal. During the ramp increase in voltage, the beam is swept gradually across the screen.

duced when the time base is too slow or is changed between proximal and distal stimuli.

The gain used in the EMG needle study must vary so that the waves of interest are displayed optimally on the screen. The amplitude of waveforms varies from 50 μV/division (div) for spontaneous activity to 1–2 mV/div for maximal motor unit activation. The time base chosen is the fastest at which individual sweeps can be clearly delineated. When sweep speeds are faster than about 16 frames per second, most observers cannot determine whether two waves are on the same sweep or on subsequent sweeps. This is termed the *flicker-fusion frequency*. At 10 ms/div, the distinction between sweeps is easily made. Since there are ten divisions on a screen, 10 ms/div is a sweep time of 100 ms or a frequency of 10 sweeps per second. If 5 ms/div is used, then each sweep takes 50 ms or a frequency of 20 sweeps per second, which is faster than the flicker-fusion frequency.

Evoked potential responses are displayed on CRTs, although data handling is substantially different than with EMGs. This is discussed in detail in Part IV on Evoked Potentials.

Digital CRT displays are now more commonly used than analog oscilloscope displays. These monitors are similar to those used for home and office computers except that they tend to have very high resolution and fast display rates, and special monitors and video cards are required for this optimal performance. The beam of electrons is directed to impact on the screen, as described above, but the display is continuous, so that the entire screen is refreshed at a rate much faster than the human eye can detect. The data are displayed in a format that appears similar to oscilloscope display but is, in fact, recreated digitally. With modern equipment, the performance of these displays is at least equal to oscilloscope displays, and the allowance for additional displayed information on the screen is an added advantage.

Screens display in color by activating different phosphors on the screen. The electron beam is the same, but if it hits one phosphor the color might be red and if it hits another the color may be yellow. In practice, the resolution of the screen is too high for the unaided eye to detect the discrepancy in position of the different colored phosphors.

Liquid Crystal Displays

Liquid crystal displays have only recently been used for neurophysiologic equipment. Their major advantages are their light weight and low-power consumption, which make them advantageous especially for portable devices. Major disadvantages include narrow viewing angle, expense that is amplified with increasing resolution, and slow refresh rates. These disadvantages will wane with time.

Liquid crystals do not melt directly from solids to liquids but rather pass through a stage in which the molecules are partially ordered. In this state, the material is translucent or cloudy, allowing the passage of light through the material but not with clarity. When exposed to a weak electric field, the translucent liquid crystal becomes turbulent, further scattering light and making the liquid crystal virtually opaque. Arrays of liquid crystals and corresponding electrical grid provide for high-resolution displays that surpass all but the best CRTs in clarity. The slow refresh rate is due to the relatively slow rate of transition of the liquid crystal material. The state of the crystal can be changed by elements other than electric fields, as can be observed if one leaves an inexpensive (one hopes) digital watch in bright sun, heat, or a strong magnetic field.

Digital Displays for Electroencephalography

Digital displays will become increasingly prevalent in the next decade, as their advantages are appreciated and their limitations are overcome. A major advantage of digital EEG recording and display is the ability

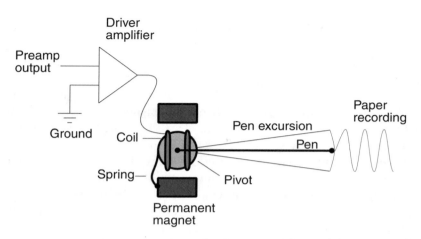

Figure 6.3 Paper display. Output from the driver amplifier is delivered to a coil attached to the pen. Current passing through the coil creates a magnetic field that makes the pen pivot within the field of the permanent magnets.

to review the same epoch of EEG in different montages, sensitivities, and even time bases. This allows for more information on field distribution of waves of interest, especially spikes. Calculations based on the digital data can also include power spectral analysis, automated spike detection, and brain mapping.

Digital display of EEG usually employs the largest available monitors. A 17-inch monitor is a minimum, and a larger monitor is preferable. Smaller displays are not able to display 16–21 channels of information adequately. The display is essentially a color CRT in which the EEG data is digitized and displayed in a format that resembles that obtained with conventional pen and paper (see the following section).

Paper Displays

Pen Electroencephalographic Display

EEG recording is usually accomplished by the movement of paper past pens whose vertical movements are governed by the amplified signal. After passage through filters and preamplifiers, the signal voltage is fed to a driver amplifier. The output is connected to a resistor and coil attached to the pen (Figure 6.3, resistor not shown). The pen coil, in turn, is mounted between poles of a permanent magnet. The passage of an amplified signal current through the coil produces a magnetic field that is oriented so that it acts on the permanent magnetic field to deflect the pen. Most of the time, a spring keeps the pen pointing in a center position, but the fluctuating electromagnetic field moves the pen from this center position. Some pen arrangements use counterbalancing electromagnets to control pen position rather than a single electromagnet and spring. Others use slightly different arrangements, but, in all of these, the basic mechanism is as described here.

Two important physical properties of EEG recording pens are inertia and nonlinearity. Inertia is caused by their weight. More torque is required to get the pen moving than to keep it moving, which results in the pen's tendency to overshoot when made to move rapidly. Overshoot is compensated for by electrical and mechanical damping. Electrical damping is accomplished by a feedback circuit to the pen driver amplifier that corrects the pen position when it overshoots its target position. Mechanical damping is accomplished by varying pen pressure. Damping is not perfect, and alterations in damping change the frequency response of the record.

Nonlinearity is largely due to the pivot mechanism that produces an arc rather than a straight vertical line (see right side of Figure 6.3). Since the signal voltage proportionately determines pen angle, the relationship between signal voltage and vertical distance from baseline to pen tip is not linear. Therefore, a signal of high amplitude can be misinterpreted as occurring at an earlier time than a signal of lower amplitude. This curved appearance is especially prominent with sharp spikes. Since precise timing is not important for most EEG interpretation, the arc distortion is not a major source of interpretive error.

Dot Matrix Printer

Dot matrix printers use a head with a linear array of small wires that impact on paper as the head moves past the paper. Although dot matrix printers have been largely replaced by newer technology for most home and office applications, they continue to be used for high-volume industrial printing and for some neurophysiologic equipment.

A few EEG machines use a dot matrix head that remains stationary as the paper travels past the head. From a distance, the paper display looks the same as that printed using conventional pens; however, there are some important differences. The most obvious difference is the presence of dots composing the lines. This does not greatly detract from visual interpretation of the recording, but there is concern that the resolution of the coarse dots may result in some loss of information. Also, there is no arc distortion, which makes high-amplitude spikes and other fast activity look perceptibly different from the pen display. Dot matrix displays are immune from inertia and therefore do not require damping.

Laser Printer

Laser printers use an electrostatic printing method closely related to that employed by modern copy machines. Plain paper is pulled across a rotating drum that is positively charged. The computer translates the intended print image into commands for a laser beam that precisely impacts on the paper and drum. Dry negatively charged toner adheres to the paper where the electrostatic charge is maintained. Heat from the drum causes the toner to adhere to the paper, producing the printed page. Laser printing is much faster than ink-jet printing and less expensive per printed page. Laser printers were once much more costly than alternative printer types, but this has changed in the past 2 years. Only recently have color laser printers become affordable.

Ink-Jet Printers

Ink-jet printers have become increasingly popular because of their low cost, high print quality, and low maintenance. The only disadvantage is the relatively low print speed, but this is not a concern for individuals who do not have high-volume printing or for computers that use print spoolers.

Ink can be sprayed onto paper in a number of ways, most commonly by heat. The print head contains many small holes. Behind the holes is a thin layer of ink in continuity with a reservoir. Behind the ink is a plate containing tiny heating elements. A command from a microprocessor tells the heating element to become hot quickly. A bubble forms as the temperature soars almost instantaneously. The bubble expands, displacing ink. The force of the expansion results in sufficient pressure to spray ink through the hole and onto the paper. The element then cools, allowing the bubble to collapse. As the bubble collapses, the area behind the opening fills with ink from the reservoir. This is the basic idea behind ink-jet or bubble-jet printers.

These printers are low cost and low maintenance because of the paucity of parts. They need electronics to decode the signal from the computer, a transport mechanism for paper, mechanics to move the head back and forth, and a print head. The entire print head is usually replaced with each cartridge. The number of moving mechanical parts is much smaller than in a laser printer. While the cost of an ink-jet printer is less than most other printers, the cost per page of printing is relatively high because of the cost of the ink cartridge.

Thermal Transfer Printers

Thermal transfer printers use heat to produce an imprint on special paper. The printing is usually of poor quality and very expensive because of paper costs. This method of printing has waned in recent years. Thermal transfer is used predominantly for ECG and strip-chart recorders. Older EMG machines use thermal transfer to print recorded traces.

7

□ □ □
□ □ □
□ □ □

Electrodes and the Patient-Electrode Interface

All neurophysiologic equipment requires electrodes. It is a common misconception that the electrodes pick up electrical activity and the equipment records it. Rather, the electrodes and the patient are integral parts of the circuit formed only in part by the recording equipment. The equipment measures current flow through a loop composed of the patient, electrodes, wires, and equipment. Since the resistance to current flow is known, the voltage fluctuations produced in the patient can be calculated. This is the essential function of the equipment.

Electrode Theory

The recorded electrical activity is generated by charge movement in brain, muscle, or nerve. The charge moves into one electrode, through the circuitry of the amplifier, and back into the patient through another electrode. Therefore, the patient and amplifier form a complete circuit loop.

Electroencephalographic and Evoked Potential Electrodes

Insertion of EEG and evoked potential electrodes into conducting gel is more complex than it seems. The skin is prepared by abrasion to remove oils and layers of dead skin that contain low levels of electrolytes. (Tissue must have electrolytes in solution to be a good conductor.) Electrolyte gel then connects the skin and electrode. The gel is essentially a malleable extension of the electrode. The gel maximizes skin contact and is required for low-resistance recording through the skin.

Electrodes may be reversible or nonreversible. The nonreversible nature of some electrodes is due to polarization of the junction between the gel and the electrode; this polarization reduces current flow through the junction. Essentially, the junction has features of a diode plus a capacitor. Current flows in only one direction (diode effect), which results in charging of the capacitance with no ability to discharge. In this situation, little current will flow and the signal will be lost, especially at low frequencies, since low frequencies have greater tendency to charge the capacitance. Reversible electrodes allow for charge to pass through the junction in both directions, although these also have small junction potentials. An electrode is reversible because either the electrode has ions in common with the gel or the electrode gel contains dissimilar ions at two valence states, allowing for mutual oxidation-reduction reactions to transfer charge.

The best known electrode-gel system is a chlorided silver (AgCl) electrode in a sodium chloride (NaCl) solution. Before using the electrodes, silver (Ag) electrodes must first be oxidized using chlorine (Cl). To do this, the electrode is placed in a NaCl solution and electric current passed through the electrode into the solution. In the solution, the NaCl is dissociated to Na^+ and Cl^-. The Cl^- binds to the Ag to form AgCl on the electrode. The current is required to impart a positive charge to the Ag so it will accept the Cl^-. Formulae for this process are as follows:

in water:

$$NaCl = Na^+ + Cl^-$$

in the electrode:

$$Ag = Ag^+ + e^-$$

at the electrode surface:

$$Ag^+ + Cl^- = AgCl$$

to clean up:

$$Na^+ + e^- + H_2O = NaOH + \tfrac{1}{2}(H_2)$$

Once the electrode has been chlorided, it is placed in a gel that contains Cl^- ions, such as NaCl, as above. Then, conduction of charge across the junction is similar to the chloriding process in forward and reverse.

Figure 7.1A is a schematic diagram of the ionic fluxes during the recording of an EEG signal. A negative charge arises from the head forcing Cl^- from the skin to the gel. Subsequently, the Cl^- combines with the Ag^+ to give AgCl and one free electron (e^-). This free electron travels to the amplifier to complete the flow of charge.

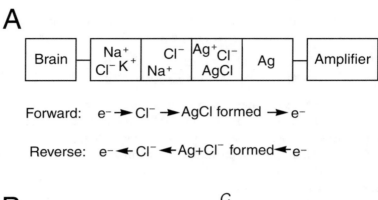

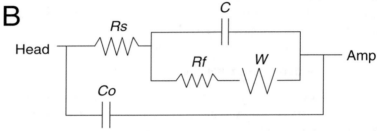

Figure 7.1 Interface between the patient and the machine. A. Ionic fluxes during the recording of EEG signals. B. Circuit simulating the interface among skin, gel, and electrode.

The functions of the skin-gel-electrode interfaces are complex but can largely be modeled by the use of circuit elements (Figure 7.1B). In Figure 7.1B, Rs is the resistance of the gel, C is the capacitance of the interface, Rf is the resistance of the chemical reaction that moved charge at the interface, W is the Warburg impedance, which is a frequency-dependent resistance, and Co is an additional element of capacitance that, in reality, is too small to be of major importance. The most important part of the circuit is the central loop made by C, Rf, and W. In a reversible surface electrode the capacitance is fairly large, and the resistance of Rf and W are small. Thus, there is little modification of the incoming signal, since the capacitor is essentially bypassed for low frequencies, and higher frequencies may be conducted through both arms of the circuit. With a nonreversible electrode, however, the resistances through Rf and W are large; therefore, current flows onto the capacitor, resulting in a build-up of charge. This essentially acts like a low-frequency filter, blocking transmission of low frequencies to the amplifier. Therefore, nonreversible electrodes are not satisfactory for recording EEG.

Electromyographic Electrodes

The design and function of needle electrodes is fairly easy to conceptualize. The needle is inserted into the muscle, where electrical activity of the muscle fibers is detected. The voltage changes of nearby fibers cause a very small amount of current to flow through a coaxial electrode and through its leads to the amplifier before completing the circuit through the reference electrode and tissue. Although the electrode impedance is fairly small, the amplifier input impedance is large, so the actual amount of current flowing into the amplifier is small.

Electrode-Amplifier Interface

When several amplifiers are connected in series, each amplifier draws little current from the preceding amplifier. This is also true of the interface between the amplifiers and the electrode connected to the signal source. In the case of EEG and EMG, electrode resistances are kept relatively low for two reasons: (1) to decrease electrical noise and (2) to make the recorded potential a true representation of the physiologic potential. Noise will be discussed in Chapter 8.

The relationship between electrode resistance and amplifier input resistance is as important as the absolute resistances. The connection of an electrode to the biological signal source can be considered to be the electrical circuit shown in Figure 7.2A, with the electrode resistance (Re) and amplifier input resistance (Rin) being in series with the signal voltage (Vs).

Current (I) flows around the circuit, so from Ohm's law:
$$Vs = I \times Req$$
and:
$$Vs = Ve + Vin$$
and also:
$$Ve = I \times Re \text{ and } Vin = I \times Rin$$

where Ve is the voltage drop across the electrode and Vin is the voltage drop across the amplifier input resistance. Remember that Vin is what will be amplified.

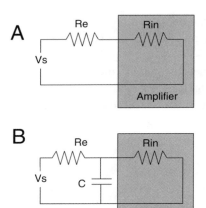

Figure 7.2 Electrode-amplifier interface. A. Simple circuit created by the electrode and amplifier. B. Circuit of electrode and amplifier with capacitance represented by the capacitor symbol (*C*). This is not a manufactured capacitor, but rather capacitance among electrode leads, tissues, and equipment. (*Vs* = signal voltage; *Re* = electrode resistance [impedance]; *Rin* = input resistance [impedance] of the amplifier.)

Dividing the second equation above by *Vs*, then rearranging:

$$\frac{Vin}{Vs} = \frac{Vs - Ve}{Vs}$$

Now, substituting in the third equation, above:

$$\frac{Vin}{Vs} = \frac{(I \times Req) - (I \times Re)}{(I \times Req)}$$

where *Req* = *Re* + *Rin*. So:

$$\frac{Vin}{Vs} = \frac{Rin}{(Re + Rin)}$$

This equation means that the ratio of the amplifier input voltage to the signal voltage approaches 1 only when *Rin* is much greater than *Re*. In general, *Rin* is kept at least two orders of magnitude (100×) greater than *Re* so that the input voltage is at least 99% of the signal voltage.

This chapter refers to the electrode and amplifier input resistance; however, it is important to remember that they are actually impedances, since impedance is frequency-dependent resistance. This implies that there must be an element of capacitance in the circuit, even though it has not been drawn in the previous diagrams (see Figure 7.2B). The capacitances come from the tissue, connecting wires, and other components of the electrical circuits. The equations for impedance would result in the same basic conceptual conclusions, but the mathematics would be much more complex.

8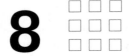

Artifacts and Noise

Signal-to-Noise Ratio

A recording is composed of signal and noise. What is signal and what is noise depends on what is being measured. For example, in conventional EEG, the signal-to-noise ratio is high, meaning that with good technique, the signal is clearly discernible from other electrical activity. In contrast, for evoked potentials, not only is the response much smaller in amplitude, but the normal EEG background is also part of the noise, which obscures the recording. Therefore, a signal-to-noise ratio is defined for the signal under study only after filtering. The signal-to-noise ratio is usually calculated for absolute amplitude. Absolute means that the signal is rectified for calculation—that is, all negative values are made positive. Signal-to-noise ratio can also be expressed in terms of power.

The best ways to maximize signal-to-noise ratio are

- Use of a careful technique
- Placing a preamplifier in the electrode junction box
- Averaging

Some important features of careful technique include (1) equal electrode impedances, so that there is no degradation of common mode rejection; (2) short electrode leads and power cords to avoid stray capacitance and inductance; and (3) proper grounding and selection of location for equipment to minimize electrical noise.

A preamplifier in the electrode junction box magnifies the signal so that it is not as susceptible to degradation by electrical interference. The effect of stray capacitance is proportionately less on a 10-mV signal than a 1-mV signal.

Averaging is the most important way to improve the signal-to-noise ratio of evoked potentials and is helpful for sensory nerve action potentials. In both of these cases, noise includes not only stray electrical activity but also biological electrical activity not associated with the stimulus. The signal-to-noise ratio improves with increasing numbers of averaged trials. If the ratio is expressed in terms of amplitude, the ratio improves by a factor of the square root of the number of samples.

$$\text{Averaged S/N ratio} = \frac{\text{Single sample S/N ratio}}{\sqrt{n}}$$

where n is the number of samples.

If the ratio is expressed in terms of power, the ratio improves in proportion to the number of samples. Table 8.1 lists signal-to-noise ratios for differing numbers of samples. The signal-to-noise ratio is the best index of clarity of recording. In general, avoiding the sources of electrical artifacts will improve the signal-to-noise ratio.

There are many potential sources of artifacts and noise in neurodiagnostic recordings. Only the basic principles are discussed in this text.

60-Hertz Noise

Two of the most important factors causing electrical noise are stray capacitance and stray inductance. The small amount of capacitance that exists among electrode wires, power lines, and tissue-gel-electrode interfaces allows a charge gradient to be built up. This is called *stray capacitance*. The charge can flow in an unpredictable manner into the amplifier or alter the response of the amplifier to the physiologic potential. Since the stray capacitance is variable and the charge movement is influenced by signal voltages or line voltages, for example, the effect is virtually impossible to predict and is seen as noise.

Stray inductance is the production of current in a wire by a surrounding magnetic field. For example, the movement of current through the wires of a light will produce a weak magnetic field. This magnetic field can induce electrons to flow in another wire, such as an electrode lead. This effect is negligible if electrode resistances are small and the signal current flow is large. However, if electrode resistances are high and the signal current flow is small, then induced current becomes a substantial fraction of the total current input to the amplifier. This is one reason that 60-Hz interference is more prominent when electrodes have high impedances (e.g., a broken wire,

Table 8.1 Averaging and Signal-to-Noise Ratio

Samples	Improvement in Signal-to-Noise Ratio
2	1.4
4	2.0
8	2.8
16	4.0
100	10.0
1,000	31.6
2,000	44.7
10,000	100.0

a loose electrode lead, or an electrode with normally high impedance, such as a microelectrode).

Common mode rejection was previously discussed as one of the most important features of EEG machines responsible for eliminating 60-Hz noise (see Chapter 4). This effect is degraded by high or unequal electrode impedances, loss of proper ground, or smear of electrode gel between the ground and an active electrode. Electrode gel smear is not detected by ensuring that electrode impedances are less than 5 kohms.

In summary, the measures that reduce 60-Hz activity are the following:

- Ensuring proper ground
- Keeping electrode impedances that are relatively low and approximately equal
- Using reversible electrodes
- Keeping power lines away from electrode leads
- Electrical shielding of room, cables, or both.

In addition to these general techniques, most equipment uses additional electronic circuitry to reduce and suppress noise.

Movement Artifact

Movement of the patient or the electrode wires during EEG or EMG recordings results in relatively high-amplitude artifacts caused by a disturbance in the junction potentials between electrode and gel or gel and skin and by movement of electrode leads.

Junction potentials are stable only as long as the electrode system is stationary. Movement disturbs the ionic gradients that have developed and causes charge to move down potential gradients. The input to the amplifier changes because the capacitance of the system had previously negated the effect of the junction potentials (i.e., the direct current shift was essentially filtered out). With time, the junction potential forms again. This process can also be perceived by the input amplifier as a slow electrical potential change. Moving electrode leads changes the amount of stray capacitance and the distribution of current caused by stray inductance.

Electrode Pops

Electrode pops are spike-like potentials that occur in an apparently random fashion and are caused by sudden changes in junction potentials. Electrode pops are made more likely if there is a high junction potential, the junction of dissimilar metals, or both. An imperceptible movement or alteration in electrode-gel interface can temporarily short out the junction potential. This sudden change in direct current potential delivered to the amplifier is seen in all channels with that electrode in common. As the stable junction potential is reestablished, the amplifier, as well as pen deflection, returns to baseline. Dissimilar metals build up large junction potentials that are subsequently discharged into the input amplifier. The discharge can cycle repetitively at irregular rates, depending on electrode and wire movement and ongoing electrocerebral activity. High electrode impedances and loose electrodes also predispose equipment to electrode pops.

9

□ □ □
□ □ □
□ □ □

Electrical Safety

The principles of electrical safety are intended to protect the patient from potentially lethal currents while obtaining optimal recording of biological signals. Line power in a hospital is supplied by three wires; the hot lead has black insulation, the neutral lead has white insulation, and the ground has green insulation. *Hot* means that there is alternating ±110 V. *Neutral* is the reference for the hot line from the power company but is not necessarily at 0 V. The *ground* is the building ground connection.

The chief concern in electrical safety is *leakage current*. Leakage current has several sources. Two of these, stray capacitance and stray inductance, are often easily detected because they also accentuate electrical noise. When dealing with leakage current, the capacitance and inductance are mainly in the power supply wires. This condition can increase the potential differences of references and grounds to much greater than 0 V. The amount of leakage current depends on the length and capacitance of the wires. Therefore, extension cords should not be used during electrophysiologic recordings. For example, a 6-foot power cord may produce up to 70 μA of leakage current. Figure 9.1 shows a diagram of a patient hooked up to a machine (Figure 9.1A) and a corresponding electrical circuit diagram of this situation (Figure 9.1B).

The delivery of leakage currents to patients is increased when a ground fault exists. This usually occurs when the ground connection of a piece of equipment is lost. The most common causes are either a broken ground wire in the power cord or loss of building ground. If the power cord wire is broken, repair is always made because the machine does not work. However, the operator may not know the ground connection is broken without specifically testing it. With the loss of building ground, especially in older buildings in which the third wire was added later, some electricians install a three-prong plug to the wall but attach the ground connection to the plug

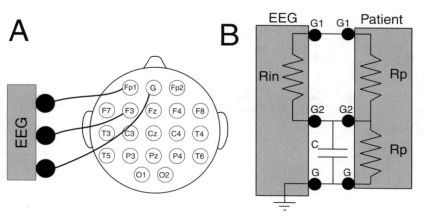

Figure 9.1 Patient-equipment interface. A. Diagram of a patient hooked up to an EEG machine. The cartoon depiction of the head is a standard diagram for indicating electrode positions. Electrode placement follows the 10–20 Electrode Placement System (see Part II). The electrode connections shown are for the first channel of the longitudinal bipolar montage. B. Equivalent electric circuit to some of the connections in A. The capacitor (C) represents the capacitance of the electrode leads and equipment; it is not a true capacitor. (Rin = input resistance [impedance] of the amplifier; Rp = resistance of patient tissues.)

box, which has only a weak connection or no connection at all to earth ground. The deleterious effect of these conditions is enhanced if a patient is attached to two pieces of electrical equipment where one is adequately grounded and the other is not. If the patient is grounded to both devices then leak current can flow from the ground wire of one machine, through the patient, and into the ground of the other machine. The practical rule based on this example is that only one ground should be attached to a patient, and all equipment attached to a patient should be connected to the same power strip and to a single ground.

Ground loops also degrade the recording of the biological signal, since they introduce the potential for greatly magnified 60-Hz interference. Basically, the loop acts like a transformer coil—that is, magnetic fields in the environment cause relatively large amounts of current to flow in the wires. Current has the potential to flow through the patient as part of this loop. The loop can be minimized by using the same outlets for all of the interconnected equipment and making sure that only one ground is used on the patient.

Table 9.1   Maximum Allowable Leakage Current

Clinical Situation	Maximum Allowed Leakage Current (μA)
Patients not connected to electrical equipment	500
Patients connected by surface electrodes to electrical apparatus (e.g., ECG or EEG)	100
Patients with a direct conductive pathway to the heart (e.g., temporary pacemaker)	10

Leakage current poses the greatest threat to patients, especially patients with a temporary pacemaker, when it is applied directly to the myocardium. Patients can be classified into three categories of electrical risk according to the amount of current that is safely applied. These categories are listed in Table 9.1.

The following is a suggested set of guidelines for electrical safety:

- Electrical equipment for patient use must be inspected regularly for safety. The inspection should include verification of proper ground and measurement of leakage current.
- All electrical equipment attached to a patient should be plugged into the same power strip to avoid ground loops and to minimize the possibility of ground faults.
- Machines should be turned on before attaching electrodes to the patient. This avoids power surges that may be transmitted through the patient. Likewise, the patient should be disconnected before the equipment is turned off.
- Use only one patient ground. This decreases the opportunity for leak currents from other machinery to pass through the patient.
- Do not use extension cords. Extension cords can increase leakage current.
- When recording EMGs, be sure the ground is on the same limb as the active electrode so that leakage currents do not flow through the heart.

II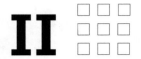

Electroencephalography

10 ⬚⬚⬚
⬚⬚⬚
⬚⬚⬚

Physiologic Basis of Electroencephalography

EEG is the recording of brain electrical activity. Some of the activity recorded by scalp electrodes is generated by action potentials of cortical neurons but most is generated by excitatory postsynaptic potentials (EPSP) and inhibitory postsynaptic potentials (IPSPs). The basic principles of synaptic transmission and nerve conduction were reviewed in Chapter 1.

Generation of Electroencephalographic Rhythms

Scalp electrodes detect charge movement only in the most superficial regions of the cerebral cortex. Electrical activity in the deep nuclei produces surface potentials of low amplitude. These potentials are overwhelmed by cortical activity. Therefore, a discussion of generation of EEG rhythms must concentrate on generation of cortical potentials.

Cortical Potentials

The cerebral cortex functions in a manner similar to most nuclei. The cortex receives input that is processed with the assistance of interneurons and creates output that is projected to other regions. The cerebral cortex differs from other nuclei mainly in the multiplicity and diversity of input and output connections (Figure 10.1). Throughout most of the cortex, the largest neurons are the source of efferent outflow. These neurons are oriented perpendicular to the cortical surface, such that dendritic arborizations are prominent in superficial layers and the soma and axon hillock are located in deeper layers. This creates a vertical columnar organization of the cortex.

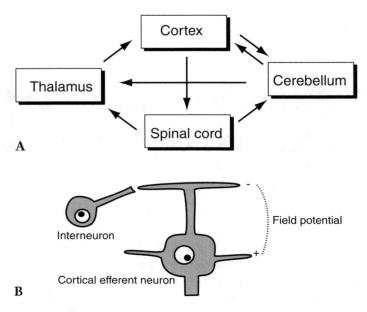

Figure 10.1 Cortical and subcortical organization. A. Efferent neurons have projections to subcortical structures as well as intracortical projections (not shown). Afferent input to the cortex comes from both deep cerebral nuclei plus ascending afferents from the brain stem and spinal cord. B. Close-up of the cortex showing synapse of an excitatory interneuron on the dendrites of a cortical efferent neuron. Depolarization of superficial dendrites results in a negative field potential in the upper layers of the cortex. Electrotonic depolarization of the soma and axon hillock results in a positive field potential in deeper layers.

Activation of thalamocortical afferents results in EPSPs and IPSPs in the interneurons and efferent neurons. Depolarization of the dendrites is conducted along the cell membrane to the axon hillock, where an efferent action potential is generated. Efferent action potentials project to nuclei in the subcortex, brain stem, spinal cord, and other cortical regions. The influx of positive ions into the efferent neuron results in a negative extracellular field potential. Electrotonic depolarization of the soma and axon hillock results in a positive field potential. Because of the vertical organization of the large efferent neurons, the negative field potential is usually superficial to the positive field potential. This is a *dipole*. While the term *dipole* is usually used to describe the orientation of epileptiform activity, virtually all electrophysiologic potentials can be represented, at least in theory, as a positive-negative dipole.

Generation of EEG rhythms has been an area of constant scientific study, yet many questions remain unanswered. We do know that rhythmicity is a characteristic of many excitable cells. The mechanism for rhythmic membrane potential oscillation can be local, within a particular neuron, or dependent on excitatory and inhibitory interactions between neurons. For example, single cells from the thalamus may demonstrate membrane potential oscillation in culture, yet slices of hippocampus may develop rhythmic cellular discharge that is dependent on neuronal interaction. In humans the thalamus is thought to be the main site of origin of EEG rhythms. Oscillation at the thalamic level activates cortical neurons. The EPSPs acting on the dendrites chiefly in layer IV (the main site of depolarization) create a dipole with negativity at layer IV and positivity at more superficial layers. As the rhythmic excitation produces multiple small dipoles around each cortical neuron, the scalp electrodes detect a small but perceptible far-field potential that represents the summed potential fluctuations. Individual rhythms probably depend on differing sites of generation with differing projections—for example, an occipital 9-Hz alpha in waking state as compared with a frontocentral 14-Hz spindle in the sleeping state. Precise loci of generation of these rhythms have not been identified.

Scalp Potentials

Scalp electrodes are not able to detect all of the charge movement occurring on the cortical surface. One estimate suggests that 6 cm^2 of cortical surface area must be synchronously activated for a potential to be recorded at the scalp. Potentials are volume-conducted through the meninges, skull, and scalp before they are picked up by the surface electrodes.

Scalp potentials are determined by the vectors of cortical activity. If the superficial layers of the cortex have a positive field potential, and the deeper layers have a negative field potential, then the vector is vertical, with the positive end pointing toward the scalp electrodes. The amplitude of the vector depends on the total area of activated cortex and the degree of synchrony between cortical neurons. Scalp electrodes are not able to record electrical activity in deep nuclei. Their effective recording depth is only a few millimeters.

Generation of Epileptiform Activity

Epileptiform activity is generated when depolarization of the cortex results in synchronous activation of many neurons. It is conceptually attractive to equate action potentials and EEG spikes, but action potentials occur normally. The abnormality in epileptiform activity is the degree of synchrony. By virtue of the nature of scalp EEG recordings, synchronous activation of many neurons is required for generation of both normal and abnormal rhythms.

Spikes and Sharp Waves

Epileptiform activity consists predominantly of spikes and sharp waves. Spikes have a duration of less than 70 ms, while sharp waves have a duration of 70–200 ms. Scalp recordings occasionally show only rhythmic slow activity or background suppression during a seizure. In this circumstance, the spikes are probably too deep within the brain to be in recording range of surface electrodes.

Spike potentials are the summation of synchronous EPSPs and action potentials in the cortex. A sustained depolarization of the neuron is associated with multiple action potentials on the crest of the depolarization. If one neuron is affected by this activation, the scalp electrodes can not detect it. But when the depolarization spreads synchronously to many neurons through associative connections, the summed field potentials are detected on the surface as a spike, with negativity at the focus. The foundation for this bursting of spike discharges is the paroxysmal depolarization shift (discussed below in the section on Paroxysmal Depolarization Shifts).

Typically, the negative end of the epileptiform dipole points toward the cortical surface. While there are extensive convolutions to the brain, the most superficial cortical tissue is oriented parallel to the skull and scalp. Therefore, spikes and sharp waves are predominantly negative to scalp electrodes.

The negative end of the dipole can be detected by several surface electrodes, although there is usually a region of maximum voltage. The distribution of the potential across the cortical surface is called a *field*. These relationships are presented in Figure 10.2.

Spikes and sharp waves are occasionally surface positive. Positive sharp waves are common in intraventricular hemorrhage of the newborn and in two normal patterns (14- and 6-Hz positive spikes and positive occipital sharp transients of sleep [POSTS]).

Paroxysmal Depolarization Shifts

Paroxysmal depolarization shifts (PDS) are extracellular field potentials characterized by waves of depolarization followed by repolarization (Figure 10.3). High-amplitude afferent input to the cortex produces

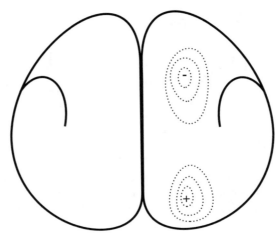

Figure 10.2 Cortical fields of a dipole. The negative and positive ends of a dipole are shown. This is the circumstance in which both ends can be seen on the surface. Usually, the positive end of the dipole is subcortical and cannot be recorded using surface electrodes. The dotted lines indicate zones of similar positivity or negativity, similar to altitude isobars on topographic maps of the earth.

depolarization of cortical neurons sufficient to trigger repetitive action potentials, which in turn contribute to the potential recorded at the surface. Repolarization due to inactivation of interneurons is followed by a brief period of hyperpolarization.

Cyclic depolarization and repolarization is believed to be the intracortical counterpart of the rhythmic spike activity seen in epilepsy. Rhythmicity is probably caused by the inability of cortical neurons to sustain prolonged high-frequency discharges. This inability is not caused by exhaustion but is a built-in mechanism of inactivation after sustained discharge. Termination of the sustained depolarization is likely accomplished by activation of potassium channels and inactivation of the calcium channels, which are at least partly responsible for the prolonged depolarization.

Ultimate termination of the epileptiform activity is probably due to inhibitory feedback to the neurons. The inhibitory neurons can exhibit a bursting similar to that seen in excitatory cortical neurons. Inhibition can suppress and ultimately stop the bursting that is feeding to other neurons. Ultimately, the repetitive activation stops, often with a time of relative suppression.

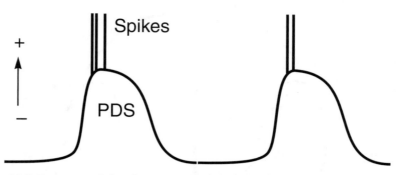

Figure 10.3 Paroxysmal depolarization shift (PDS). An electrode is in a pyramidal tract neuron. The slow waves are the PDSs. The vertical lines represent action potentials superimposed on the PDS when the membrane potential reaches threshold.

The above discussion of seizure activity applies for focal spikes. However, for primary generalized epilepsies, the generator is not thought to be cortical with intracortical projections. Rather, the generator is probably a loop between the thalamus and cortex, with oscillation around that circuit that is not inhibited as it normally should be. This loop is anatomically similar to that thought to be responsible for sleep spindles, which might explain why this type of seizure activity is particularly activated during sleep.

No clear explanation is available for the discrepancy between the electrocerebral discharge of absence seizures and the relatively modest clinical manifestations. I believe that this points out clearly that EEG patterns represent the fraction of electrical activity that is synchronous, and that much more activity is undoubtedly present that lacks the synchrony to be detected on the surface. In fact, if there were no synchrony at all, the EEG would be virtually flat. For absence seizures, selected thalamocortical neurons are activated in synchrony, but inhibitory influences continue to prohibit entrainment of many cortical neurons. When patients with absence epilepsy develop a generalized tonic-clonic seizure, this inhibitory mechanism has broken down, allowing for involvement of more neurons and greater disturbance in cerebral function than with absence seizures alone.

11 □□□ □□□ □□□

Technical Requirements for Electroencephalography

In 1994, the American Electroencephalographic Society published guidelines for performance of EEGs and evoked potentials, which will be referred to here as the *Guidelines* (American Electroencephalographic Society, 1994). This section summarizes the essentials of the technical requirements and offers suggestions for optimizing the acquisition of data.

Electroencephalographic Equipment

Although at least eight channels of EEG are needed to sample activity from broad regions of the brain, 16 channels are preferable and are now considered the real minimum for EEG. Sixteen channels allow the development of an accurate topographic map of EEG activity across both hemispheres but do not provide for the measurement of other physiologic functions. A seventeenth channel is usually needed for the ECG, and additional channels are often useful to record other physiologic functions, such as eye movements and respiration. Eye movement potentials are often detected on EEG channels and can be misinterpreted as frontal slow-wave activity. Respiratory movement produces periodic artifacts on the EEG channel. These artifacts are best identified by simultaneously monitoring these physiologic functions.

The equipment available to record EEG activity changed substantially in recent years. Digital EEG recording and data manipulation have become popular in concert with the availability of low-cost, high-performance microcomputers. Direct recording from individual electrodes provides the opportunity to inspect the same waveform in several different montages, since montages are created during playback. Further, paperless recordings are more environmentally sound and reduce storage needs.

In summary, if one is buying equipment for a diagnostic laboratory, 16 channels are the minimum and 21 channels are desirable. Factors to consider in buying an EEG machine include the following:

- Price: Cost considerations do not justify the purchase of an eight- or ten-channel machine. This is false economy. The difference in cost between an eight- and a 16-channel machine is more than offset by technician and physician time involved in obtaining an EEG of limited diagnostic use.
- Portability: The demand to transport hospital-based EEG machines to special care units is increasing. Such machines must be easy to move and constructed to withstand the movement.
- Technician familiarity: It is preferable for all machines in one laboratory to be of the same brand and even of the same series. Technicians alternating between brands are more likely to make mistakes and are less efficient.
- Service: EEG machines frequently need service. Poor service support is an absolute contraindication to purchasing a machine. For many busy laboratories, service is a more important factor than performance specifications.
- Digital versus paper display: This is personal preference, but eventually paperless EEG machines will replace conventional pen recorders. While hesitation to buy was reasonable when the technology was still in development, state-of-the-art machines are now adequate for routine clinical use.

Recommended Electrodes and Montages

Electrodes

The *Guidelines* recommends electrodes that do not attenuate frequencies between 0.5 and 70.0 Hz. Silver–silver chloride electrodes were among the first to be used because they produced little polarization. However, silver–silver chloride electrodes are expensive and have to be chlorided. Modern amplifiers have a very high input impedance and allow the use of other electrode materials. High impedance reduces the flow of current and reduces the opportunity for electrode polarization.

Surface Electrodes

Surface electrodes are used routinely for almost all EEG studies. Surface electrodes are disks that are fixed to the skin with electrode gel, which is a viscous solution containing ions that can carry charge. The gel acts as a malleable extension of the electrode. Details of the function of electrodes are presented in Chapter 7.

Application of surface electrodes using electrode gel involves the following steps:

1. Locate positions for electrodes using the 10–20 Electrode Placement System, which is explained later in the section on Electrode Position.
2. Separate strands of hair over the electrode positions using the wooden end of a cotton-tipped applicator.
3. Clean dead skin and dirt from the region with an agent such as Omni-Prep (D. O. Weaver Co., Denver, CO) using the cotton-tip applicator.
4. Scoop some gel into the electrode.
5. Place the electrode in position over the skin.
6. Put a 2″ × 2″ gauze pad over the electrode and push it firmly onto the head. (This provides a good seal that prevents the electrode from falling off in all but the most vigorous head movements.)

Application of electrodes with collodion involves the following steps:

1. Prepare the head as mentioned for electrode gel.
2. Place the electrode on the scalp.
3. Place a piece of gauze soaked with collodion over the electrode.
4. Use compressed air to dry the collodion.
5. Insert a blunt-tipped needle into the cup and scrape the skin to lower electrode impedance.
6. Inject electrolyte into the cup of the electrode using the blunt-tipped needle.

Each method has its advantages. Collodion provides a more secure attachment and is more suitable for long-term recordings. Electrode gel is easier to apply and remove, and is suitable for most routine office and hospital recordings.

Needle Electrodes

Needle electrodes offer no advantages over conventional surface electrodes and should not be used for routine studies unless recording cannot be accomplished any other way. The risk of infection to the patient and technician is unacceptably high.

Sphenoidal Electrodes

Sphenoidal electrodes are used to evaluate patients with suspected temporal lobe seizures. They are inserted adjacent to the zygoma until they reach the base of the skull. Sphenoidal electrodes should be placed only by physicians who are trained in their insertion and experienced in interpretation of the recorded potentials.

Subdural Strip Electrodes

Subdural strip electrodes are used to evaluate patients for epilepsy surgery. A burr hole or small craniotomy is performed and the electrode strips are placed overlying the cortex, usually in the area immediately overlying the suspected seizure focus. The purpose is to map the anatomical extent of the focus. Subdural strip electrodes should only be used by investigators experienced in their placement and recording interpretation and then only for preoperative evaluation before surgery for epilepsy.

Depth Electrodes

Depth electrodes are used to localize a seizure focus in patients being evaluated for surgery. Each electrode probe inserted into the brain is actually an array of small electrodes from which individual recordings are made. The position of the electrode is determined by skull radiographs and by correlation with computerized tomography. Depth electrodes should only be used by physicians trained in their insertion and recording interpretation.

Electrode Position

Electrodes should be placed according to the 10–20 Electrode Placement System, as recommended by the International Federation of Societies for EEG and Clinical Neurophysiology. This system uses 21 electrodes placed at positions that are measured at 10% and 20% of head circumference (Figure 11.1).

The terminology of electrode position is based on a key letter that indicates the brain region and a number that specifies the exact position. The key letters are *F* for frontal, *Fp* for frontopolar, *C* for central, *T* for temporal, *P* for parietal, *O* for occipital, and *A* for auricular (ear). The numbers indicate the electrodes within the specified region. Odd numbers are on the left and even numbers are on the right. In general, lower numbers are anterior and higher numbers are posterior. Midline electrodes are indicated by *z* instead of by a number.

The head is measured in the following manner:

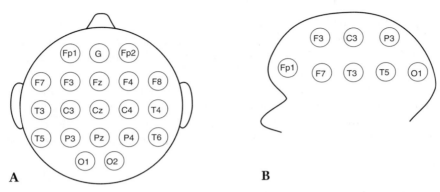

Figure 11.1 10–20 Electrode Placement System. A. Top view. This diagram is similar to that seen on EEG paper. The nose is at the top, with the lateral protrusions representing ears. Circles with letters indicate electrodes and are meant more as indicators of relative positions than exact positions. B. Side view. See text for details.

1. Measure the distance from nasion to inion across the vertex. Mark a line at 50% of this distance.
2. Measure the distance between the preauricular points, just in front of the ear. Mark a line at 50% of this distance. The intersection of this line with that of step 1 is Cz.
3. Lay the measuring tape from nasion to inion through Cz. Mark 10% of this distance above the nasion for Fpz and above the inion for Oz. Fz is 20% of this distance above Fpz. Pz is 20% of this distance above Oz.
4. Lay the tape between the preauricular points through Cz. T3 is 10% of this distance above the left preauricular point, and T4 is 10% above the right preauricular point. C3 is 20% of this distance above T3, and C4 is 20% of this distance above T4.
5. Lay the tape from Fpz to Oz through T3. Fp1 is 10% of this distance, F7 is 20% posterior to Fp1. O1 is 10% anterior to Oz, and T5 is 20% anterior to O1. Measure in the same manner for Fp2, F8, O2, and T6 over the right hemisphere.
6. Lay the tape from Fp1 to O1 through C3. F3 is half the distance between Fp1 and C3, P3 is half the distance between C3 and O1. Repeat for the right, with the tape from Fp2 to O2 through C4. F4 is half the distance between Fp2 and C4, and P4 is half the distance between C4 and O2.

7. Lay the tape from F7 to F8 through Fz, P3, and F4 to ensure that the distance between electrodes is equal. Then lay the tape from T5 to T6 through Pz, P3, and P4 to also ensure equal interelectrode distances.

Abbreviations for special electrodes, such as *Sp* for sphenoidal and *Naso* for nasopharyngeal, are less standardized and may vary between laboratories. Subdural strip and depth electrodes often use both numbers and letters. The letter generally indicates the array, and the numbers indicate which electrode in the array.

Montages

The sequence of electrodes being recorded at one time is called a *montage*. All montages fall into one of two categories, bipolar or referential (Figure 11.2). Referential means that the reference for each electrode is in common with other electrodes; for example, each electrode may be referenced to the ipsilateral ear. An average reference means that each electrode is compared to the average potential of every electrode. Bipolar means that the reference for one channel is the active for the next; for example, in the longitudinal bipolar montage, channel 1 is Fp1-F3. This means that Fp1 is the active electrode and F3 is the reference. Channel 2 is F3-C3, so that F3 is now the active electrode and C3 is the reference.

For all channels, negativity in the active input produces an upward deflection of the pen on the paper. Negativity at the reference produces downward deflection. Details of localization are discussed in the Chapter 12. The *Guidelines* recommends the following principles in designing montages:

- Record at least eight channels.
- Use the full 21 electrode placement of the 10–20 system.
- Every routine recording session should include at least one montage from each of the following groups: referential, longitudinal bipolar, and transverse bipolar.
- Label each montage on the recording.
- Use simple montages that allow easy visualization of the spatial orientation of waveforms—for example, bipolar montages should be in straight lines with equal interelectrode distances.
- List the anterior and left-sided channels before posterior and right-sided channels.
- Use at least some montages that are commonly used in other laboratories.
- Remember that negativity in the active electrode of each channel produces an upward deflection of the pen.

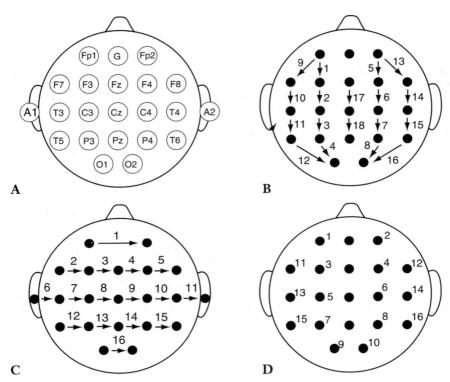

Figure 11.2 Bipolar and referential montages. A. Electrode positions. B. Longitudinal bipolar montage. C. Transverse bipolar montage. D. Referential montage. Only the active input (G1) is shown. The electrodes can be referenced to the ear or to an average. For all of these, the number near the electrode position indicates channel number. The line represents the comparison of two adjacent electrodes in bipolar montages. G1 is anterior, left, or both of G2.

The recommended 16-channel montages for routine use in adults are shown in Table 11.1. Additional channels, when available, are used for monitoring other biological functions, such as ECG, eye movements, respirations, and EMG, or for recording from the midline.

Technical Requirements for Electroencephalography

Montages selected for children are age-dependent. The entire 10–20 electrode placement can be used in term newborns but is not rou-

Table 11.1   Recommended Montages for Routine
Electroencephalogram in Adults*

Channel Number	LB	TB	Ave	Ref
1	Fp1-F3	Fp1-Fp2	Fp1-Ave	Fp1-A1
2	F3-C3	F7-F3	Fp2-Ave	Fp2-A2
3	C3-P3	F3-Fz	F3-Ave	F3-A1
4	P3-O1	Fz-F4	F4-Ave	F4-A2
5	Fp2-F4	F4-F8	C3-Ave	C3-A1
6	F4-C4	A1-T3	C4-Ave	C4-A2
7	C4-P4	T3-C3	P3-Ave	P3-A1
8	P4-O2	C3-Cz	P4-Ave	P4-A2
9	Fp1-F7	Cz-C4	O1-Ave	O1-A1
10	F7-T3	C4-T4	O2-Ave	O2-A2
11	T3-T5	T4-A2	F7-Ave	F7-A1
12	T5-O1	T5-P3	F8-Ave	F8-A2
13	Fp2-F8	P3-Pz	T3-Ave	T3-A1
14	F8-T4	Pz-P4	T4-Ave	T4-A2
15	T4-T6	P4-T6	T5-Ave	T5-A1
16	T6-O2	O1-O2	T6-Ave	T6-A2
17	Fz-Cz	Fz-Cz	Fz-Ave	Fz-A1
18	Cz-Oz	Cz-Pz	Pz-Ave	Pz-A2

LB = longitudinal bipolar; TB = transverse bipolar; Ave = average reference; Ref = ear reference.
*These montages are for a 16-channel machine. If a seventeenth channel is available, it is usually used for ECG. If 21 channels are available, additional channels are particularly useful for the LB montage. Extra channels may be Fz-Cz, Cz-Pz, and eye leads.
Source: American Electroencephalographic Society. Guidelines in EEG, evoked potentials, and polysomnography. J Clin Neurophysiol 1994;11:30.

tinely needed. Monitoring noncerebral functions such as ECG and respiration are essential in all newborns and special montages must be used when only 16 channels are available. Specific recommendations for neonatal EEG are presented in Chapter 18.

Routine Electroencephalography

All EEG recordings should be clearly labeled with the patient's name, age, recording date, identification number, and name of the technologist performing the recording. This should be done before the record leaves the recording room to avoid mixing up patients' records. A fact sheet accompanying the record should include the reason for the study, time of last seizure (if applicable), technical summary, and annotation of regions to which the technician wants to call particular attention. Current medications should also be listed. The technical summary will include exact time of recording, state(s) of the patient, page numbers of activation methods used, sedative doses, and findings of note reported by the technician.

Calibration

Two phases of calibration are performed before starting the study. The first is square-wave calibration and the second is biological calibration (Biocal).

Square-Wave Calibration

In square-wave calibration, a square-wave pulse is delivered to the inputs of each amplifier. The pulse is 50 µV amplitude and alternates on and off at 1-second intervals. The waveform is modified by the preset filters and recorded on paper. Sample square-wave calibration recordings are shown in Figure 11.3.

The low-frequency filter (LFF) transforms the plateau of the square wave into an exponential decay. The high-frequency filter (HFF) slightly rounds off the peak of the calibration pulse signal. For educational purposes, I recommend trying several different high- and low-frequency filter settings during the calibration test to see the effect of filter changes on the record. It is also instructive to change filter settings during the recording of EEG activity, at a time that will not interfere with clinical interpretation.

The time constant (TC) of the LFF can be measured from the square-wave calibration page. As was discussed in Part I, TC is equal to the time it takes for a potential to fall to $1/e$ of the original value, where e is the base of natural logarithms (approximately 2.7). Therefore, TC will be the time taken to decay to 37% of peak value or approximately one-third of the peak voltage.

It is difficult to estimate the setting of the HFF from the square-wave calibration; however, electroencephalographers should have an idea of what

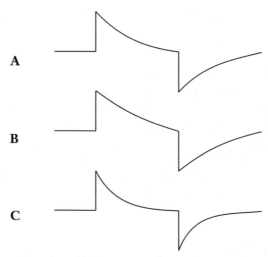

Figure 11.3 Square-wave calibration signals. A 50-μV square wave was delivered and the response recorded. A. Normal response. B. Increased time constant of the low-frequency filter. The potential decays slower than normal. C. Decreased time constant of the low-frequency filter. The potential decays faster than normal.

the peak should look like. If the HFF is set too low, there will be a slow roll-off on the peak of the calibration pulse. If the HFF is set too high, the wave will appear too peaked and may even show overshoot, as if there is too little pen damping.

Biological Calibration

Biological calibration, or *Biocal,* assesses the response of the amplifiers, filters, and the recording apparatus on a complex biological signal. Electrodes Fp1 and O2 are connected to all amplifier inputs. The recordings from all channels should be identical (Figure 11.4).

Pen Pressure and Damping

Mechanical writing instruments have two inherent limitations, inertia and friction. Even when the filters are set properly, the frequency response may be inaccurate because of these mechanical factors. The physical mass of the pen produces inertia that slows its response time to sudden changes of signal voltage. Inertia is partially compensated for by con-

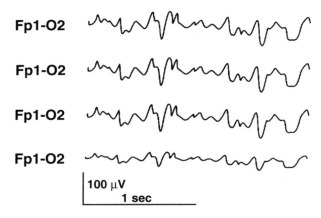

Figure 11.4 Biocalibration signals. Four channels are shown, all of which have the same input, that is Fp1-O2. The trace from every channel should be identical; however, the last channel has a smaller amplitude response. This smaller response indicates unequal amplification and should be corrected before performing the study.

trol mechanisms in the pen drive mechanism. Friction is also compensated by EEG machine electronics, but excessive pressure of the pen on the paper results in a sluggish response. This is the main reason that electroencephalographers and technicians need a visual memory of what a calibration pulse looks like with proper filter settings.

The same inertia that inhibits pen movement also promotes excessive pen movement (overshoot). Overshoot is minimized by the pen control mechanism; this minimization is termed *damping*. When damping is not sufficient, normal waveforms may look like spike discharges (Figure 11.5). These effects are minimized with proper setting of pen pressure and damping. The manuals provided with the EEG machines give instructions on setting the damping and pen pressure.

Sensitivity

The recording sensitivity is initially set at 7 µV/mm and subsequently adjusted depending on the amplitude of the EEG activity. Movement artifact and other noncerebral transients may exceed maximal pen excursion, but electrocerebral activity may not. Important waveforms may be missed when sensitivity is set too low.

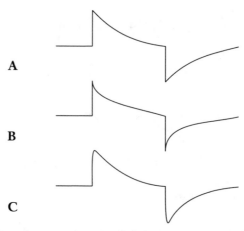

Figure 11.5 Pen damping. A. Normal damping. B. Under damping. Note the overshoot in the deflection on the rising phase of the calibration pulse. C. Overdamping. Note the blunted response at the rising phase of the calibration pulse.

For children, the sensitivity is often reduced to 10–15 μV/mm because EEG amplitude is high in both the awake and sleep states. The elderly often have low-voltage EEG activity, and increased sensitivity is required.

Studies performed for the determination of cerebral death are started at 7 μV/mm but the sensitivity is always increased to 2 μV/mm (see Chapter 17).

Duration of Recording

A routine EEG should include at least 20 minutes of relatively artifact-free record. Longer duration recordings are often helpful in neonates, so that transitions between states can be identified. The *Guidelines* recommends 30 minutes of recording for cerebral death studies.

Filters

The standard filter settings for routine EEG are LFF = 1 Hz and HFF = 70 Hz. The LFF setting of 1 Hz corresponds to a TC of 0.16 seconds. See Part I for a detailed discussion of filters. If the LFF is set higher than 1 Hz, there will be attenuation and distortion of some slow waves. Slow waves have an increased number of phases and are composed of faster frequencies. Technicians should be discouraged from turning up the LFF, especially when there is an abundance of slow activity. If the HFF is set too low, then faster activity is blunted, and spikes and sharp waves may be impossible to identify.

The 60-Hz filter should not be needed in most laboratories. Two important features to minimize 60-Hz artifact are careful selection of equipment location and adequate grounding. Shielding of the room is desirable but usually not essential and cannot completely abolish artifact induced by a strong electromagnetic field. Studies in a special care unit usually require use of the 60-Hz filter. Sources of artifact include ventilators, intravenous infusion pumps, air beds, heating or cooling blankets, and monitoring equipment.

Activation Methods

The performance and interpretation of records obtained with activation methods are discussed in detail in Chapter 14. Hyperventilation, photic stimulation, and sleep may activate epileptiform activity. After an initial period of recording in the relaxed, wakeful state, the patient is asked to hyperventilate for 3 minutes. If absence seizures are suspected, the patient is asked to hyperventilate for 5 minutes. Hyperventilation is not performed in elderly individuals or in patients with advanced atherosclerotic disease because of concern for vasoconstriction with resultant cardiac or cerebral hypoperfusion.

Photic stimulation is performed on older children and adults of all ages. Photic stimulation of sleeping infants is probably of limited clinical value.

Sleep is not considered by some to be a true activation method, because it is a transition between natural states. However, sleep helps to promote epileptiform activity, and in routine EEG sleep frequently has to be induced by sedatives or sleep deprivation. In this sense, sleep is an activation method. Sleep recordings are routinely indicated in all patients being evaluated for seizures but are not helpful in patients being evaluated for encephalopathy. The mechanism of sleep is not important. There is no convincing evidence that natural sleep, sedated sleep, and sleep deprivation differ in their ability to promote epileptiform activity.

Telephone Transmission Electroencephalography

Telephone transmission of EEG is useful and accurate with certain caveats. The interpreter must be aware of several sources of artifact from public telephone lines and the equipment required to transform the data into a form for transmission.

The EEG signal is carried from one institution to another across a single telephone line. Therefore, the signal is multiplexed. Multiplexing means that the line carries brief samples of each channel in turn. A voltage measurement of channel 1 is followed by channel 2, then channel 3, and so on.

After the last channel, an additional channel is often transmitted for error checking and comment information. Then voltage for channel 1 is transmitted, and the cycle begins again. At the receiving end, the multiplexed signal is reconstructed into separate channels and displayed on EEG paper.

The *Guidelines* recommends that telephone transmission EEGs be performed in accordance with the guidelines for routine EEGs. In addition they make the following recommendations:

- Manufacturers of telephone transmission EEG equipment must provide specifications on frequency response, noise, and crosstalk. The equipment should be checked periodically to ensure that these specifications are continually met.
- The equipment should indicate if there is difficulty with transmission at either station or in the telephone transmission itself.
- Integrity of transmission should be checked before and after each recording.
- The record should be labeled as already described. In addition, the record should indicate that it is a telephone transmission recording.
- A paper recording should be made at both the transmitting and receiving stations, for accurate relay of information on physiologic state, activity, and artifacts.
- The EEG from both transmitting and receiving stations should be stored for future comparison.
- The technicians at the transmitting and receiving stations should be well trained not only in routine EEG but also in the techniques and problems associated with telephone transmission EEGs.
- Telephone transmission EEG cannot be used as a confirmatory test for determination of brain death.

Technicians at outside facilities are seldom as well trained and supervised as technicians in the home EEG laboratory. Therefore, there is greater opportunity for technical error. Many outside facilities use electrode caps. These caps fit snugly on the head. There are several problems with electrode caps: (1) impedances are usually higher than with normally applied electrodes, (2) the cap may not be positioned perfectly on the head, and (3) the relative positions of the electrodes differ between patients because of head size.

The Electroencephalographic Laboratory

EEGs can be performed in virtually any patient care area of a hospital, but routine studies are best performed in a central EEG laboratory.

Because sleep is a requisite part of many studies, the EEG laboratory should be located in a quiet area. Many experts recommend locating the EEG machine in a room adjacent to the patient room, so that technician and equipment noise do not interfere with performance of the study. In practice, this isolation is not usually needed for routine studies.

All laboratory outlets should accept a three-prong plug and be properly grounded. Improper grounding is the most common cause of shock hazard. All equipment attached to a single patient must be grounded to a common point that is functioning well (see Chapter 9).

Electrical shielding is usually not necessary and should not be installed routinely. Excessive interference is more likely to result from improper grounding or electrode problems than from the environment. With adequate grounding and the use of bipolar montages, good recordings can be made in most facilities.

Electroencephalographic Reports and Record Keeping

The Electroencephalographic Report

The EEG report must be complete, clear, and concise (Figure 11.6). It should be no longer than one page not including representative samples of the record. Every record must have the following information: patient name, hospital or laboratory unit number, EEG record number, date of study, age, sex, reason for study, current medications, time of last seizure (if applicable), description of the record, interpretation, and name of the electroencephalographer.

Description of the Record

The description is the body of the report. This section is not read by many referring physicians but will be used by neurologists who may want the evidence supporting the final impression. It will also be used for comparison with future studies. The essential elements of the description include state of the patient, including state transitions during the study, description of the background and reactivity, and response to activation methods.

A description of a normal record might read as follows:

EEG #1 The recording began with the patient in the awake state and was characterized by a posterior dominant rhythm of 10 Hz that reacted to eye opening. Hyperventilation for 3 minutes produced symmetric slowing. Photic stimulation produced a driving response at flash fre-

ST. NOWHERE'S HOSPITAL
NEURODIAGNOSTIC LABORATORY

Patient: Jane Q. Doe
Hospital number: 12345
Study: EEG wake and sleep
Requested by: Jim Public, M.D.
Date: 2/1/97
Clinical: 32F with new-onset tonic-clonic seizures
Medications: Dilantin 300 qhs
Notes: Last seizure 1/1/97

Description: The recording begins with the patient in the awake state and is characterized by a posterior dominant rhythm of 10 Hz that reacts to eye opening. There is an anterior-posterior gradient, with faster frequencies from the frontal lobe. Photic stimulation resulted in a driving response at flash frequencies of 7–14 Hz. Hyperventilation produced symmetric buildup of slow activity. The patient was sedated with 1 g of chloral hydrate, and stage 2 sleep was obtained. The sleeping state was characterized by well-formed sleep spindles and vertex waves. No focal or epileptiform activity was seen.

Impression: Normal awake and sleep EEG

Figure 11.6 Normal EEG report.

quencies of 9–18/sec. The patient was sedated with 1 g of chloral hydrate and stage 2 sleep was obtained. The sleeping state was characterized by symmetric sleep spindles, vertex waves, and slow activity in the theta and delta range.

A description of an abnormal record might read as follows:

EEG #2 The recording began with the patient in the awake state and was characterized by a posterior dominant rhythm of 9 Hz that reacted to eye opening. Posterior slow waves of youth are superimposed on the record. During the waking state, generalized 3-per-second spike-wave complexes were seen with maxima in the frontal regions. Duration of the discharges was 2–7 seconds. Hyperventilation augmented the spike-wave complexes. Photic stimulation produced a driving response at flash frequencies of 7–15/sec. The patient was sedated with 2 g of chloral hydrate and became drowsy, but stage 2 sleep was not obtained.

The description is the location for any abnormalities or irregularities in the record. For example, a single spike may be seen that does not recur during the record. A conservative reader will hesitate to interpret a record as abnormal on the basis of a single spike. Therefore, the description may include the following passage:

EEG #3 . . . During the waking state, a single spike was observed with maximal negativity at C3. The spike did not recur during the record . . .

The final impression of this recording would be normal. If a future EEG showed more obvious epileptiform activity, the interpreter could look back at this report and conclude that the spike was consistent with the patient's known seizure disorder.

Interpretation

For the referring physician, the interpretation is the most important part of the report. First, state whether the record is normal or abnormal, then summarize the abnormalities, and conclude with the clinical implications of the abnormalities. Interpretations for the EEGs described above are as follows:

EEG #1 Normal awake and sleep EEG.
EEG #2 Abnormal EEG because of generalized 3-per-second spike-wave complexes. This is consistent with a seizure disorder of the generalized type.

Ordinarily, the EEG interpretation should provide a definitive diagnosis that requires no further interpretation by the clinician. Sometimes the EEG interpretation can be further refined by clinical data, however. Usually, the clinical neurophysiologist does not know the patient but is in the best position to interpret the clinical significance of the EEG. Some examples are the following:

Finding #1 Spike focus in a patient with partial complex seizures.
Impression #1 This is an abnormal study because of a spike focus in the right anterior temporal region. This is consistent with a partial seizure disorder.

Finding #2 Sharp wave focus in a patient with a behavioral disorder. Impression #2 This is an abnormal study because of a sharp-wave focus in the left posterior temporal region. While this could be consistent with a seizure disorder, patients without clinical seizures can manifest this pattern.

Electroencephalographic Recordkeeping

The *Guidelines* gives few recommendations regarding keeping EEG records and reports. With paper displays, it is not practical to permanently keep the entirety of every EEG record. Options to archive records include microfilming the entire record or saving representative paper sheets. One advantage of digital EEG is that long storage can be accomplished in very little space using optical disks and other high-capacity digital media.

The EEG report should be kept indefinitely. Hospital-based laboratories must follow institutional and state requirements for record keeping.

12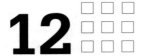

Electroencephalography Basics

Clinical Indications for Electroencephalography

EEG studies are most useful for diagnosis and classification of seizures, encephalopathy, encephalitis, and brain death. Modern imaging techniques have reduced the usefulness of EEG in the evaluation of headache and focal neurologic disturbances.

Basic Interpretation

Specific EEG waveforms are rarely normal or abnormal, with the exception of certain epileptiform discharges. The EEG is interpreted in the context of the patient's age and awake-sleep state. For example, slow activity is normal in sleep stages 3 and 4 and abnormal in an awake adult. Visual analysis of EEG recordings seems automatic for the experienced electroencephalographer. The analysis is based on a foundation that usually includes the following starting points:

1. Note the patient's age, clinical state, medication list, and the reason for ordering the EEG.
2. Examine the composition of frequencies and their topographic organization (e.g., occipital alpha or frontal delta).
3. Examine the right-to-left symmetry of EEG patterns.
4. Examine changes in EEG background activity during the recording that are associated with stimulation and state changes (e.g., drowsiness, sleep, flash, hyperventilation).
5. Note abnormal waveforms such as spikes. Question if these could be normal waveforms.

EEG interpretation is subjective and difficult. Electroencephalographers need to have a conservative bias. An EEG should not be called abnormal, if there is reasonable doubt. More harm is usually done by a false-positive interpretation than by a false-negative interpretation. Finally, do not hesitate to consult EEG texts when reviewing records that are difficult to interpret. For future reference, it may be helpful to cite supporting documentation in the impression.

Electroencephalographic Rhythms

EEG rhythms are classified into four frequency bands (Table 12.1). No individual band is normal or abnormal by definition. All are interpreted in the context of the topographic location and age and conscious state of the patient.

Alpha Rhythms

The alpha rhythm is usually seen in normal, relaxed individuals who are awake with their eyes closed. It is approximately 10 Hz in adults with the maximum voltage originating from the occipital electrodes, O1 and O2. The term *alpha rhythm* is used by some physiologists to signify any posterior dominant rhythm regardless of frequency, but this is an improper use of the term.

In children, the dominant occipital rhythm is slower in frequency and may not attain the minimal 8.5 Hz until 12 years of age. Slower frequencies in a 12-year-old would be interpreted as abnormal and would most likely indicate a diffuse encephalopathy or, if unilateral, suggest a structural lesion.

The posterior dominant rhythm is suppressed by eye opening and promptly returns when the eyes are closed. This reactivity of the posterior alpha rhythm should be routinely tested during an EEG recording. The alpha rhythm is suppressed if the patient is tense during the recording. The lack of alpha rhythm should not be interpreted as abnormal in this situation. Other EEG features that suggest a tense state include frequent eye blinks and muscle artifact in frontal and temporal leads.

The amplitude of the posterior dominant alpha rhythm is 15–50 µV in young adults. Older individuals often have lower amplitude, but the frequency is the same. Low amplitude should not be interpreted as abnormal if the frequency composition is normal. Slowing of the posterior dominant rhythm is not a normal part of aging. Amplitude asymmetries of the poste-

Table 12.1 Electroencephalographic Rhythms

Rhythm	Description	Normal	Abnormal
Alpha	8–13 Hz	Posterior dominant rhythm in older children and adults	Diffuse alpha in alpha coma Can signify seizure activity, especially in neonates
Beta	>13 Hz	Normal in sleep, especially in infants and young children	Drug-induced frontal beta Breach rhythm over a skull defect
Theta	4–7 Hz	Drowsiness and sleep Posterior slow waves of youth may have a theta component	Temporal theta in the elderly Focal theta activity over a structural lesion.
Delta	<4 Hz	Sleep	Intermittent rhythmic delta activity Polymorphic delta activity with focal lesions
Spikes and sharp waves	Spike: 27–70 ms duration Sharp wave: 70–200 ms duration	Vertex waves and frontal sharp transients in neonates Positive occipital sharp transients of sleep Benign epileptiform transients of sleep 6/sec phantom spike and wave, 14-and-6 positive spikes	Focal and generalized epileptiform activity

rior dominant rhythm are common. The amplitude is usually higher from the nondominant hemisphere, but the difference should not exceed 50%.

A prominent alpha rhythm can be recorded during anesthesia and coma, but the distribution is different from the normal posterior alpha rhythm. In anesthesia and coma, the alpha rhythm is generalized with an anterior predominance. This alpha activity is invariant and monotonous, lacking the usual modulation in frequency and amplitude of an occipital alpha. The appearance of alpha coma in a patient signifies a poor prognosis for good neurologic recovery.

Beta Rhythms

EEG activity with frequencies faster than 13 Hz occurs in all individuals but is usually of low amplitude and often overlooked in favor of slower frequencies during wakefulness and sleep. Beta activity is normally distributed maximally over the frontal and central regions. A low-amplitude high-frequency beta is especially prominent during normal sleep in infants and children and is enhanced by several sedatives, especially barbiturates and benzodiazepines. In some children the beta activity is so prominent as to dominate the record.

People with hyperthyroidism may accelerate their posterior rhythm from 10 to 14 Hz or more. This is technically in the beta range, but the rhythm continues to react like an occipital, awake, resting rhythm and should be considered no different than the alpha rhythm in this context.

Alterations in the frequency, amplitude, and abundance of beta activity should be commented on in the description of the record but interpreted with caution. Marked asymmetry in beta activity suggests the possibility of a structural lesion on the side lacking the beta. Focal, high-amplitude beta activity (termed a *breach rhythm*) can be recorded over a skull defect, such as a burr hole and fracture site.

Theta Rhythms

EEG activity with a frequency between 4 Hz and 8 Hz is seen in normal drowsiness and sleep and during wakefulness in young children. Theta is also present in normal waking adults, but the content is small and the amplitude is low. The detection of this theta usually requires high-sensitivity recordings or digital frequency analysis.

Posterior slow waves of youth may be in the theta or delta range. Theta activity in the temporal region in older individuals has been ascribed to vascular disease. While the significance of temporal theta is controversial, I suspect that it is not part of normal aging. I suggest commenting on the presence of temporal theta in the body of the report and interpreting it as a mild abnormality.

Delta Rhythms

Delta activity is not normally recorded in the awake adult but is a prominent feature of sleep and becomes increasingly abundant during the progress from stage 2 to stage 4 sleep. Focal polymorphic delta activity may be recorded over localized regions of cerebral damage. Intermittent rhythmic delta activity is recorded when there is dysfunction of the relays between the deep gray matter and cortex. This activity has a frontal predominance in adults and is called frontal intermittent rhythmic delta activity, while in children the activity has an occipital predominance and is called occipital rhythmic delta activity or posterior intermittent rhythmic delta activity.

Spikes and Sharp Waves

The mechanisms of generation of spikes and sharp waves were discussed in Chapter 10. Spikes are usually surface negative. The positive end of the dipole is occasionally detected on the cortical surface distant from the region of greatest negativity.

Spikes and sharp waves usually indicate epileptiform activity; however, sharp waves are normal in certain situations, such as in newborns. Spikes and sharp waves are also seen overlying structural lesions, even in the absence of seizures. Interpretation of spikes and sharp waves is discussed in detail in Chapter 15.

Slow Waves

EEG patterns can take two forms: (1) slow background rhythms and (2) slow waves superimposed on the background. A posterior dominant rhythm of 7 Hz is abnormally slow and is consistent with an encephalopathy. In contrast, focal slow waves in the theta and delta range superimposed on an otherwise normal background suggest a structural lesion. Interpretation of slow waves is discussed in detail in Chapter 16.

Localization

Interpretation of the EEG depends on accurate localization of recorded electrical activity. Every potential has a field, although the extent of the field may not be within range or resolution limits of the electrodes. A field consists of a positive pole, a negative pole, and a distribution of the potential throughout the brain.

Localization is easiest with the average reference montage. In this montage, the reference for each channel is the average potential for all electrodes on the scalp, which approaches electrical neutrality.

Figure 12.1 shows stylized recordings from a portion of an average reference montage. Each surface electrode is referenced to a computed average of

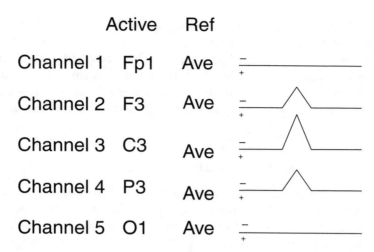

	Active	Ref
Channel 1	Fp1	Ave
Channel 2	F3	Ave
Channel 3	C3	Ave
Channel 4	P3	Ave
Channel 5	O1	Ave

Figure 12.1 Spike localization in an average reference montage. These are the left parasagittal leads of the average reference montage. Data are simulated.

potentials from all electrodes. By convention, negativity at the active electrode gives an upward deflection on routine EEG. The spike has maximal potential in the region of the C3 electrode (channel 3), with some spread of the potential to adjacent electrodes (channels 2 and 4). The potential is not recorded from distant electrodes (channels 1 and 5). Localization on an average reference montage is relatively straightforward.

On first inspection, bipolar montages make visual analysis more complex, but they facilitate precise spatial localization. The same spike as shown in Figure 12.1 is shown in Figure 12.2 for the left parasagittal portion of the longitudinal bipolar montage.

For the same spike as described for the average reference montage, channel 2 shows a downward deflection because of negativity at C3, the reference electrode. Channel 3 shows an upward deflection, because C3 is the active electrode. The smaller spike at channel 1 also points down because of a lesser negativity at F3. Likewise, the small spike at channel 4 is upward because of negativity at P3. The appearance of this recording is that spikes point toward each other. The electrode where the direction of deflection changes is the most negative location of the spike. Bipolar montages can also allow for location of spikes even between F3 and C3, the spike will point downward in channel 1 and upward in channel 3. Since the negativity is approximately equal in F3 and C3, there will be virtually no deflection in channel 2.

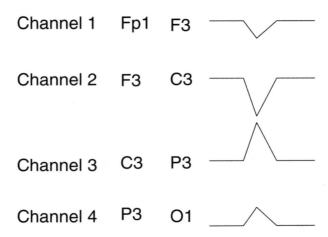

Figure 12.2 Spike localization in a longitudinal bipolar montage. These are the left parasagittal channels of the longitudinal bipolar montage. Data are simulated and at the same localization as the spike demonstrated in Figure 12.1.

Slow waves can be localized by polarity. Slow waves, however, are usually not as stereotyped as spikes. Therefore, localization depends more on absolute amplitude than polarity. The exception to this rule is differentiation of eye movement artifact from slow activity in the frontal lobes, which is discussed in detail in Chapter 13.

13 ⬜⬜⬜ ⬜⬜⬜ ⬜⬜⬜

Normal Electroencephalographic Patterns

Waking Rhythms

Normal Adult

Fast frequencies dominate the normal adult EEG in the awake, relaxed state when the eyes are closed. A posterior alpha rhythm is recorded with highest amplitude from the O1 and O2 electrodes (Figure 13.1). A central alpha rhythm may also be recorded, but it is usually of lower amplitude than that recorded from the occipital region. The background activity from the anterior region is composed predominantly of low-voltage, fast activity with superimposed eye movement artifact. Rhythmic beta may be recorded in the frontal and central regions, especially when sedatives are used. Drug-enhanced beta is more commonly seen after benzodiazepine and barbiturate sedation than following chloral hydrate. Theta and delta are not prominent in the normal awake adult EEG. However, digital frequency analysis shows a small amount of bihemispheric theta in most patients.

The occipital-predominant alpha is attenuated when the eyes are opened, or when the patient is tense. An indication of patient tenseness is the recording of EMG activity in scalp muscles. EMG activity is faster in frequency and sharper in configuration than EEG activity.

The posterior dominant rhythm is usually symmetric, but asymmetries of up to 25% are often seen. Asymmetry should not be interpreted as abnormal unless it is at least 50%. The amplitude from the left hemisphere is often less than the right, so this should be considered when interpreting abnormalities.

With increasing age in adults, the alpha may be lower in amplitude and less well organized. While slowing of the background is common in the

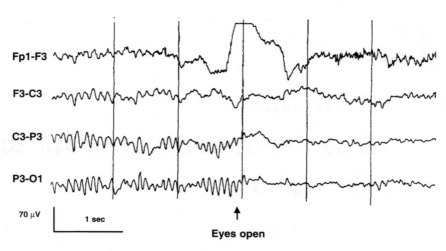

Figure 13.1 Normal EEG. Posterior dominant alpha rhythm of about 10–11 Hz. Only the first four channels of the longitudinal bipolar montage are shown.

elderly, it is still abnormal. I use a rigid cutoff of 8 Hz; any less than this is described as abnormal at any adult age.

Normal Child

Normal EEG patterns vary with age. The amplitude of potentials in children is generally greater than in adults. This applies not only to the posterior alpha but also especially to the frontal beta, which may be further enhanced by sedatives. Beta activity can be large enough to impair evaluation of other frequencies.

Theta activity is more prominent in children than in adults. Adolescents with 10-Hz posterior dominant rhythms will often have some bihemispheric theta that should be considered normal if the background is otherwise normal and the theta does not appear rhythmic.

Maturation of the Posterior Dominant Rhythm

The posterior dominant rhythm in the awake infant is approximately 4 Hz. The rhythm becomes faster with age, reaching the normal adult frequency of approximately 10 Hz by 10 years. This maturation is

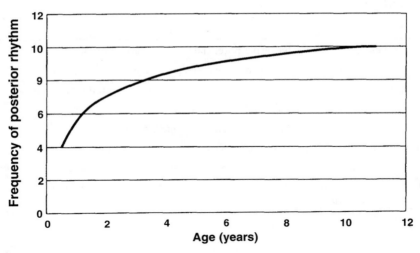

Figure 13.2 Maturation of the posterior dominant rhythm. Graph of frequency of the waking posterior dominant rhythm as a function of age.

shown in Figure 13.2. The amplitude gradually increases, such that by age 10 years the alpha is often in the range of 50–100 μV. In adults, the alpha amplitude gradually declines with increasing age.

Slow Waves of Youth

Slow waves of youth are in the delta range and are superimposed on the normal posterior dominant rhythm. They are seen primarily in the waking state and occasionally in light drowsiness. Slow waves of youth may be differentiated from pathologic slow waves by the otherwise normal background and their reactivity to eye opening. Slow waves of youth decrease with increasing age, and are not seen after the age of 30 years.

Sleeping Rhythms

Sleep promotes some epileptiform activity and is used as an activation method. However, the morphology of epileptiform discharges may look different in sleep than they look in the waking state. Sleep patterns differ in children and adults and are discussed in the next section.

Table 13.1   Sleep Rhythms

Pattern	Description
Vertex waves	Negative potentials with a maximum at Cz
	Occur in stage 2 sleep and during arousal
Sleep spindles	11- to 14-Hz waves of 1- to 2-sec duration
	Maximum at C3 and C4
	Most prominent in stage 2 sleep
K complexes	Fusion of a vertex wave and sleep spindle
	Prominent in stage 2 sleep and partial arousal
Positive occipital sharp transients of sleep	Positive potentials with maximum at O1 and O2

Normal Adult Sleep Patterns

The posterior dominant rhythm of relaxed waking state attenuates with drowsiness. As the alpha disappears, theta activity appears from both hemispheres. This is commonly referred to as stage 1 sleep (see the section on sleep stages later in this chapter). Stage 2 sleep occurs when sleep spindles and vertex waves appear. These are the most common sleep stages seen in routine EEG. Deeper stages of sleep are rarely seen in routine daytime EEG. Below is a detailed description of sleep patterns and stages (Table 13.1 also provides a description of sleep rhythms).

Vertex Waves

Vertex waves are surface negative potentials with maximum amplitude on either side of the midline (C3 and C4). They are most common in stage 2 sleep and often appear at times of partial arousal. The vertex waves are a diphasic sharp wave with an initial negative deflection followed by a positive deflection. The sharp wave may be followed by a slow wave or a spindle, the latter being termed a *K complex.*

The vertex waves can be asymmetric, especially in children, and high amplitude in younger patients. The asymmetry should be interpreted as abnormal if more than 25% and if consistent between the hemispheres. Vertex waves first appear at approximately 8 weeks of age. In children, vertex waves that appear in trains may be mistaken for seizure activity.

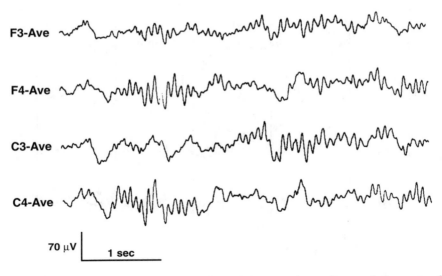

Figure 13.3 Sleep spindles. The high frequency waveforms have a frontocentral predominance and are most prominent in stage 2 sleep.

Sleep Spindles

Sleep spindles are rhythmic 11- to 14-Hz waves whose duration is typically 1–2 seconds (with a minimum 0.5 sec) and whose amplitude is at least 25 μV (Figure 13.3). They are most prominent in the central regions during stage 2 sleep. Unlike vertex waves, the maximum amplitude of sleep spindles is typically seen lateral to the midline (in the region of C3 and C4). Asymmetry in the abundance of sleep spindles is normal unless sleep spindles fail to appear from one hemisphere.

K Complexes

K complexes are formed by the fusion of sleep spindles and vertex waves (Figure 13.4). They are most commonly seen in stage 2 sleep and during partial arousal. They have no special significance beyond their individual elements.

Positive Occipital Sharp Transients of Sleep

Positive occipital sharp transients of sleep are surface positive potentials with maxima at O1 and O2. They may occur as single waves or in

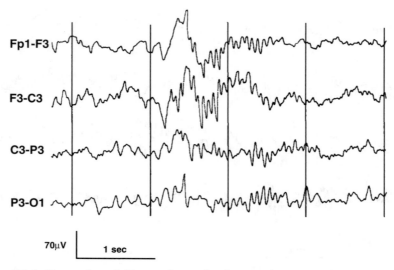

Figure 13.4 K complex. A K complex is the fusion of a vertex wave with a sleep spindle and is most prominent in stage 2 sleep.

trains. They resemble lambda waves, except that they are present only in the sleeping state, whereas lambda waves are present only in the waking state with eyes open.

While positive occipital sharp transients of sleep may be related to a replaying of visual information, this hypothesis is not universally accepted. They are not seen in patients who are blind or severely visually impaired.

Positive occipital sharp transients of sleep are not a constant feature of sleep and have no diagnostic significance, unless they are absent from only one side. This asymmetry is unlikely to be the only sign of focal abnormality in an EEG record.

Sleep Stages

Stage 1

Sleep stage 1 is subdivided into stages 1A and 1B. Stage 1A is light drowsiness, characterized by attenuation of the alpha, slight slowing of the background, and spread of the alpha anteriorly. Stage 1B is characterized by less than 20% alpha with a predominance of slow activity in the theta range. Vertex waves may be seen in stage 1B, but are usually a sign of stage 2. Differentiation of 1A and 1B is not important for routine EEG.

Stage 2

Stage 2 sleep is characterized by sleep spindles, vertex waves, increased theta, and the appearance of delta. However, less than 20% of the record contains delta. Since some vertex waves can be seen in stage 1B, the primary differentiating feature is the appearance of sleep spindles.

Stage 3

Stage 3 sleep is characterized by increasing delta content and reduction in faster frequencies. Delta comprises 20–50% of the record.

Stage 4

Stage 4 sleep is characterized by a further increase in delta content, so that delta comprises more than 50% of the record. Vertex waves and sleep spindles are less prominent and are often absent.

Rapid Eye Movement Sleep

Rapid eye movement (REM) sleep is characterized by a low-voltage background composed of predominantly fast frequencies. It can be difficult to distinguish REM sleep from light drowsiness. Rhythmic 6–8 Hz activity, which is called *sawtooth waves* because of its unusual morphology, may appear in the frontal regions and vertex.

Typically, REM sleep follows after progression from sleep stages 1 through 4. Progression from drowsiness to REM sleep without passing through other stages (termed *REM-onset sleep*) occurs in patients with narcolepsy, after sleep deprivation, and after alcohol- or drug-induced REM-deprivation sleep.

The features of REM sleep that distinguish it from drowsiness are the following:

- Rapid and chaotic eye movements (drowsiness is associated with slow roving eye movements)
- Hypotonia as measured by submental EMG
- An irregular respiratory rate

Sequence of Sleep Stages

The sequence of sleep stages for a normal adult is discussed in Part V. The cycle of sleep stages is repeated approximately three to four times per night, although there may not be progression to deeper stages with every cycle. Usually REM sleep occurs after at least one sleep cycle and increases in duration during subsequent cycles. Respiratory pattern is usually regular in all sleep stages except REM. Submental EMG activity declines progressively as sleep becomes deeper until disappearing during REM sleep.

Changes in Sleep Stages with Age

Sleep patterns in children, after the neonatal period, are similar to those in adults. Neonatal sleep patterns are detailed in Chapter 18.

A child normally has identifiable sleep patterns by 1 year of age. Sleep spindles are present by 2 months of age and vertex waves by 5 months of age, although initial vertex waves have a blunted morphology. By 2 years of age, sleep spindles and vertex waves are abundant, sharp in configuration, and high in amplitude. Clusters of vertex waves may be mistaken for epileptiform activity. Later in childhood, vertex waves are less abundant but still high in amplitude. Sleep patterns continue to evolve throughout adult life, as the total hours of sleep decline and the number of awakenings during sleep increases. Stages 3 and 4 become shorter, producing a reduced latency of REM sleep.

Normal Noncerebral Potentials

Noncerebral potentials can obscure normal cerebral potentials and can be mistaken for physiologic potentials. Noncerebral potentials are of two types: (1) noncerebral potentials of physiologic origin, and (2) electrical artifact (Table 13.2). The most prominent noncerebral physiologic potentials are from eye movement.

Eye Movement

Eye movement artifact is seen in anterior leads in virtually all records. The eye is polarized with the cornea positive relative to the fundus. Therefore, when the eye rotates to look down, the leads over the frontal region are close to the negative end of the ocular dipole. This effect is most prominent for Fp1, Fp2, F3, and F4. The reverse is true with upward gaze, as the frontal leads are close to the positive end of the dipole. With lateral gaze, the electrodes most affected are F7 and F8. For example, with left gaze, F7 becomes more positive while F8 becomes more negative.

Differentiating eye movement artifact from electrocerebral activity is usually not difficult. First, eye movements have a stereotypic pattern that looks different from most abnormal frontal slow activity, which is usually

Table 13.2 Normal Noncerebral Potentials

Pattern	Description
Eye movement	Eye is polarized with the cornea positive to the fundus Appearance dependent on the montage and direction of eye movement Differentiated from cerebral activity with the help of eye leads
Muscle artifact	Very brief activity with a temporal predominance when awake Abates with relaxation and opening of the mouth
ECG	Fast activity seen especially with ear reference Identified by comparison with an ECG channel
Glossokinetic artifact	Tongue is negative at the tip as compared with the base Talking can exacerbate Best differentiated using infraorbital electrodes and asking the patient to make intentional lingual movements
Movement artifact (two types)	Slow activity due to change in orientation of the electrode leads Fast activity if movement produces changes in junction potentials
Machine artifact	Usually high-frequency artifact with a nonphysiologic periodicity Usually no localization

more polymorphic. The onset of slow waves caused by eye movement is rapid with a slower decay. Also, eye movement waveforms are typically superimposed on a normal low-voltage, high-frequency background. Abnormal frontal delta activity is usually associated with increased theta activity and reduced beta activity in the frontal regions. If identification is in doubt, eye leads should be placed to definitively distinguish between cerebral and eye activity.

Eye leads can be placed in several ways. The two most common methods are shown in Figure 13.5. We use the method shown in Figure 13.5A. Electrodes are placed above and lateral to the right eye and below and lateral to the left eye. These electrodes are referenced to an average or ear electrode. With upward gaze, the positive end of the dipole rotates toward the right lead but away from the left. This causes pen deflections of opposite polarity in the recording. With left gaze, the positive cornea rotates toward the left lead but away from the right. Again, the pen deflections will be in

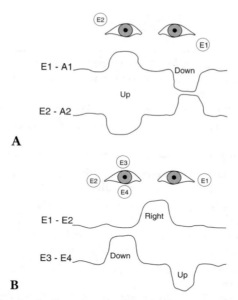

Figure 13.5 Eye lead placement. These leads help differentiate between eye movement and frontal slow activity. A. Method used in our laboratory. B. Alternative method.

opposite directions. These electrode derivations will detect slow activity in the frontal lobes, but this slow activity will not reverse between the two sides. Therefore, in these channels, slow activity that is opposite in polarity is of ocular origin, while slow activity that is of the same polarity on both sides is most likely of cerebral origin.

The method shown in Figure 13.5B of eye movement detection allows for precise determination of direction of gaze. Vertical gaze can be distinguished from horizontal gaze. This is seldom of interest on routine EEG testing.

Muscle Artifact

EMG activity is a frequent contaminant of EEG recordings. It is most prominent in the awake state and is characterized by fast, short-duration spikes in the temporal and frontal regions (Figure 13.6). Amplitude is approximately 50 µV. EMG activity is due to discharge of motor units in the temporalis and frontalis muscles. Distinction from spikes of cerebral origin is usually not difficult.

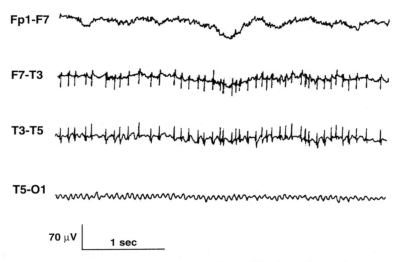

Figure 13.6 Muscle artifact. Fast activity in lateral leads is the surface recording of motor unit potentials.

- EMG activity is very fast. In fact, the predominant frequency is much faster than the high frequency filter setting of 70 Hz.
- EMG activity is not followed by a slow wave.
- EMG is most prominent in the waking, tense state and disappears with relaxed wakefulness and sleep. In contrast, epileptiform activity is often best seen in drowsiness and sleep.
- EMG activity can often be attenuated by asking the patient to open his mouth. While the masseter and pterygoid muscles do not contribute much to surface EMG activity, this relaxation promotes decreased activation of scalp muscles as well.

Electrocardiogram Artifact

ECG artifact is a frequent contaminant of EEG recordings and can be mistaken for epileptiform activity. It is most prominent with high sensitivities, ear reference montages, and in ICU recordings (Figure 13.7). Recording of ECG on a separate channel prevents confusion. If there is no extra channel, the technician should sacrifice a channel during part of the recording, especially if sharp waveforms are seen.

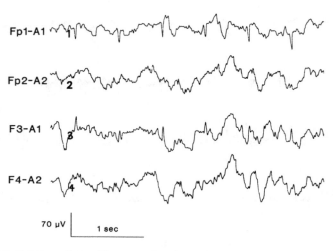

Figure 13.7 ECG artifact. The periodic sharp waves in channels 1 and 3 are due to contamination by EMG. This is most common in ear reference montages. A separate EMG channel was recorded but is not shown.

Glossokinetic Artifact

Glossokinetic artifact is due to tongue movement. The tongue is a dipole with the tip negative with respect to the base. Tongue movements in the waking state are seen in the EEG as delta activity and can be mistaken for pathologic frontal delta activity. Glossokinetic activity disappears with drowsiness and sleep.

Differentiation of glossokinetic artifact from electrocerebral slow activity can be difficult and may require technician observation. It is usually concurrent with muscle artifact of the temporalis and frontalis. If there is still any doubt, electrodes should be placed below the orbits. These electrodes are too distant to detect electrocerebral activity but will pick up slow activity due to tongue or eye movement. The patient can be asked to say "la, la, la" so that the potential field and appearance of glossokinetic artifact can be identified.

Movement Artifact

Movement artifact was briefly discussed in Part I. There are two sources of movement artifact: electrode-gel interface and electrode leads.

Electrode-Gel Interface

A diffusion potential is established at the interface between the electrode and the gel, which is caused by movement of ions between the two substances. The concept is similar to the creation of a resting membrane potential in cell membranes. When there is movement of the electrodes, the junction is disturbed, and the junction potential discharges, injecting current through the electrode into the input amplifier. This is interpreted by the amplifier as a voltage pulse. This type of movement artifact looks like a brief spike followed by a gradual decay toward zero. During the pulse, the responsiveness of the amplifier may be reduced, since the amount of current flow from the artifact can be sufficient to overload the input amplifier. If there is no further movement, a new equilibrium is established.

Electrode Leads

The flow of electrons through electrical lines creates a weak magnetic field. Magnetic fields in turn can influence the flow of electrons through conductors (i.e., they can induce current). This interaction between current and magnetic fields is termed *inductance* and is the physical basis for inductors, which were discussed in Chapter 2. Inductance is also important for the generation of noise.

Electrode leads are unshielded and therefore susceptible to the effects of ambient magnetic fields. These magnetic fields are created by current in nearby power lines and equipment. Magnetic fields then induce current to flow through the electrode leads. This mechanism is termed *stray inductance* because the inductance is not intentional within the machinery. The induced current flows through the electrode leads just as signal current does. The amplifier cannot distinguish between signal and noise, so both are amplified. Since line power is 60 Hz, this creates 60-Hz interference.

The other major source of 60-Hz interference is *stray capacitance.* There is a small amount of capacitance between electrode leads and between leads and power lines. A charge can build up across this capacitance. The capacitance will change with electrode lead movement, thereby altering the built-up potential. Also, alternating current in power lines can create a small capacitive current in electrode leads, thereby creating 60-Hz interference.

The differential amplifier will reject much of the 60-Hz interference; however, the rejection is incomplete under the following conditions:

- If electrodes are affected unequally by stray inductance and stray capacitance (because of difference in lead position and proximity to electrical wires)
- If there are unequal electrode impedances
- If there is electrode movement

When the electrodes are stable, stray inductance can cause 60-cycle interference that is rejected by the differential amplifiers. When there is electrode movement, however, the orientation of the electrode leads in space is altered. This produces a sudden change in induced current. The transient alteration in current is interpreted by the amplifier as a voltage shift.

Machine Artifact

Machine artifact is discussed in more detail in the section on 60-Hz Interference in Chapter 8. It is not normal but is a frequent accompaniment to otherwise normal EEG recordings. The opportunity for machine artifact is greatest in the ICU. Figure 13.8 shows the artifact created by the motor of an air bed. The artifact disappears after the bed is unplugged. Machine artifact is usually interpreted as normal, with a comment about the artifact in the report. If artifact obscures much of the recording such that interpretation of the EEG background is impossible, the interpretation should state something along the lines that the EEG is a "technically unsatisfactory study because of electrical artifact. Clinical interpretation cannot be rendered on the basis of this recording."

Normal Variant Patterns

Table 13.3 describes normal variant patterns in EEG recording.

Mu Rhythm

Mu rhythm is not a common feature of normal EEGs. It is a run of negative wicket-shaped spikes with an approximate frequency of 10 Hz and a duration ranging from less than 1 second to many seconds. The negativity is maximal in the rolandic regions, mainly C3 and C4. Mu has the appearance of a centrally located alpha rhythm but is usually slightly faster than the patient's alpha rhythm. It is blocked by movement of the contralateral extremity: this is the key to identification. In fact, mu can be blocked by

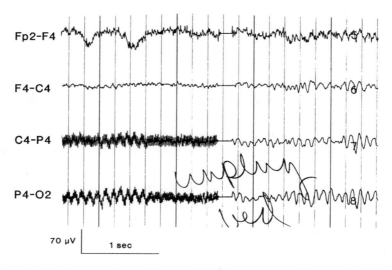

Figure 13.8 Machine artifact. The very high-frequency artifact on the left side of the trace was from an air bed. Unplugging the bed abolished the artifact.

merely thinking about limb movement. The technician should ask the patient to move a limb to verify the waveform.

Lambda Waves

Lambda waves are normal positive waves that appear over the occipital region when the patient is looking at a picture or pattern. Lambda waves indicate visual exploration and are blocked by eye closing. They are called lambda waves because of their resemblance to the Greek lowercase letter lambda (λ).

Wicket Spikes

Wicket spikes are sharply contoured waves that are most prominent in the temporal regions during drowsiness and light sleep. They are differentiated from true spikes by the absence of a following slow wave, normal background activity, and occurrence in a series of waves at 6–10 per second. Wicket spikes are more common with increasing age.

Table 13.3 Normal Variant Patterns

Pattern	Description
Mu rhythm	Wicket-shaped spikes at 10 Hz Duration <1 sec Prominent in C3 and C4 Blocked when even thinking about limb movement
Lambda waves	Positive occipital waves when patient is looking at a pattern Blocked by eye closure
Wicket spikes	Temporal sharp waves and spikes during drowsiness and light sleep
14-and-6 positive spikes	Sharply contoured rhythm with temporal predominance at 6 or 14 Hz during drowsiness and light sleep
Benign epileptiform transients of sleep	Small spike-like potentials in temporal region during drowsiness and light sleep
Slow alpha variant	Subharmonic variant of posterior dominant alpha rhythm 4–5 Hz
Rhythmic temporal theta of drowsiness	Trains of sharply contoured theta waves Temporal predominance in drowsiness
Mittens	Fusion of a sleep spindle and a vertex wave, especially in stage 2 sleep

14-and-6 Positive Spikes

The 14-and-6 positive spike rhythm is a sharply contoured, positive waveform that occurs mainly in drowsiness and light sleep. The distribution can be widespread but reaches highest amplitude over the posterior temporal region. At times, the rhythm has the appearance of 14 Hz, and at others it appears to be 6 Hz. Both frequencies may not occur together or in a particular patient during a single recording. The 6-Hz component predominates in young children, and the 14-Hz frequency predominates in older children.

Although 14-and-6 positive spikes have been reported in association with many pathologic conditions, the association is weak and the incidence is probably not different than in normal individuals. The 14-and-6 pattern should be described in the body of the EEG report but not interpreted as abnormal. One exception is in metabolic encephalopathies, such as hepatic coma. In this situation, the presence of 14-and-6 positive spikes is not considered normal; however, in these patients the background is abnormal, as well.

Benign Epileptiform Transients of Sleep

Benign epileptiform transients of sleep (BETS) are very small spike-like potentials that occur in the temporal regions during drowsiness and light sleep. They are less than 50 µV with a duration of less than 15 ms. Also called small sharp spikes, benign epileptiform transients of sleep are differentiated from epileptogenic spikes by their small amplitude, short duration, lack of slow wave, and normal EEG background.

Slow Alpha Variant

The slow alpha variant is a subharmonic of the normal alpha rhythm. The frequency is 4–5 Hz and the wave is usually notched, so that the native 10-Hz alpha rhythm can be identified.

Differentiation of the slow alpha variant from a diffuse encephalopathy is made by looking for the notching and examining the background activity. Most conditions that would slow the posterior dominant rhythm to 4–5 Hz in an adult would be associated with a poorly organized background with theta from more frontal and central regions.

Rhythmic Temporal Theta of Drowsiness

Rhythmic temporal theta of drowsiness has been called the *psychomotor variant*. This term is not preferred because the psychiatric implication is inappropriate. The rhythm consists of trains of sharply contoured waves in the theta range (Figure 13.9). They are most prominent in the temporal region but are also present in central regions. As the name suggests, the rhythm is seen mainly in drowsiness but may also be seen in relaxed wakefulness.

Rhythmic temporal theta of drowsiness is differentiated from seizure activity by the normal background before and after the train and by the absence of typical frequency progression that characterizes most seizure discharges.

Mittens

Mittens are waveforms that are occasionally mistaken for spike-wave complexes. A sleep spindle and a vertex wave are partially fused,

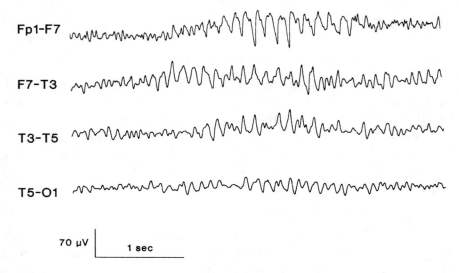

Figure 13.9 Rhythmic temporal theta of drowsiness (psychomotor variant).

such that the last wave of the spindle is superimposed on the rising phase of the vertex wave. The voltage summation gives the last spindle wave a taller, faster appearance, which simulates a spike. The name is derived from the appearance of a mitten; the thumb is the fused spindle wave, and the hand portion is the slow component of the vertex wave.

14 □□□ □□□ □□□

Activation Methods

Activation methods are used to bring out epileptiform discharges in patients with suspected seizure disorders. Hyperventilation and photic stimulation are routinely used during EEG. Sleep is not considered by some neurophysiologists to be a true activation method, but it certainly aids in evoking epileptiform discharges.

Hyperventilation

The most predictable use of hyperventilation is to activate the three-per-second spike and wave discharge of primary generalized epilepsy. In some patients, discharges are seen only during hyperventilation. The patient is asked to mouth-breathe deeply for approximately 3 minutes. If there is suspicion of absence seizures, the patient should hyperventilate for 5 minutes.

The normal response to hyperventilation is generalized slowing of the background activity to the theta range in both hemispheres. Absence of slowing is not abnormal and depends on patient effort, age (children are more likely to show slowing than adults), and time from last meal (hypoglycemia may augment slowing). Movement artifact may contaminate the record, especially in the posterior leads, as a result of head movement with chest excursions. Normal slow activity may have a notched appearance and should not be interpreted as epileptiform. The epileptiform discharges activated by hyperventilation are usually not subtle.

Hyperventilation should not be performed in patients with cerebrovascular disease or intracranial hemorrhage. Hypocapnia and alkalosis may cause vasospasm and impair cerebral perfusion.

The mechanism by which hyperventilation activates epileptiform activity is not completely known. The effect of hyperventilation-induced alkalosis and hypocapnia on the caliber of cerebral vessels is probably not important in the genesis of epileptiform discharges. The development of slow activity and disinhibition of spikes and slow waves may be due to depression of activity of the reticular activating system.

Photic Stimulation

Photic stimulation is more likely to activate epileptiform discharges in patients with primary rather than secondary epilepsy. A strobe light is placed in front of the patient's closed eyes. The light delivers trains of flashes at specified rates. These routines are programmed in most EEG machines. General guidelines for performing photic stimulation include the following:

- Train duration of 10 seconds
- Trains delivered every 20 seconds
- Initial flash rate of 3/sec
- Higher frequency for each successive train (e.g., we use the following flash rates in our laboratory: 3, 5, 7, 9, 11, 13, 15, 18, 20, 24, and 30 per second)

If a discharge is activated at a specified frequency, the technician should repeat that frequency at the completion of the photic stimulation routine.

Normal responses to photic stimulation include the visual evoked response, the driving response, and the photomyoclonic response.

Normal Photic Response

A visual evoked response can be seen in occipital leads at flash frequencies of less than 7/sec (Figure 14.1). This response is the same as the flash-induced visual evoked potential discussed in Chapter 34 but is much more variable because the response is not averaged. A driving response is seen at flash frequencies of 7/sec and greater (Figure 14.2). The two responses look alike but are distinguished by their temporal relation to the stimulus. The visual evoked response occurs approximately 100 ms after the stimulus, and the driving response is exactly time-locked to the stimulus.

The absence of visual evoked and driving responses is not abnormal unless it is well developed on one side and absent on the other. Such asymmetry suggests an abnormality affecting either the projections from the lateral geniculate to the cortex or the calcarine cortex itself.

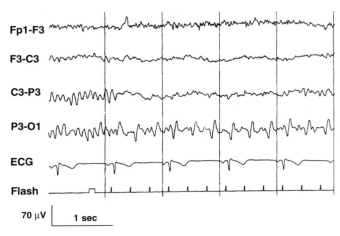

Figure 14.1 Photic evoked potential. Note the lag between the stimulus and the peak of the evoked potential in channel 4. This lag and the response only at low frequencies differentiates the evoked response from the driving response.

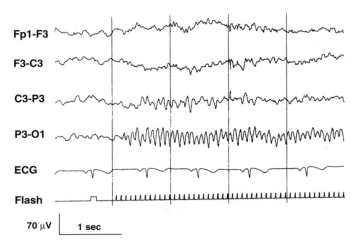

Figure 14.2 Photic driving response. The driving response is time-locked to the flash, without the lag that characterizes the evoked response. Also, the driving response is present at faster frequencies.

Photomyoclonic Response

The photomyoclonic response is caused by repeated contraction of frontal muscles that are time-locked to the flash stimulus with a delay of 50–60 ms. The discharges are suppressed by eye opening and disappear with neuromuscular blockade. Muscle activity that may have the appearance of seizure discharges appears in the anterior leads. Factors that help distinguish a photomyoclonic response from a photoconvulsive discharge are the following:

- The photomyoclonic response is anterior, whereas photoconvulsive responses are posterior or generalized.
- The photomyoclonic response stops promptly at the end of the stimulus train, whereas the photoconvulsive response typically outlasts the stimulus.
- The spikes that make up the photomyoclonic response are much faster than those of cerebral origin. The synchrony of muscle fiber discharges is much greater than that of neuronal discharges.
- The photomyoclonic response has the same frequency as the flash, whereas photoconvulsive discharges are often slower, in the range of 3/sec.

The photomyoclonic response is enhanced in patients undergoing alcohol or barbiturate withdrawal and should be considered as a nonspecific, normal response despite unconfirmed reports of an association with seizures and psychiatric disorders.

Photoconvulsive Response

The photoconvulsive response is characterized by spike-wave complexes during photic stimulation (Figure 14.3). The discharge is usually activated only by a few specific flash frequencies. It never begins with the first flash and usually ends before the flash ends. The correlation of a photoconvulsive discharge with seizures is greatest if the discharges continue after the end of flash train.

Sleep

The frequency of interictal epileptiform discharges is often increased during drowsiness and light sleep. Therefore, patients being evaluated for a seizure disorder should be studied both when awake and when asleep.

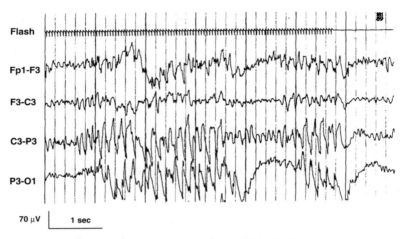

Figure 14.3 Photoconvulsive response. Note that the discharge is not time-locked to the stimulus and outlasts the train of flashes.

Sleep is also helpful in identifying potentials that are seen in the waking state. For example, subtle sharp transients may be evident in the waking state that are not clearly epileptiform. During sleep, the spikes may be activated into definite epileptiform activity. Conversely, sharp transients that disappear during sleep are unlikely to be epileptiform. They may be normal waveforms with unusually sharp contours or artifact.

Since most routine EEG recordings are performed in the waking state, sedation or sleep deprivation is often necessary. There is no convincing evidence that spontaneous sleep, sedated sleep, and sleep by deprivation differ in their ability to evoke epileptiform activity.

Sedated Sleep

Chloral hydrate is commonly used for sedation because it is safe to use in outpatients and does not produce the widespread beta activity that is characteristic of benzodiazepines and barbiturates. The usual oral dose for adults is 1 g, with a single repeat if needed. The dose for children is 25 mg/kg, which may be repeated up to 75 mg/kg. The major side effects of chloral hydrate in adults are confusion and ataxia. Therefore, all outpatients who are sedated must have an attendant who will look after them and drive them home. Children can have confusion and ataxia but may alternatively develop an agitated delirium.

Barbiturates are an alternative to chloral hydrate and are especially useful in patients with a history of agitation from chloral hydrate. Intravenous administration of short-acting barbiturates has been advocated by some investigators for the detection of focal epileptiform activity; however, this is not routine practice.

Sleep Deprivation

Sleep deprivation involves keeping the patient awake for 24 hours prior to the recording. After arising one day, the patient does not sleep until the EEG is performed the following morning. The patient is discouraged from drinking caffeine-containing beverages. Patients who adhere to the sleep deprivation regimen usually fall asleep during the recording. Unfortunately, patients often progress quickly into stage 3 or 4 sleep, missing the transition from wakefulness through drowsiness into light sleep. This progression is most important for detection of spikes. Therefore, it is helpful to keep the patient awake and watch the drowsy pattern for epileptiform activity. Sleep deprivation for 24 hours probably does not evoke spikes in normal individuals. Therefore, concern over false positives is small.

The relative merit of sleep deprivation compared to sedated sleep is controversial. Literature can be found to support the use or nonuse of this activation method. I personally believe the balance of the evidence supports increased diagnostic sensitivity with sleep deprivation. Since this is a noninvasive procedure, although not easy for the patient, it is reasonable to perform this study, especially if a good sedated sleep study cannot be obtained.

Withdrawal of Anticonvulsants

Inpatient EEG monitoring is discussed in detail in Chapter 20. During monitoring, electroencephalographers use a variety of methods to provoke seizures, one of these is the withdrawal of anticonvulsants, thus increasing the likelihood of having seizures. Although anticonvulsants probably do not suppress interictal electrical activity, the withdrawal of anticonvulsants may have a psychological effect in promoting pseudoseizures, thereby facilitating differentiation from epileptic seizures.

15 Spikes and Sharp Waves

Definition and Identification

Spikes and sharp waves are transients that stand out from the background. Spikes are usually surface negative and have a duration of 20–70 ms. Sharp waves are also usually surface negative but have a duration of 70–200 ms. Pointed potentials with a duration of less than 20 ms are usually not of cerebral origin. The negative pole of spikes and sharp waves is distributed across a region of the cortex. The distribution is called a *potential field*. This field is not directly comparable to the field potentials recorded by intracortical electrodes. The positive end of the spike dipole is occasionally visible on the surface, usually indicating that the dipole is oriented horizontally.

Table 15.1 lists criteria for differentiating spikes from nonspike potentials. Major pitfalls include misinterpreting sharply contoured slow waves and pointed waves of background rhythms. Theta activity occurs normally in drowsiness and in children. The theta is polymorphic, and multiple waves occasionally sum to give a sharp appearance. A sharp wave should not be considered abnormal unless it stands out from the background and is reproducible. The alpha rhythm may occasionally appear sharp, even though the pointed component is positive. Positive polarity helps to distinguish this waveform from a spike potential. The sharp component occurs in step with the other waves comprising the alpha rhythm, indicating that it is merely a sharply contoured alpha wave and not a pathologic spike.

In general, more harm is done by overinterpretation than by underinterpretation of EEG. If you are uncertain whether a potential is abnormal, consider it to be normal. Questionable findings should be described in the body of the report to facilitate comparison with future studies.

When spike potentials are seen in studies requested for nonseizure indications, it is not helpful to interpret the record as "consistent with a seizure

Table 15.1 Differentiation Between Spike and Nonspike Potentials*

Spike	Nonspike
Stereotyped	Vary in morphology
Stand out from background	Embedded in background
Rising phase is fastest	May be slower in the rising phase than in the falling phase
Usually followed by a slow wave	Usually not followed by a slow wave
Defined potential field	Often a single electrode
Activated by sleep	No change with sleep

*In addition to this differentiation, it is important to distinguish pathologic from non-pathologic sharp waveforms, especially normal sharp waves in neonates, vertex waves, lambda waves, 14- and 6-Hz positive spikes, mu rhythm, and artifacts.

disorder." Instead, interpret the record as follows: "This is an abnormal study because of a spike focus in the left posterior temporal region. Spikes are not always associated with a seizure disorder." If there is no textbook interpretation, the clinician should interpret the findings in the context of the clinical situation. Table 15.2 shows clinical disorders frequently characterized by spikes on EEG. Specific disorders are discussed below.

When Spikes and Sharp Waves Are Normal

Most spikes and sharp waves are abnormal in adults. Several physiologic spike-like potentials may be recorded, however. These include vertex waves, occipital lambda waves, 14- and 6-Hz positive spikes, wicket spikes, benign epileptiform transients of sleep, positive occipital sharp transients of sleep, and six-per-second phantom spike and wave. These are discussed in Chapter 13.

Generalized Spike-Wave Discharge

Spike-wave complexes correlate better than single spike discharges with clinical seizures. Generalized spike-wave discharges fall into four categories: (1) three-per-second spike-wave complex, (2) slow spike-wave complex, (3) fast spike-wave complex, and (4) six-per-second spike wave complex (Table 15.3).

Table 15.2   Electroencephalographic Patterns with Selected
Disorders That Frequently Demonstrate Spikes

Disorder	Electroencephalogram Pattern
Rolandic epilepsy	Stereotyped spikes, often with triphasic appearance, followed by a slow wave Independent discharges with maxima near C3 and C4 Activated by sleep Otherwise normal background
Occipital epilepsy	Unilateral or bilateral high-amplitude occipital spikes, which are increased by light sleep and suppressed by eye opening Rapid discharge from the same regions during a seizure
Absence epilepsy	Classic three-per-second spike-wave or polyspike-wave complex Increased by hyperventilation Less well organized in sleep.
Subacute sclerosing panencephalitis	Periodic high-amplitude bursts of sharp waves, often with an irregular delta wave superimposed Synchronous between hemispheres Duration of 0.5–2.0 secs Many seconds to a minute or more between bursts
Creutzfeldt-Jakob	Periodic complexes with a frequency of 0.5–2.0/sec Maximal anteriorly Abnormal background, with low voltage slowing Periodic complexes abate during sleep
Anoxic encephalopathy	From normal to isoelectric depending on severity Common patterns include burst suppression and a periodic pattern that resembles Creutzfeldt-Jakob disease Alpha coma is a diffuse nonreactive alpha activity with a frontocentral prominence; these latter patterns indicate a poor prognosis
Herpes simplex encephalitis	Generalized slowing with a frontotemporal predominance Periodic complexes of sharp waves or sharply contoured slow waves, which appear irregularly High amplitude frequency of 0.2–1.0/sec
Arbovirus encephalitis	Slowing in the theta and delta range with little intra- or interhemispheric synchrony Few faster frequencies.
Lennox-Gastaut syndrome	Slow spike-wave complex Slow background in many Increasing disorganization during sleep
Juvenile myoclonic epilepsy	Generalized polyspike discharges followed by a slow wave Higher amplitude in the frontal region Otherwise normal background

Table 15.2 *(continued)*

Disorder	Electroencephalogram Pattern
Complex partial seizures	Various patterns depending on site of origin of epileptiform activity May be unilateral temporal or frontal spikes Focal slowing or no discharge recordable with surface electrodes
Simple partial seizures	Midline spikes with a prominent negative phase or biphasic in most patients Occasional patients may have a positive prominence on surface electroencephalogram This pattern correlates with focal motor seizures
Generalized tonic-clonic seizures	Generalized polyspike discharge that often, but not invariably, has a slow wave Ictal activity often is high-frequency spikes without obvious slow waves

Three-Per-Second Spike-Wave Complex

The three-per-second spike-wave complex is usually equated with absence seizures. Although there is a strong correlation between the two, a patient with a three-per-second spike-wave complex may exhibit other seizure types, including generalized tonic-clonic seizures. The interpretation of such records should read: "This is an abnormal study because of three-per-second spike-wave complexes. This is consistent with a seizure disorder of the generalized type."

Characteristics of the Three-Per-Second Spike-Wave Complex

The three-per-second spike-wave complex is synchronous from the two hemispheres, with the highest amplitude over the midline frontal region. The lowest amplitudes are in the temporal and occipital regions. The frequency changes slightly during the course of the discharge, beginning close to 4/sec and declining to 2.5/sec. Immediately following the discharge, the record quickly returns to normal (Figure 15.1). The spike component may have a double spike or polyspike appearance.

The three-per-second spike-wave complex is promoted by hyperventilation. If absence epilepsy is considered, the patient should be asked to hyperventilate for 5 minutes instead of the usual 3 minutes. Children with absence become symptomatic if the discharge lasts longer than 5 seconds.

Table 15.3   Spike Interpretation of Generalized Spikes

Type	Electroencephalogram Features	Clinical Features
Burst suppression	Bursts of slow waves with superimposed sharp waves, interspersed on periods of relative flattening	Severe encephalopathy from anesthesia, anoxia, or other diffuse causes
Three-per-second spike-wave	Spike or polyspike complexes between 2.5/sec and 4/sec Increased by hyperventilation	Generalized epilepsy May be seen in relatives of clinically affected patients
Six-per-second (phantom) spike wave	Small spike-wave complexes May have a frontal or occipital predominance	If frontal, associated with generalized tonic-clonic seizures If occipital, usually not associated with seizures
Hypsarrhythmia	High-voltage bursts of theta and delta with multifocal sharp waves superimposed, interspersed by relative suppression	Seen in patients with infantile spasms
Slow spike-wave	Spike-wave pattern resembling the three-per-second variety but at 1–2/sec and often with asymmetry and less interhemispheric synchrony	Lennox-Gastaut syndrome Generalized seizures, often tonic; may be atypical absence, atonic, or myoclonic

During the discharge, the technician should ask the patient a question. The patient with absence seizure often answers after the discharge. The question and response should be noted on the record.

The three-per-second discharge is less well organized during sleep than during the waking state. Its appearance is more polyspike in configuration and the spike-wave interval is less regular.

Clinical Correlations of the Three-per-Second Spike-Wave Complex

The three-per-second spike-wave discharge correlates well with primary generalized epilepsy. Factors that should make the clinician doubt the diagnosis of primary generalized epilepsy include (1) abnormal background on EEG, (2) clearly focal discharges, or (3) history of slow neurologic development or an abnormal neurologic examination.

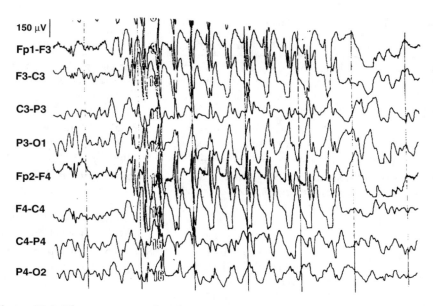

Figure 15.1 Three-per-second spike-wave complex. This is a typical discharge occurring during hyperventilation. Multiple episodes occurred during the recording.

The spike component of the three-per-second spike-wave complex is polyspike in some patients. Patients with this polyspike pattern are more likely to exhibit myoclonus.

Treatment of absence epilepsy often abolishes the interictal discharge. This is different from most focal epilepsies, in which interictal spiking persists despite good seizure control.

Slow Spike-Wave Complex

The slow spike-wave complex is frequently associated clinically with the Lennox-Gastaut syndrome. It also has been called *petit mal variant*. The term is misleading and should not be used.

The frequency of the slow spike-wave complex is 2.5/sec or less, and its morphology is less stereotyped than the three-per-second complex. The duration of the slow spike is usually more than 70 ms, which is technically a sharp wave. The complex is generalized and synchronous across both hemispheres, with the highest amplitude in the midline frontal region.

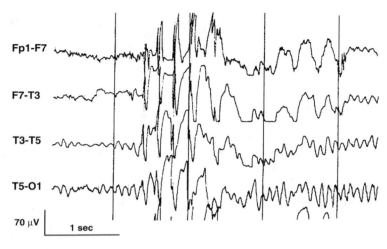

Figure 15.2 Fast spike-wave complex. The patient has juvenile myoclonic epilepsy.

During sleep, the slow spike-wave activity may be continuous. This may not indicate status epilepticus but rather represents activation of the interictal activity with sleep.

Lennox-Gastaut syndrome manifests the slow spike-wave complex. The slow spike-wave complex is usually an interictal pattern but may be ictal as well. Since these patients have a mixed seizure disorder, ictal events may be characterized by patterns other than the slow spike-wave complex. Atonic seizures are characterized by generalized spikes during the myoclonus, followed by the slow spike-wave pattern during the atonic phase. Atonic seizures are most characteristic of the Lennox-Gastaut syndrome. Akinetic seizures are characterized by the slow spike-wave discharge throughout the seizure. Tonic seizures also occur in Lennox-Gastaut syndrome and are characterized by rapid spike activity or desynchronization rather than the slow spike-wave complex.

Fast Spike-Wave Complex

The fast spike-wave complex has a frequency of 4–5/sec and is characterized by slow waves (Figure 15.2). Maximal amplitude is in the frontocentral region. Patients have generalized tonic-clonic seizures with or without myoclonus. Absence seizures are rare. This is the most common pattern seen in patients with idiopathic generalized tonic-clonic seizures. The discharge is not as stereotyped and synchronous as the three-per-second spike-wave complex.

Six-Per-Second Hertz (Phantom) Spike-Wave Complex

The six-per-second phantom spike-wave pattern is characterized by brief trains of small spike-wave complexes that are distributed diffusely over both hemispheres. They are most common during the waking and drowsy states and disappear during sleep.

The six-per-second spike-wave complex may have frontal or occipital predominance. Frontal predominance is frequently associated with generalized tonic-clonic seizures, whereas occipital predominance is usually not associated with clinical seizures. Hughes (1980) provided the acronyms WHAM and FOLD. WHAM stands for *w*aking record, *h*igh amplitude, *a*nterior, *m*ales; FOLD stands for *f*emales, *o*ccipital, *l*ow amplitude, *d*rowsy. WHAM is associated with seizures, FOLD is not.

This rhythm is differentiated from the 14- and 6-Hz positive spikes not only by the polarity but also by the more widespread distribution and the occurrence in wakefulness. Both rhythms may occur in the same patient. The six-per-second spike-wave complex is interpreted as abnormal and the different clinical implications should be emphasized in the report.

Hypsarrhythmia

Hypsarrhythmia is seen in children with infantile spasms. High-voltage bursts of theta and delta waves have multifocal sharp waves superimposed (Figure 15.3). The bursts are separated by periods of relative suppression. In some circumstances, flattening of the EEG may be an ictal sign, indicating that there has been sudden desynchronization of the record.

Focal Spikes

Focal spikes often indicate a focal seizure disorder. Frontocentral discharges may be seen in patients with simple partial seizures. Temporal or frontal spikes may be seen in patients with complex partial seizures. Normal focal spike-wave complexes include 14- and 6-Hz positive spikes, subclinical rhythmic electrographic discharge of adults, and wicket spikes (Table 15.4).

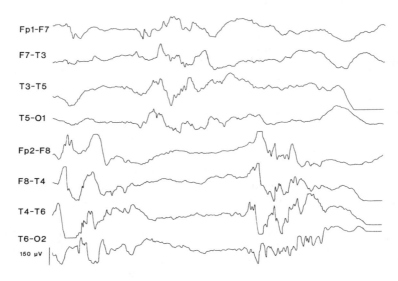

Figure 15.3 Hypsarrhythmia. This is a sleeping record in a patient with infantile spasms. During the waking state, the periods of suppression are not as prominent.

Focal spikes are diagnosed only if the spike is consistent, has a definable field, and cannot be explained by artifact. A single spike during the course of a recording should not be interpreted as abnormal. Also, great caution should be exercised when interpreting a spike that is seen from a single electrode (remember that a single electrode may be represented on more than one channel in a montage).

Focal Spikes Associated with Epilepsy

Focal spikes are associated with partial seizures and the benign epilepsies of childhood. Partial seizures are subdivided into simple and complex, based on the symptomatology. Benign epilepsies of childhood are associated with focal and generalized seizures.

During simple partial seizures, the EEG usually shows prominent spiking over the involved cortex, but in some patients, there is localized slowing that may become generalized. A typical pattern would be left central spikes in a patient who presents with focal seizures affecting the right arm. Occasionally, the sharp component of the discharge may be subtle or missing

Table 15.4   Spike Interpretation of Focal Spikes

Type	Electroencephalogram Features	Clinical Features
Rolandic spikes	Spike and slow wave complex Often triphasic and fast Maximal at C3 and C4	Benign rolandic epilepsy May be seen in subjects without seizures
Occipital spikes	Negative-prominent or biphasic spikes over the occipital region Unilateral or independent bilateral discharges	May be benign occipital epilepsy, but occipital spikes are not always benign May be seen in blindness
Parietal sharp waves	Sharp waves or spikes in the parietal region Can be activated by forehead taps	Often associated with versive (head and eye movement) or sensory seizures
Temporal sharp waves	Sharp waves in the temporal region Anterior temporal: F7, F8 Midtemporal: T3, T4 Posterior temporal: T5, T6	Anterior temporal sharp waves often associated with partial-complex seizures Midtemporal sharp waves associated with seizures and with psychological complaints Posterior temporal sharp waves associated with seizures in the majority of patients, often generalized tonic-clonic. Also associated with psychological complaints
Periodic lateralized epileptiform discharges	Unilateral or bilateral independent sharp and slow wave complexes at 1–2/sec	Any destructive process Often anoxia, herpes simplex encephalitis, stroke, tumor

altogether. The epileptiform activity may occur in deep layers of cortex and subcortical structures, so that the spike potentials are not projected to surface electrodes. Alternatively, there may not be sufficient synchrony to produce a spike detectable on the surface.

During complex partial seizures, the EEG usually shows focal spikes in the temporal or frontal region. Routine EEG may not detect the spikes if they originate in cortex that is not directly underlying the surface electrodes. Sphenoidal, nasopharyngeal, or depth electrodes may be needed to identify these discharges.

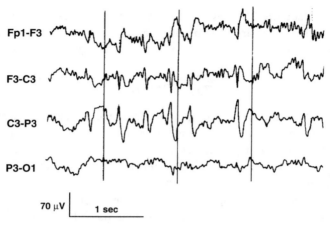

Figure 15.4 Central spikes. The patient has rolandic epilepsy.

Benign Focal Epilepsies of Childhood

Benign focal epilepsies of childhood are termed *benign* because they are age-related and seldom persist into adult life. There are two types: rolandic and occipital.

Rolandic Epilepsy

Rolandic epilepsy is characterized by interictal discharges arising from the central regions, localized near electrodes C3 and C4. The interictal discharges are independent and augmented by sleep. Relatives of patients with rolandic epilepsy may have the EEG abnormality as a genetic marker without clinical seizures.

The discharges of rolandic epilepsy are so characteristic in location and pattern that they are seldom confused with other pathologic activity (Figure 15.4). Independent central spikes are seen on an otherwise normal background. This must be differentiated from multifocal spikes, however.

Occipital Epilepsy

Occipital epilepsy is characterized by interictal sharp waves with predominance at O1 and O2. Rolandic and occipital epilepsy may occur in the same families, and relatives with no history of seizures may have either occipital or rolandic discharges on EEG.

During the seizure, the EEG shows two- to three-per-second spike-wave discharges with predominance in the occipital region. The interictal discharge may be blocked by photic stimulation or eye opening.

Focal Sharp Waves Without Clinical Seizures

Patients with no clinical evidence of seizure activity are occasionally found to have focal spikes or sharp waves. Some of these are children who are genetic carriers of benign focal epilepsies, in other patients there is no explanation. The interpretation of these records is controversial. Some electroencephalographers believe that all abnormal sharp activity is potentially epileptogenic and should be interpreted as such. Unfortunately, this may result in unneeded use of antiepileptic drugs. Patients should be treated with antiepileptic drugs based on clinical presentation rather than on EEG findings. The old adage is still valid: "Treat the patient, not the EEG."

Approximately 3% of normal individuals exhibit epileptiform activity on EEG. The proportion is somewhat higher in children than adults. Approximately 25% of these discharges are focal. Some of these patients will go on to develop seizures; however, these patients should not be treated with anticonvulsants without clinical evidence of convulsive activity. Of patients with seizures, approximately 50% will show abnormalities on an EEG, but this percentage differs dramatically on the clinical setting. Patients with absence epilepsy are more likely to have abnormal EEG than patients with complex partial seizures, for example.

Children with behavioral disturbances have been reported to have an increased incidence of focal sharp waves and spikes. The implication of these waveforms is controversial. Some investigators believe that the spikes may have contributed to the behavioral disturbance by interfering with normal social and intellectual development. Others believe that the spikes are incidental and should not be treated. The spikes are probably a reflection of brain dysfunction, which correlates with the behavioral disorder rather than being the cause of the disturbance.

Subclinical rhythmic electrographic discharge of adults (SREDA) is sharply contoured rhythmic theta activity with prominence in the centroparietal region. This pattern is seen in older patients and has no definite clinical correlate. This is not an ictal discharge. Patients with this finding are said to be at increased risk for cerebrovascular disease, but the association is not convincing. This rhythm is not found in normal younger individuals and is probably an abnormal pattern. The report should reflect the nonspecific clinical implications, however.

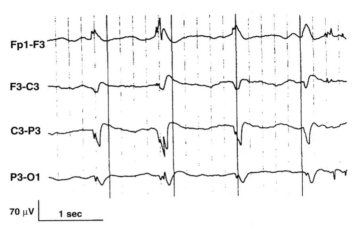

Figure 15.5 Periodic lateralized epileptiform discharges. The patient has hypoxic encephalopathy. The contralateral side showed a similar pattern, although there was no synchrony between the hemispheres.

Some patients with congenital blindness may exhibit occipital spikes. These should not be interpreted as epileptiform.

Periodic Patterns

Periodic Lateralized Epileptiform Discharges

Periodic lateralized epileptiform discharges (PLEDs) are high-amplitude sharp waves that recur at a rate of 0.5–3.0/sec (Figure 15.5). They are prominent over one hemisphere or one region. When bilateral, they are independent, thereby keeping the term *lateralized*.

PLEDs are a sign of parenchymal destruction and are most commonly seen in strokes. Other important causes include head injury, abscess, encephalitis, hypoxic encephalopathy, brain tumors, and other focal cerebral lesions. It is impossible to distinguish definitively between causes on the basis of waveform. Of the encephalitides, herpes simplex most commonly produces PLEDs. Other viral infections produce slowing without PLEDs.

The PLEDs have an amplitude of 100–300 μV. An early negative component is followed by a positive wave. The discharge may be complex, with additional sharp and slow components superimposed on the waveform.

Patients with PLEDs may have myoclonic jerks that are either synchronous with the PLEDs or independent. When the jerks are independent, the generator for the myoclonus is probably deep. Even when they are synchronous, the generator is probably subcortical. The cortical discharge reflects projections from the deep generator.

Periodic Pattern with Herpes Simplex Encephalitis

The EEG usually shows PLEDs at some time in the course of herpes simplex encephalitis. Initially, there may be only slow activity in the theta range and subsequently in the delta range. The PLEDs are sharply contoured slow waves with a frequency of 2–4 Hz. The duration of each wave is often more than 50 ms. This relatively slow frequency of repetition helps to differentiate PLEDs in herpes encephalitis from the higher frequency discharges of subacute sclerosing panencephalitis (SSPE).

Neonates with herpes encephalitis may have necrosis that is not confined or even most prominent in the temporal region. These patients often do not have PLEDs. The EEG may show a poorly organized background with slow activity in the delta range predominating.

Periodic Pattern with Anoxic Encephalopathy

Patients with hypoxic-ischemic encephalopathy have disorganization of the background with diffuse slowing and suppression. Periodic sharp waves are often seen and may predominate in the record. They look similar to PLEDs, except that they are synchronous between the hemispheres. Patients may have myoclonus associated with the discharges. These probably represent the extreme of the burst-suppression pattern, seen often in patients with hypoxic encephalopathy.

Burst Suppression

The burst-suppression pattern occurs in patients with severe encephalopathies. The finding is not specific as to etiology but is most often seen in patients with hypoxic-ischemic damage and in barbiturate coma.

The burst-suppression pattern seen in patients with barbiturate coma is very similar to that seen in the 29-week-gestation newborn. Bursts of slow waves with superimposed sharp activity are superimposed on a very suppressed background. The background is not flat, but rather is very low voltage, composed of a mixture of frequencies.

Periodic Pattern with Subacute Sclerosing Panencephalitis

SSPE has almost disappeared as a result of measles immunization. Periodic complexes are seen in most patients at an intermediate stage. Early on, there may be only mild slowing, with disorganization of the background. Late in the course, the periodic complexes may completely disappear, leaving the recording virtually isoelectric. The discharges are slow waves with sharp components. The duration of the complex is up to 3 seconds, and the interval between complexes is 5–15 seconds. The background during the interval is disorganized and generally suppressed. Myoclonus is typically synchronous with the discharge.

The EEG in SSPE resembles burst suppression. The background is usually more suppressed with burst suppression than with SSPE. The two patterns are more easily differentiated by clinical presentation. Patients with burst suppression usually have a known history of hypoxia or severe metabolic derangement. Patients with SSPE have a typical history of a progressive neurologic disorder with intellectual deterioration and seizures. SSPE is very rare.

Periodic Pattern with Creutzfeldt-Jakob Disease

Creutzfeldt-Jakob disease is characterized by periodic complexes composed of a sharp wave or sharply contoured slow wave. The interval between discharges is 500–2,000 ms. The discharges are maximal in the anterior regions and may occasionally be unilateral. Only rarely are the discharges predominant posteriorly, and they are commonly associated with blindness. The discharges may or may not be temporally locked to myoclonus. These discharges are superimposed on an abnormal background, characterized by low-voltage slowing in the theta and delta voltage range. The periodic complexes abate during sleep.

Early in the course, the periodic complexes cannot be seen, and the only finding may be focal or generalized slowing. Approximately 10–15% of patients may not show the periodic pattern during their course.

16 Slow Activity

Slowing may be generalized or focal. Generalized slow activity usually indicates encephalopathy. Focal slow activity usually indicates a structural lesion.

Generalized Slowing

Slowing of the Posterior Dominant Rhythm

A posterior dominant rhythm of less than 8.5 Hz is always abnormal in adults. Such slowing is usually bilateral and is often interpreted as indicating a diffuse encephalopathy. Bilateral occipital lesions may also result in loss of the posterior alpha rhythm. These lesions may result in cortical blindness. Figure 16.1 shows focal slowing superimposed on a generalized slow background.

Slow Activity Superimposed on the Waking Background

Theta and delta activity in waking records are usually abnormal. An important exception is the occipital delta of posterior slow waves of youth, which is discussed in Chapter 13. Waking records contain a small amount of theta, but this is usually overshadowed by alpha and faster frequencies. Patients with low-voltage records may seem to have excessive theta if the gain is increased, but at a normal gain of 7 µV/mm, the theta is not prominent.

Generalized Slowing in Sleep Recordings

EEG frequencies during sleep are generally slower than in the waking state. EEG activity is very slow during the deeper stages of sleep

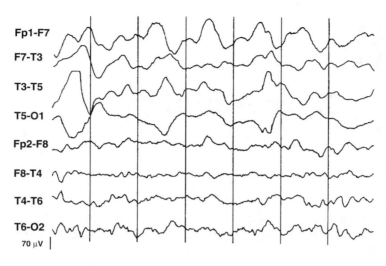

Fp1-F7	
F7-T3	
T3-T5	
T5-O1	
Fp2-F8	
F8-T4	
T4-T6	
T6-O2	
70 μV	

Figure 16.1   Generalized and focal slowing. The record shows slowing to be most prominent from the left hemisphere, although both hemispheres are slow.

(stages 3 and 4) with virtual abolition of normal fast frequencies. These deep-sleep stages may be misinterpreted as an encephalopathy. Encephalopathy should be diagnosed during sleep only if the background is nonreactive and incompatible with any stage of the sleep cycle. Even then, a waking record should be examined if at all possible.

Conversely, normal sleeping activity does not rule out an encephalopathy. It is possible to have abnormal slowing during the waking state and normal sleep patterns. Therefore, the diagnosis of encephalopathy cannot be excluded if only a normal sleeping record is provided. The EEG report should reflect these limitations on interpretation of encephalopathy in the sleeping state. The report might read, "Normal sleeping EEG. Encephalopathy is difficult to diagnose in the sleeping state. A waking record should be obtained if clinically indicated."

Focal Slowing

Focal slowing usually correlates with focal structural lesions of the hemispheres. The slowing usually overlies the lesion but does not always correlate precisely. The slowing is irregular and composed of delta activity with theta activity superimposed. It is termed *polymorphic delta activity* (PDA) because of the variability in waveform morphology. Faster frequencies meld with the slow activity. For reasons that are unclear, PDA may not be continuous, but instead may punctuate an otherwise normal EEG background.

The neurophysiologic substrate of PDA is not understood completely. In general, PDA is interpreted as being due to an abnormality in the white matter relays between the cortex and subcortical nuclei.

PDA is the most common finding in focal structural lesions such as tumors, contusion, hemorrhage, infarction, and abscess. The presence of focal spikes or sharp waves without another disturbance on the background is seldom a sign of a focal parenchymal lesion. Focal slowing is nonspecific, there are no characteristics that distinguish one cause from another. Complicated migraine and postictal state may cause focal slowing.

Intermittent Rhythmic Delta Activity

Intermittent rhythmic delta activity is always a sign of cerebral dysfunction. The distribution across the hemispheres depends on the age of the patient. In adults, the activity is predominantly frontal (i.e., frontal intermittent rhythmic delta activity [FIRDA]). In children, the activity is more commonly posterior (i.e., posterior intermittent rhythmic delta activity [PIRDA]) or occipital intermittent rhythmic delta activity (OIRDA). The frequency of the slow wave is approximately 2.5/sec in all of these patterns. Intermittent rhythm delta activity is augmented by eye closure or hyperventilation, but attenuated by stimulation or by non-rapid eye movement (non-REM) sleep. FIRDA reappears in REM sleep.

Intermittent rhythmic delta activity is thought to be caused by a disconnection of activity between the deep nuclei and cerebral cortex. The EEG pattern should be interpreted as showing cerebral dysfunction without implications for localization. There are no major diagnostic differences between FIRDA and PIRDA. FIRDA implies dysfunction of deep gray matter. PIRDA can occur in children with absence epilepsy. Causes include midline tumors, metabolic encephalopathies, degenerative disorders, and some infections. FIRDA is differentiated from PDA by the latter's lack of reactivity to stimuli and continuous appearance.

Seizures That Manifest as Rhythmic Slow Waves

Seizures occasionally manifest on routine EEG as rhythmic slow waves. Presumably, the spike component is either very small in amplitude or not projected to the cortical surface.

Differentiating epileptiform slow waves from FIRDA, PIRDA, and PDA can be difficult. Epileptiform slow activity interferes with the normal background, whereas FIRDA may be associated with an otherwise near-normal background. Epileptiform slow activity is differentiated from PDA by the stereotypic nature of the epileptiform activity. Epileptiform waves tend to be smoother, and if the discharges are bilateral, there is usually a high degree of interhemispheric synchrony.

Focal Loss of Electroencephalographic Patterns

Focal attenuation of EEG activity, especially loss of beta activity, usually indicates a structural lesion. Occipital lesions can cause unilateral loss of the posterior alpha. Unilateral lesions may also disrupt sleep patterns so that sleep spindles, vertex waves, or both are not seen from the affected hemisphere.

Unilateral suppression is commonly seen with subdural hematomas. Caution is required in these cases in which the background from the opposite hemisphere may be slow due to either trauma or midline shift with compression. In this situation, the electroencephalographer may focus attention on the side of higher amplitude with prominent slow activity and erroneously interpret the affected side as desynchronized.

17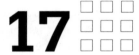

Brain Death Studies

Guidelines for Determination of Brain Death

The guidelines for determination of brain death (BD) are based on the consensus of the Medical Consultants on the Diagnosis of Death to the President's Commission for the Study of Ethical Problems in Medicine and Biomedical and Behavioral Research, hereafter referred to as the President's Commission. For BD, the patient must meet the following criteria:

- Cessation of all brain functions
- Recovery not possible
- Known cause of coma

Clinical examination for BD should show the following:

- No pupillary reflexes
- No corneal responses
- No response to auditory or visual stimuli
- No response to "doll's head maneuver"
- No response to ice water calorics
- No respiratory efforts with apnea testing

The clinician must ensure that the absence of responsiveness is not due to drug intoxication, metabolic disturbance, or neuromuscular blockade, however. Therefore, it should be ensured that the patient has the following:

- A temperature greater than or equal to 90°F
- Systolic blood pressure greater than or equal to 80 mm Hg
- No toxic levels of central nervous system depressants
- No neuromuscular blockage

Patients being evaluated for BD will frequently be hypothermic and hypotensive; therefore, maintenance using warming blankets and pressors is often required. Evidence against neuromuscular blockade can be the presence of tendon reflexes, the presence of primitive responses to nociceptive stimulation, or the response of the muscle to electrical stimulation of motor nerves.

The guidelines for determination of BD indicate that there should be a period of observation, with documentation of examinations for BD before and after this period. If the cause of coma is not anoxia, the period of observation must be 12 hours. If the cause is anoxia, the period of observation is 24 hours.

The period of observation can be shortened if there is a confirmatory test. These tests include the following:

- EEG
- Brain stem auditory-evoked potential
- Radionucleotide flow study
- Angiogram

Recently, transcranial Doppler has also been studied as a confirmatory text for BD. Since BD is a complex legal issue and the President's Commission did not specifically mention transcranial Doppler, this technique should not be used until the clinician can be assured that its use for determination of BD is accepted medical practice.

If a confirmatory test is performed and is consistent with BD, the period of observation can be reduced to 6 hours if the cause is not anoxia. The period of observation can be reduced to 12 hours if the cause is anoxia.

In general, BD should be established on the basis of clinical findings alone. Some patients with no clinical evidence of cerebral or brainstem activity will have evidence of EEG activity but otherwise fulfill the clinical criteria for BD. The literature is not clear on what to do in this situation. The probability of meaningful neurologic recovery is virtually nonexistent if the patient has no evidence of cerebral or brain stem function throughout an appropriate period of observation, regardless of the results of a confirmatory test.

Guidelines for Brain Death in Children

The 1981 President's Commission did not make specific recommendations for the determination of BD in children. The only specific comment recommended "caution in children under the age of five years."

The Task Force for Brain Death in Children (1987) subsequently provided recommendations that are increasingly used. The recommendations follow those outlined for adults above except for the following:

- Do not declare a patient who is under the age of 7 days brain dead. Clinical and EEG criteria are not established for this early period.
- If the patient is between 7 days and 2 months of age, perform two examinations and two EEGs 48 hours apart to determine BD.
- If the patient is between 2 months and 1 year of age, perform two examinations and two EEGs 24 hours apart to determine BD.
- If the patient is older than 1 year of age, perform two examinations 12 hours apart without a confirmatory test. The observation period can be 6 hours if a single EEG is done.

Despite these recommendations, most pediatricians do not feel comfortable declaring BD without a confirmatory test.

Electroencephalography for Brain Death

Technical standards include the following recommendations:

- Use a minimum of eight scalp electrodes covering all brain regions. This is usually a reduced version of the 10–20 Electrode Placement System. The following electrodes are recommended as a minimum: Fp1, Fp2, C3, C4, O1, O2, T3, T4.
- Use interelectrode distances of at least 10 cm. This allows for better detection of low-amplitude EEG activity. A minimal montage would be the following:

Channel Number	Montage
1	Fp1-C3
2	C3-O1
3	Fp2-C4
4	C4-O2
5	Fp1-T3
6	T3-O1
7	Fp2-T4
8	T4-O2

- Use interelectrode impedances that are no greater than 10 kohms but no less than 100 ohms. Too low an impedance occurs with electrode-gel smear. The amplitude of recorded electrocerebral activity will be excessively low if the impedance is low.
- Use a sensitivity of 2 μV/mm during most of the recording.
- Use a low-frequency filter setting of 1 Hz and a high-frequency filter setting of 30 Hz.
- Use ECG monitoring and other physiologic monitoring if necessary. Monitoring of chest-wall motion may be needed if there is apparent slow activity in the record. Electrodes on the dorsum of the hand may aid in identification of artifact.
- Record reactivity of the EEG to auditory, visual, and tactile stimuli.
- Use a recording time of at least 30 minutes, most of which must be relatively artifact-free.
- Remember that the integrity of the system must be tested. Touching of the electrodes with a cotton swab produces high-amplitude artifact on the EEG recording, ensuring that failure to detect activity is not due to technical problems.
- Recording should be made by a qualified technologist.

Brain Death Studies in Adults

BD studies should be performed in the period of observation between the two extensive neurologic examinations. All of the above recommendations should be followed. All of the physiologic parameters set forth by the President's Commission should also be followed, however. These are (1) systolic blood pressure of at least 80 mm Hg, (2) temperature of 90°F or greater, and (3) no sedatives or neuromuscular blockers.

Brain Death Studies in Children

BD studies in children are performed in the same manner as BD studies in adults. More physiologic monitoring is often required in children's studies, however. Because of small body size, respiratory movement artifact is relatively greater, and a chest-wall sensor is desirable. An ECG channel is desirable for adult BD studies but is even more important for BD studies in children. At high sensitivities, ECG artifact can be the predominant potential in the record.

18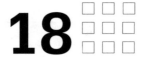

Neonatal Electroencephalography

Technical Requirements

Recording Procedures

Neonatal EEG must be performed according to the guidelines for routine EEG in adults and children outlined in Chapter 11. The sensitivities and filter settings are the same as those used for adult EEGs. At the initial sensitivity of 7 µV/mm, pen excursion is usually excessive, and sensitivity reduction is needed.

The *Guidelines* (American Electroencephalographic Society, 1994) recommends that at least three physiologic parameters be monitored, respirations, eye movements, and ECG. Respirations can be rapid and produce an artifact that mimics slow activity in the EEG. ECG monitoring is useful to identify ECG and pulse artifacts. Eye-movement recordings and submental EMG help in identifying wake and sleep states. These parameters are measured using procedures described in Chapter 13.

Newborns spend most of their day sleeping, and sedation is usually not required. The electrodes should be placed before the baby is fed. Most newborns fall asleep immediately after being fed. The newborn should be aroused late during the study to observe arousal and the waking state.

Electrode impedance must be less than 10 kohm. The absolute impedance is not as important as consistency between impedances. If impedances are greater than 5 kohm, impedance checks for mismatch should be performed.

Photic stimulation is of little benefit in newborns and is not routinely performed. Driving responses are not consistent, and photoconvulsive discharges are rare at this age. Hyperventilation is not performed.

Table 18.1   Recommended Montages for Neonatal Electroencephalography*

Channel Number	Longitudinal Bipolar	Ear Reference	Newborn Montage
1	Fp1-F3	Fp1-A1	Fp1-C3
2	F3-C3	Fp2-A2	C3-O1
3	C3-P3	F3-A1	Fp1-T3
4	Fp2-F4	F4-A2	T3-O1
5	C4-C4	C3-A1	Fp2-C4
6	C4-P4	C4-A2	C4-O2
7	F7-T3	P3-A1	Fp2-T4
8	T3-T5	P4-A2	T4-O2
9	T5-O1	O1-A1	T3-C3
10	F8-T4	O2-A2	C3-Cz
11	T4-T6	T3-A1	Cz-C4
12	T6-O2	T4-A2	C4-T4
13	ECG/EMG	ECG/EMG	ECG/EMG
14	Resp	Resp	Resp
15	Left EOM	Left EOM	Left EOM
16	Right EOM	Right EOM	Right EOM

ECG = electrocardiogram; EOM = extraocular movement; EMG = submental electromyogram; Resp = respiration.
*Newborn montage differs from longitudinal bipolar in that there are double electrode distances and one channel includes vertex derivations.
Source: Recommendations are from American Electroencephalographic Society. Guidelines in EEG, evoked potentials and polysomnography. J Clin Neurophysiol 1994;11:2–27.

Montages

A recommended montage for newborns includes a truncated version of the adult longitudinal bipolar montage plus recording of several physiologic functions (Table 18.1). If fewer non-EEG channels are required, the bipolar montage may be more complete. The full longitudinal bipolar montage can be used if the recording is made using a 21-channel machine. The placement of many electrodes on a small head increases the chance for electrode-gel smear with electrical contact between electrodes, however. Since the longitudinal bipolar montage used by most machines does not record activity at the vertex, additional channels that allow a longitudinal or transverse view of the central area and vertex are desirable.

Guidelines for Interpretation of Neonatal Electroencephalography

Accurate interpretation of neonatal EEG requires knowledge of the newborn's gestational age, postnatal age, physiologic state, and reactivity. Conceptional age is the sum of gestational age and postnatal age. A term newborn is at least 38 weeks' gestational age. Younger newborns are considered to be premature. The gestational, postnatal, and conceptional ages should be indicated on all neonatal EEG recordings.

Neonatal EEG is unfamiliar to most adult neurologists but is facilitated by the following guidelines:

- Examine the frequency composition and distribution of the background. Is the background appropriate for the conceptional age and physiologic state?
- Look for left-right asymmetries in the background. Is one side suppressed in comparison with the other? Does one side have excessive delta activity in comparison with the other?
- Look for sharp waves and spikes. Are they unifocal or multifocal? Unilateral or bihemispheric? Are they in the frontal or temporal region? Are they single or repetitive?
- Look for possible epileptiform activity. Are there episodic suppressions due to desynchronization? Is there a stereotypic rhythm? Monomorphic alpha in neonates is usually a subcortically generated seizure discharge.
- Look for changes in background with changes in state. An invariant pattern may be abnormal.
- Can a possible abnormality be explained by a normal rhythm?

Normal Neonatal Electroencephalography

Wake and Sleep Cycle in Neonates

Normal term patterns of EEG activity are seen by 38 weeks' conceptional age. At term, two stages of sleep are identified, *quiet sleep* (QS) and *active sleep* (AS). QS is characterized clinically by the absence of movement and regular respiration. AS is characterized by small eye and body movements and less regular respirations. AS is the equivalent of rapid eye movement (REM) sleep, and QS is considered the equivalent of non-REM sleep.

Two EEG patterns are associated with QS. One is slow-wave sleep, in which continuous delta activity predominates, and the other is *tracé alternant* (TA), in which there are alternating periods of relative quiescence and bursts of sharply contoured theta activity. These bursts may be 3–6 seconds long. The interburst activity ranges from 5 seconds to almost 15 seconds. The TA pattern must be distinguished from a pathologic burst suppression and from the normal discontinuous pattern of premature infants. The EEG in AS is characterized by theta activity with some delta and beta activity superimposed. During the course of a long sleep, the first AS period is higher amplitude than subsequent AS periods. The later AS periods have more theta and less delta.

Maturation of the Electroencephalogram

The preceding characteristics of EEG are only true for term infants. The EEG background matures quickly from 29 weeks to 38 weeks. In general, the background becomes more continuous, and wake-sleep states become distinct as the brain becomes more mature (Table 18.2).

Twenty-Two to Twenty-Nine Weeks' Conceptional Age

The EEG shows long periods of low-voltage activity punctuated by short bursts of higher voltage activity. The bursts are composed of mixed frequencies. Sharply contoured theta and faster frequencies can give the normal bursts an epileptiform appearance, but this appearance is normal. The interburst intervals may last up to 2 minutes, although intervals of less than 1 minute are more typical. When the bursts first develop, there is poor synchrony between the hemispheres. With full development, there is good interhemispheric synchrony.

The alternating bursts and low-voltage activity are termed discontinuous, and the pattern is called *tracé discontinu* (TD). This pattern appears similar to the burst suppression pattern seen in some older patients with encephalopathy. The two are differentiated easily by knowledge of the conceptional age, but otherwise only with difficulty.

Twenty-Nine to Thirty-One Weeks' Conceptional Age

The interburst intervals of the TD pattern are now shorter in duration and less regular. The interburst periods have a higher amplitude than in younger premature infants. Sleep stages are more differentiated than in younger neonates, and TD is seen prominently in QS.

Table 18.2   Neonatal Electroencephalography Maturation

Conceptional Age	Electroencephalographic Findings
22–29 wks	Long periods of low-voltage activity with short bursts of higher voltage mixed-frequency bursts that contain sharply contoured theta with faster frequencies Interburst interval may be 2 mins
29–31 wks	Still a discontinuous pattern but interburst intervals are shorter Appearance of delta brushes
32–34 wks	Discontinuous pattern in quiet and active sleep Appearance of multifocal sharp transients
34–37 wks	Discontinuous pattern in quiet sleep but progressively shorter interburst intervals Active sleep (REM) is almost continuous Less multifocal sharp transients Appearance of frontal sharp transients
38–40 wks	Tracé alternant pattern in non-REM sleep, with burst-to-interburst ratio of 1:1 May be a continuous slow wave pattern Less frontal sharp transients

REM = rapid eye movement.

Delta brushes are prominent at this age. These are composed of a slow component in the delta range with superimposed fast rhythmic activity in the alpha or beta range. Delta brushes are most prominent in central and occipital regions and are seen best in AS. Delta brushes resemble sleep spindles but are physiologically different. Sleep spindles are not prominent in REM sleep and are minimal in the occipital regions. Also, the disappearance of delta brush later in development and the subsequent development of frontal spindles argue against a common physiologic substrate.

Thirty-Two to Thirty-Four Weeks' Conceptional Age

The EEG during QS is still discontinuous, although the intervals of quiescence are shorter and less pronounced. Delta brushes are still present, and the spindle component is of higher frequency. Slow waves in the delta range are seen in posterior leads. AS is still discontinuous. Chin EMG is reduced during AS but is not a reliable indicator of state.

Multifocal sharp transients appear at this stage, occurring in the wake and sleep states. They are differentiated from pathologic spikes by their widespread distribution and lack of repetitive discharge.

Thirty-Four to Thirty-Seven Weeks' Conceptional Age

Non-REM sleep (QS) is still discontinuous, but the interburst intervals are progressively shorter. The burst to interburst time ratios are 1 to 2 and 1 to 3. REM sleep (AS) is virtually continuous, with delta predominating posteriorly and theta and faster frequencies anteriorly. For the first time, EMG becomes a reliable indicator of state, with low amplitude in REM sleep.

Multifocal sharp transients are less prominent and are replaced by frontal sharp transients (encoches frontales). These are of higher voltage than multifocal sharp transients. The EEG is more reactive to external stimuli than at earlier ages. Stimulation causes attenuation of the background and frequently is followed by a change in state.

Thirty-Eight to Forty Weeks' Conceptional Age

Term infants have good differentiation between REM sleep, non-REM sleep, and wakefulness. During non-REM sleep, the discontinuous pattern now has a burst to interburst ratio of about 1 to 1. This is the mature TA pattern (Figure 18.1). Non-REM sleep may be characterized by a continuous slow wave pattern rather than TA. This pattern is occasionally misinterpreted as encephalopathy in neonatal EEG.

Frontal sharp transients are less prominent but may be seen until 2 months of age. Delta brushes are absent.

Abnormal Neonatal Electroencephalographic Patterns

Abnormal neonatal EEG patterns can be classified into abnormalities of maturation, epileptiform activity, and background abnormalities. Lombroso's classification, based on these three categories, is shown in Table 18.3. This combined numeric and alphabetic scheme can be used but does not substitute for a narrative impression.

Abnormalities of Electroencephalographic Maturation

Dysmature means that the EEG patterns are not appropriate for the conceptional age. For example, a discontinuous pattern with an inter-

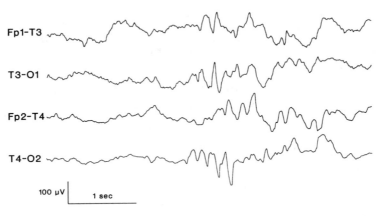

Figure 18.1 Tracé alternant pattern in a newborn. This pattern differs from premature patterns or burst suppression by the lack of profound suppression and the short interval between bursts.

burst interval of 1 minute is normal in a 29-week conceptional age neonate. This same pattern would be indicative of encephalopathy in a term infant, however. Persistent dysmaturity is associated with poor neurologic outcome. Transient dysmaturity may be due to non-neurologic causes and is not necessarily associated with brain damage.

Visual analysis of neonatal EEG allows detection of only great discrepancies in EEG maturity. Quantitative analysis can detect more subtle dysmaturity; however, this is seldom necessary.

Abnormalities of state are difficult to diagnose in routine neonatal EEG. An invariant pattern is abnormal, but state change may not necessarily be captured during a 20-minute routine EEG.

Epileptiform Activity in Neonates

Epileptiform activity may be focal, multifocal, or generalized (rarely). Immaturity in cerebral myelination usually does not allow for generalization of epileptiform activity.

Focal discharges occur usually in central region, more often on the right than on the left. The discharges may occur singly or in trains at 5–10/sec. Focal epileptiform activity is differentiated from normal frontal sharp transients and multifocal sharp transients by consistent lateralization. Also, normal sharp transients never occur in trains. The focal discharges occasionally have a smooth contour and could be confused with an alpha or theta rhythm. Sustained rhythmic activity is never normal in neonates of any conception-

Table 18.3 Lombroso's Classification of Abnormal Neonatal Electroencephalogram Patterns

Abnormal electroencephalogram patterns in term infants

I. Background abnormalities

    I-T-1 Inactive or isoelectric pattern

    I-T-2 Paroxysmal or burst-suppression pattern

    I-T-3 Low-voltage pattern through all states

    I-T-4 Interhemispheric amplitude asymmetry

    I-T-5 Positive sharp waves

    I-T-6 Diffuse delta pattern

II. Ictal abnormalities

    II-T-1 Focal or unifocal ictal patterns

    II-T-2 Focal pseudo-beta-alpha-theta-delta ictal patterns

    II-T-3 Multifocal ictal pattern with abnormal background

    II-T-4 Low-frequency discharge pattern on low-amplitude background

    II-T-5 Lack of electroencephalographic discharges during clinical seizures

III. Abnormalities of states or maturation

    III-1 No recognizable states

    III-2 Changes in percentage of time of sleep state

    III-3 Abnormal maturation of sleep cycles and electroencephalogram

    III-4 Patterns of dysmaturity

Abnormal electroencephalographic patterns in preterm infants

I. Abnormalities of background in preterm newborns

    I-P-1 Inactive or isoelectric pattern

    I-P-2 Paroxysmal or burst-suppression pattern

    I-P-3 Low-voltage pattern through all states

    I-P-4 Interhemispheric amplitude asymmetry

    I-P-5 Positive sharp waves

II. Ictal electroencephalographic abnormalities in premature infants

    II-P-1 Focal ictal patterns

    II-P-2 Focal pseudo-beta-alpha-theta-delta ictal patterns

    II-P-3 Multifocal ictal pattern

    II-P-4 Low-frequency ictal pattern

T = term; P = preterm.

Source: CT Lombroso. Neonatal Electroencephalography. In E Niedermeyer, FH Lopes daSilva (eds), Electroencephalography: Basic Principles, Clinical Applications, and Related Fields. Baltimore: Urban and Schwartzenberg, 1987;725.

al age, however. The rhythm must be differentiated from the fast component of delta brushes by the absence of an underlying slow wave and duration of the discharge.

Focal discharges are usually associated with focal clonic seizures. The location of the focus may not necessarily correlate well with the clinical seizure activity. The prognosis for favorable neurologic outcome is good, since focal discharges in neonates do not necessarily indicate a structural lesion.

Most focal sharp waves are surface negative. Surface-positive waves are seen in some neonates with intracerebral hemorrhage. If the sharp wave is followed by a slow wave, the hemorrhage is most likely subarachnoid. If the sharp wave is not followed by a slow component, the hemorrhage may still be subarachnoid, but is more likely intraventricular, subependymal, or intraparenchymal. The specificity of positive sharp waves for hemorrhage is controversial, however.

Multifocal discharges are usually associated with an abnormal background, characterized by disorganization or suppression. The spikes can be single or multiple, occurring in trains similar to those of unifocal discharges. The prognosis for good neurologic outcome is poorer for multifocal discharges than unifocal discharges. Seizures are usually clonic and may be subtle. The chief differential diagnosis for multifocal discharges is normal multifocal sharp transients. The abnormal background is key to differentiation between these patterns.

Pseudo-beta-alpha-theta-delta is a descriptive term for a discharge that begins at 8–12/sec and gradually slows to 0.5–3.0/sec. The discharge may have a sharp appearance but alternatively may have a smooth contour. This is an ictal pattern, with typical seizures being tonic, myoclonic, or subtle. The pseudo-beta-alpha-theta-delta rhythm usually indicates a poor prognosis and is commonly seen in patients with perinatal asphyxia. The evolution of changing frequency is common, especially to frequencies that are a subharmonic of the original frequencies.

Rarely, neonates may manifest seizures without any perceptible alteration in the background. The generator of epileptiform is probably subcortical, and the discharges are not projected to the surface. These infants usually have severe brain damage, explaining the lack of rostral projection of the activity.

Background Abnormalities in Neonates

Background abnormalities include excessive slow activity, low voltage, isoelectric recording, burst suppression pattern, and asymmetries. Excessive slow activity is difficult to discern, since neonates have prominent delta activity already. Some infants with brain damage may have widespread delta, however. The slow background is present in wake and sleep states and reacts poorly to exogenous stimuli. This pattern is differentiated from normal delta activity by its widespread distribution and lack of reactivity. Normal delta is prominent anteriorly and is attenuated by exogenous stimuli.

Amplitude asymmetries are significant only if they approach 50% or more. The asymmetry usually indicates focal cerebral damage in the region of suppressed voltage. A common pitfall is misinterpretation of asymmetries due to extracranial hematomas or fluid collections. Subdural hematomas may suppress activity from one or both sides.

The isoelectric EEG is a confirmatory test for brain death. Guidelines for determination of brain death are presented in Chapter 17.

The low-voltage record is unusual in neonates and suggests abnormalities in generation of electrical activity in the cortex. The technician needs to ensure that non-REM sleep is recorded, since normal REM sleep has a low-voltage background. Bilateral subdural hematomas may also produce bilateral attenuation of the background.

19

Quantitative Electroencephalographic Analysis

Quantitative EEG has been at the forefront of EEG research for many years, but only recently has the technology fallen into the grasp of most practicing neurophysiologists. The introduction of personal computer–based EEG systems has allowed data manipulation that can now occur in almost real time (i.e., at time of acquisition). There are both advantages and disadvantages to this technology. There is the potential for sifting out data that were elusive from visual analysis alone, and with adequate EEG-analysis algorithms, preliminary interpretation can be rendered by a computer, such as is allowed by ECG machines. The computerized analysis accentuates some features of the data that may or may not be important for diagnosis of the patient's condition, however, and digital analysis results in loss of some interpretive power because of the reliance on data analysis rather than visual analysis. It is attractive to consider all numerical data as objective, and thereby believable and significant. When a neurophysiologist reads an EEG, more factors are considered and weighted than can be calculated using precise parameters. Therefore, in a sense some data are lost with digital manipulation.

With these limitations in mind, quantitative analysis is useful in selected clinical situations as an adjunct to, not a replacement for, visual analysis. Quantitative analysis begins with analog-to-digital conversion as discussed in Chapter 5.

Digital Electroencephalographic Analysis

Digital EEG analysis begins with analog-to-digital signal conversion as described in Chapter 5. The signal from each channel is converted independently, and the digitized data are then manipulated. Montages are created by the user during viewing of the EEG. For example, the first channel of the longitudinal bipolar montage, Fp1-F3, is derived by subtracting the data points from the F3 electrode from the data points of the Fp1 electrode.

Filtering is also performed during the data analysis, since the signal is recorded with a broad frequency response. Digital filters are discussed in Chapter 3. Digital filters consist of calculations on the digital data, thereby de-emphasizing selected frequencies and frequency ranges. Although the calculations are precise, it is important to remember that data will be lost if the filters are used incorrectly.

Spike Detection

For outpatient routine EEG, the neurophysiologist reviews the entire record, every page and every epoch. For long-term monitoring, however, review of the EEG at the recorded time base is impossible. One option is to review the record in its entirety faster than patient data are acquired. This improves the ease of record review but is impractical when recordings are performed over a number of days. In these circumstances, ictal events are reviewed directly, and spike-detection software is used to isolate discharges that are possibly indicative of interictal activity. The exact calculations are complex, but spike detection essentially involves determination of waves of electrocerebral origin that have a specific upstroke, duration, and downstroke and are relatively free from artifact.

After analysis of a long epoch, the neurophysiologist is provided with a series of spike candidates, many of which, on review, are determined to be artifact or normal electrocerebral potentials. A spike focus can be identified if a consistent discharge is identified that is thought to represent interictal activity.

Analysis of spike detection records is not easy and should be performed only by individuals trained in analysis and interpretation of these recordings.

Power Spectral Analysis

Power spectral analysis was one of the first applications of digital EEG. This involves separation of the EEG into fundamental frequencies and determining the amount of each frequency in the record. The data are displayed as power as a function of frequency. Power spectral analysis was discussed in Chapter 5. Power spectral analysis has been used for decades and was prompted by the first efforts of automated signal analysis. Although digital EEG analysis has added some quantitative data for the neurophysiologist, visual analysis remains the cornerstone of EEG interpretation.

Power spectral analysis is usually used in EEG for giving a visual impression of frequency content (e.g., determination of encephalopathy or sleep state). Almost all modern EEG machines have power spectral analysis as a display option. One of the most helpful display methods uses a color scale to show the relative amount of frequencies in various bands for successive epochs. For example, the display bars during the awake state may be predominantly red and yellow, indicating faster frequencies, whereas in the sleeping state they may be predominantly blue and green, indicating slower frequencies.

Brain Mapping

Brain mapping simply means the display of frequency data topographically (i.e., making a frequency map of the cortical surface from data obtained by routine EEG recording). The type of display is variable and to a certain extent customizable for the individual clinician.

Brain mapping and other methods of quantitative EEG are not helpful for routine EEG studies. Brain mapping is most helpful for detecting small asymmetries that would suggest a structural lesion. In this regard, digital analysis is more sensitive than visual analysis for detecting subtle differences. Still, this technique is no substitute for magnetic resonance imaging and computed tomography. Part of the limitation of quantitative EEG is that much of the map is interpolated data, with relatively few solid data points. Also, the ability to assign gray scales and colors to the display allows for not only detection of important subtle differences but also emphasis of minor differences that may not be clinically important.

Interpolation is performed by calculating a value for each topographic point that is a weighted sum of the voltage values for surrounding electrodes. For example, calculations for a point halfway between F3 and C3 would give equal weight to F3 and C3 but would also include contributions from Fz, Cz, F7 and T3 at a lower weight. Various types of calculations can be performed, including interpolation of raw voltage or interpolation of power for specific frequency bands.

Brain mapping may be helpful for patients with seizures and patients with dementia. In seizures, brain mapping can aid in the identification of areas of increased epileptiform activity indicative of a focus. In dementia, quantitative EEG can increase the sensitivity of routine EEG to detect mild slowing suggestive of an organic dementia rather than pseudodementia.

Cerebrovascular disease has been studied by quantitative EEG because the changes in EEG are immediate in contrast with most imaging studies. Although this is academically interesting, EEG information does not now have a clinical use in the setting of acute stroke. In the future, there may be a role for quantitative EEG, since protocols for treatment of acute stroke may rely on an assessment of the physiologic function of the hemisphere at the time of the event and after.

Quantitative EEG during surgery is a major use of these techniques and is discussed in Chapter 20.

20

Electroencephalogram Monitoring

Telemetric Monitoring for Seizures

The two main reasons for telemetric EEG recording are to differentiate seizures from nonepileptic events and for evaluation of a seizure focus before epilepsy surgery. Many patients have unusual spells that defy clinical diagnosis on the basis of history and exam only. These are not all pseudoseizures. We have diagnosed arrhythmia, myoclonus, motor tics, and variations on normal behavior that were not necessarily pseudoseizures. Children particularly may have staring spells while awake or episodes during sleep that can be difficult to separate from seizure activity. Telemetric recording with simultaneous video monitoring is the best method for detection of these conditions. Ambulatory EEG monitoring, discussed below in the section on Ambulatory EEG Monitoring is a less expensive alternative with less diagnostic sensitivity.

EEG equipment must fulfill the technical requirements already discussed for EEG in Chapter 11. In addition, facility for storage of the voluminous data must be available. There are several methods, each with advantages and disadvantages. Paper print-out of the entire recording is difficult to review and environmentally unsound. Such a method should be discarded. Videotape is an excellent medium, since the EEG can be directly associated with behavior. This method is relatively inexpensive, the main disadvantage being the relatively short lifetime of the magnetic tape. Data errors should be expected with tape that is about 10 years old. The difficulty with random access of data is relatively minor, in my opinion.

Optical disks and recordable compact disks provide for data storage that is much longer lived than videotape and is fairly inexpensive. Digital disk media will be the data storage method for routine EEGs in the future. Data are easily and quickly read by the computer for analysis. The computer can jump to areas of interest. We use a combination of videotape and optical disk, with a prearranged montage on the split screen and a time signal fed to the optical disk. During an epoch of interest, the computer can instantly jump to the disk to obtain EEG that corresponds to the event recorded on tape. The display on the split video screen lacks the resolution for precise visual analysis.

Ambulatory Electroencephalogram Monitoring

Ambulatory EEG monitoring has improved in recent years, capitalizing on the advances in computer analysis. Yet, the most important aspect of review remains direct visual inspection of the record. With an increase in the availability of telemetric EEG recording, there is still a role for ambulatory monitoring, since it is cheaper and can be performed while the patient attends to his or her normal tasks. The disadvantages are, of course, the inability to observe an event and the possibility of not having a recorder returned. Abusive handling of the recorders has also been a problem for us.

Electrodes are placed with collodion, and the system is tested by the technician. Modern units provide eight channels of EEG, and monitoring of other physiologic functions is also possible on many units. The cassette records for an entire 24-hour period. If no events occur during that time, we occasionally change the tape and batteries and refresh the electrodes, allowing the patient to have another day of recording.

Artifacts identified with ambulatory EEG are greater than with telemetric EEG, since the patients are more active, and the neurophysiologist cannot look at the recording setup to see a potential source of artifact during the recording. For example, periodic rhythmic slow waves from the occipital region in one patient were found to be a movement artifact produced by the habit he had of shaking a pen in his hand.

When the tape is returned, the neurophysiologist scans the tape at an accelerated speed, between 20 and 60 times normal. Areas of interest should be reviewed at normal speed. Special attention is given to recording before and after press of the event marker. Analysis of the data is aided by audio monitoring. Spikes, "pops," and other sharply contoured waves have fairly distinctive sounds and can aid in identification of areas that need to be reviewed at slower speeds.

Digital analysis of ambulatory EEG has been of less help than it has for telemetric EEG because of the greater artifacts. In general, visual analysis remains the cornerstone of ambulatory EEG interpretation.

Ambulatory monitoring is more difficult for the neurophysiologist than digital EEG recording and should be performed only by clinicians trained and experienced in this modality.

Intensive Care Unit Monitoring

Intensive care unit (ICU) monitoring is primarily helpful for patients with seizures and coma. Patients with seizures may have brisk epileptiform activity that is not manifest as overt convulsive activity. Nonconvulsive seizures are probably underdiagnosed, especially after stroke and anoxia. Modern bedside monitors allow for recording of various physiologic parameters, including ECG, blood pressure, PaO_2, and respirations. EEG is just another electrical measurement and can be accomplished often at relatively little expense using generic plug-in modules or special EEG modules available from the manufacturer.

EEG display is commonly two or four channels, the former being adequate for most applications. Data would be too voluminous for recording in its entirety, so some type of data reduction is performed. We have used power spectral analysis, which produces a series of overlapping spectra, one trace for each epoch and one for each channel. It is easy to review the data for an entire shift and determine whether there had been any major state change or other alteration in background.

For ICU monitoring that can persist for days, collodion is the preferential electrode application method. The technicians must make a habit of rounding on the monitored patient(s) each morning and evening, ensuring integrity of the system and adequacy of electrode impedances.

Marketing of EEG monitor equipment has frequently emphasized the ability of non-neurophysiologists to interpret the data. I believe that a patient who requires ICU and EEG monitoring has a neurologic condition that merits expertise of a specialist in both neurology and neurophysiologic monitoring.

Intraoperative Monitoring

EEG monitoring has been used during surgery for years, especially during carotid endarterectomies. The most common technique has been to record eight- or 16-channel EEG throughout the entire recording and have the record analyzed after surgery by the neurophysiologist. If the technician identifies an abnormality, the surgeon is notified. Such information can alter surgical approach, use of a shunt, or other technical factors. If there is any doubt about the interpretation, the neurophysiologist must be available to review the EEG and provide instant interpretation to the surgical team.

Quantitative EEG analysis has been used during EEG monitoring for two main reasons. First, with digital analysis, parameters can be set that the technician can follow. Asking the technician to make a clinical judgment on visual inspection alone is difficult. In addition, quantitative EEG analysis can detect subtle differences in cerebral activity that might go unnoticed by the technician or neurophysiologist.

In intraoperative monitoring, the patient is prepared for EEG in the routine manner, although for surgical monitoring, collodion is recommended rather than conventional paste. Collodion provides better adherence of the electrodes and more stable electrode impedances. We begin the recording before induction and follow the progression through sedation and anesthesia, not pausing even during the nonvascular portion of the surgery. This has resulted in the detection of changes that were not instantly related to the surgery but, nevertheless, altered surgical approach. For example, loss of waves from the ipsilateral hemisphere during closing prompted ultrasound evaluation in the operating room, with subsequent reopening of the vessel and repair. In contrast, another case was identified as having suppression of EEG patterns contralateral to the operated side during surgery. Although the operated side retained good flow, the patient had a clinical infarction affecting the contralateral hemisphere.

Although there are different EEG effects of sedative and anesthetic agents, during anesthesia the EEG patterns are remarkably similar. During sedation, suppression of the posterior dominant rhythm and appearance of beta activity from the frontal regions are first seen. The beta increases in amplitude but slows in frequency and is often accompanied by frontal intermittent rhythmic delta activity (FIRDA). Widespread slow waves in the delta range are superimposed on this faster activity.

If the patient has had a stroke, the background may not be symmetric to begin with, and this asymmetry has to be considered in interpreting the intraoperative EEG. After infarction, the high-frequency activity may be less prominent or absent, and there may be polymorphic delta activity in the waking state that persists into anesthesia. If FIRDA was seen preoperatively, it will be impossible to identify from normal frontal delta during anesthesia.

Reduction in cerebral blood flow during surgery may reduce the amplitude of all frequencies from the hemisphere on the operated side, however the change should not be greater than 25–50%. Profound suppression of activity, especially when sudden, indicates a severe reduction in cerebral blood flow, which should be brought to the attention of the surgeon. Prominent reduction in EEG activity is a predictor of clinical appearance of deficit referable to that hemisphere after recovery from anesthesia.

Quantitative EEG monitoring requires that the EEG record be good and relatively free from artifact. One of the disadvantages of all quantitative EEG analyses is that integrity of the data is not obvious. If an EEG is of poor technical quality, it is obvious to the neurophysiologist on first inspection. If technically poor data are subjected to digital transformations and calculations, however, the poor quality of the studies may not be evident.

21

Troubleshooting in Electroencephalography

The most common difficulties encountered in routine EEG are related to noise, occurring when electrical activity of noncerebral origin contaminates the record. Other causes of poor EEG recordings are improper configuration of the EEG machine, improper electrode position, and unequal electrode impedances.

Noise

The most common sources of noise are muscle electrical activity, movement artifact, electrode pops, and 60-cycle interference. These are considered individually.

Electrode "Pops"

Electrode "pops" are caused by a periodic discharge of a junction potential, either at the electrode-gel interface or at the junction of dissimilar metals. The electrode, lead wire, and plug-in terminal are not necessarily of the same composition. When the junction potential suddenly discharges, current flows into the amplifier, producing a large fluctuation in recorded voltage. Current flow quickly stops when the discharge exhausts the potential difference. This brief surge of current produces the "pop." Hair pins may cause electrode pops by the same mechanism.

Electrode pops are promoted by high electrode impedance, poor skin preparation, damaged electrodes or leads, contact with other metallic objects, and head movement.

60-Hertz Interference

Line voltage causes 60-Hz interference. Stray inductance and stray capacitance are described above in Part I. The differential amplifier rejects most of the 60-Hz interference; however, this rejection can be degraded by unequal electrode impedances.

In the hospital or office EEG laboratory, 60-Hz interference is minimized by careful selection of equipment location, grounding and, occasionally, by electrical shielding of the room. Therefore, use of the 60-Hz filter should not be needed. Portable studies in the intensive care unit may have significant contamination of the record by 60-Hz interference because of ventilators, intravenous (IV) infusion pumps, air beds, heating/cooling blankets, and monitoring equipment. To minimize these sources of noise, the following procedures may be helpful:

- Unplug IV pumps. Most pumps have battery backup for at least 1 hour. While on battery power, the direct current power supply will not interfere with the EEG in the same manner as the alternating current line power. Most modern pumps fill a reservoir periodically and then slowly empty the reservoir into the patient. Most of the artifact arises during the brief filling period. This will not be interpreted as cerebral activity if the technician notes pump activity on the record.
- Disconnect the ECG monitor. The ECG monitor not only adds noise by virtue of its line voltage, but its patient ground also prevents the EEG technician from placing a patient ground that is connected to the EEG machine. This would create a ground-loop with potential for injury to the patient. If cardiac monitoring is essential, one channel of the EEG can be dedicated to ECG.
- Heating and cooling blankets can virtually always be disconnected for the duration of the study. The recirculating water blankets produce much less artifact than electric blankets or radiant heaters.
- Ventilator artifact is uncommon, but movement artifact from chest-wall motion is not. If regular slow activity is seen in the EEG, activity from a chest-wall expansion sensor should be recorded for at least part of the study. Technicians will occasionally mark the record by hand, drawing an "X" with each respiration. Although this may be helpful, it allows a potential for error.

Air beds are a relatively new cause of noise (see Figure 13.8). The line power can cause 60-Hz interference, but more commonly the blower motor creates a high-frequency artifact that can occasionally obscure the record. In most beds, the blower cannot be stopped without deflation of the mattress. Although some beds have battery backup, this does not solve the high-frequency interference. If absolutely necessary, the bed can usually be deflated for the duration of the recording with no adverse effects on the patient. In our practice, this has seldom been necessary.

Before performing any of these maneuvers, the technician must check with the physician or nurse directly responsible for the patient's care.

Electrode Position

For routine EEG, 21 leads are placed on the head. Great potential for error exists in placement of the leads, especially if the technician does not measure the head. Also, there are only a limited number of lead colors, so switched leads can easily occur. Often, there is no obvious clue to misplaced electrodes. Error should be suspected if a field distribution does not make sense. Examples include a spike with no clear dipole distribution, a slow wave that reverses inappropriately, or alpha activity seen anteriorly that can be attributed to only one electrode. In this latter case, the interpreter must be sure that there is no skull defect in the region of a properly placed electrode that could also cause this anomaly.

Misplaced electrodes are common in institutions where leads are placed by technicians not well trained in EEG. For example, in our practice of telephone-transmission EEG recordings, we have seen a record in which a well-modulated alpha was seen in anterior channels, and apparent eye-movement artifact was seen posteriorly. The technician in the outside hospital had placed an electrode cap backward on the patient's head.

Electrical Safety

General principles of electrical safety are discussed in detail in Part I. A few issues are specifically germane to EEG. Of all EEG procedures, portable recordings in the intensive care unit pose the greatest risk to the patient. Leak current can flow from the EEG machine through the patient into other electrodes and grounds.

The danger is greatest if the patient has a temporary pacemaker, where an externally grounded device has a lead within the heart. ECG grounds are the most common route for flow of leak current. If a patient already has a ground, the ground electrode on the EEG machine should not be placed on the patient. This precludes testing of electrode impedance in some EEG machines and increases noise. Acceptable recordings are usually possible, however. Alternatively, the leads to the cardiac monitor can be temporarily disconnected and the EEG ground placed normally, but, of course, this is done only with the permission of the treating physician. Cardiac monitoring can be performed during the recording by using a channel on the EEG machine. Alternatively, a small battery-powered cardiac monitor may be used, since this does not provide a route for exit of leak current.

III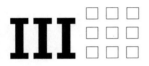

Nerve Conduction Studies and Electromyography

22 Basic Principles of Nerve Conduction Studies and Electromyography

Neurophysiologic evaluation of nerve and muscle consists of nerve conduction studies (NCSs) and EMG. NCS consists of nerve conduction velocity, F wave, H reflex, blink reflex, repetitive stimulation, paired stimulation, and sympathetic skin response. EMG consists of routine EMG, single-fiber EMG, and fiber-density determination. These techniques are discussed after a presentation of basic principles.

Equipment Required for Nerve Conduction Studies and Electromyography

Most modern EMG equipment is composed of a microcomputer with added software and hardware. The core computer is a central processing unit. Output is displayed on a video display and on paper. Storage devices almost always include a hard disk drive and floppy disk drive. Some systems add additional storage with tape drives or optical disk. The reduction in the cost of compact disc recording will make this a major method of data storage in the near future. Data entry is done by a keyboard and mouse. Microphones are used with voice recognition technology to facilitate hands-free commands. Added hardware includes an analog-to-digital (A/D) input board and stimulator board. The A/D board takes the analog signal and converts it into a digital signal for analysis by the computer. A/D conversion is discussed in detail in Chapter 5.

Software is tailored to the procedure and includes routines for performing and interpreting routine NCSs, EMGs, and special testing of neuromuscular function. The same equipment is often capable of performing evoked potentials, but this software is usually separate from the EMG software.

Filters used in EMG machines are often digital, meaning that calculations are performed on digitized data rather than filtering the raw signal.

Electrodes are plugged into a box that transmits signals to a preamplifier that, in turn, transmits signals to the main unit by a shielded cable. The signal is amplified, digitized, filtered, and displayed on the screen. The oscilloscope display is divided in both the horizontal and vertical axes. The horizontal axis (time) has ten divisions representing seconds per division (sec/div); the vertical axis (voltage) has eight or ten divisions representing volts per division (volts/div). Tables 22.1 and 22.2 show recommended stimulating and recording settings for routine NCSs and EMG, respectively.

Machines

Many different machines are available for routine NCSs and EMG. Years ago, averaging, trace storage, and repetitive stimulation capability were add-ons, but they are now part of the minimum capability of commercial EMG machines. Every machine should have the capability for the following:

- Running display of data
- Storage of multiple traces
- Averaging
- Paper printout of calculated data and traces
- Repetitive stimulation
- Paired stimuli

Table 22.1   Stimulus and Recording Parameters for Nerve Conduction Studies*

Parameter	Motor NCV	Sensory NCV	F Wave	H Reflex
Gain	2 mV/division	20 µV/division	200 µV/division	200 µV/division
Time base	2 ms/division	1 ms/division	10 ms/division	10 ms/division
LFF	10 Hz	10 Hz	10 Hz	10 Hz
HFF	32 kHz	2 kHz	32 kHz	32 kHz
Stimulus duration	0.2 ms	0.1 ms	0.2 ms	0.2 ms

NCV = nerve conduction velocity; LFF = low-frequency filter; HFF = high-frequency filter.
*Available gain and filter settings differ between machines. Not all machines are able to provide the 32 kHz HFF setting. A lower setting is acceptable for most studies, although the waveform may be altered significantly. The main effect of a lower HFF setting is on amplitude. Minimal latency is virtually unaffected. The HFF settings for the F wave and H reflex are not as critical as for motor and sensory waves.

Table 22.2 Stimulus and Recording Parameters for Electromyography*

Parameter	Resting	Motor Unit	Recruitment	Single Fiber
Gain	50 μV/division	200 μV/division	1 mV/division	0.2–1.0 mV/division
Time base	10 ms/division	10 ms/division	10 ms/division	0.5–1.0 ms/division
LFF	10 Hz	10 Hz	10 Hz	500 Hz
HFF	32 kHz	32 kHz	32 kHz	32 kHz

LFF = low-frequency filter; HFF = high-frequency filter.
*The HFF setting can be as low as 10 kHz for single-fiber EMG. An HFF of 20 kHz is acceptable for resting, motor unit, and recruitment recordings.

In addition, desirable but not essential features may include the following:

- Alternative data manipulation, including transformation, subtraction, and re-filtering
- Long-term data storage on a removable medium
- Ability to generate the report using the machine's printer

Averaging is helpful especially for sensory conduction studies. The sensory nerve action potential is occasionally of low amplitude, and baseline noise can cause difficulty in the determination of latency. Averaging provides a smooth waveform that is easier to interpret.

Electrodes

Surface electrodes are used for routine NCSs. The electrodes are stainless steel, silver, or (occasionally) gold disks soldered to multistrand conducting wire (Figure 22.1). The impedance is very low and the charge movement small; therefore the use of silver–silver chloride electrodes (as used in EEG) is not necessary. Electrode gel is needed to reduce impedance and prevent artifact, because skin surface is irregular and hair interferes with conduction. The gel is a malleable extension of the electrode, allowing electrical continuity between the ionic milieu of the skin and the electrode. Gel is also needed to reduce the impedance of the stimulating electrodes. The stimulus voltage passing through a high impedance can create sufficient heat to cause local tissue injury.

Ring electrodes are tight coils of stainless steel used to record or to stimulate sensory action potentials from fingers. The coil is coated with

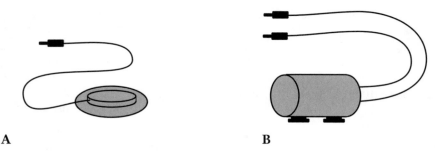

A   **B**

Figure 22.1 Electrodes. Diagrammatic representation of types of electrodes used in nerve conduction studies. A. Disk electrode soldered to multistrand conducting wire. B. Bar electrode with two surface electrodes attached to the skin.

conducting gel, wrapped around the finger, and cinched with a rubber or plastic fastener.

Needle electrodes (see Chapter 11) are needles that are insulated except at the tip. The needle electrodes are inserted into the muscle to directly record muscle fiber and motor unit activity. Needle electrodes are usually reserved for EMG but may be helpful when recording from some nerves. Needle electrodes should not generally be used for stimulation because their high impedance can result in sufficient heat to damage tissue.

Surface electrodes are used in EMG for a ground and for reference to a monopolar needle electrode. Surface references are not needed in coaxial electrodes, because the reference is the barrel of the needle.

Principles of Nerve and Muscle Physiology

The theory needed to explain the generation of EMG activity is simpler than that needed to explain the generation of EEG activity. The important components of the motor system are

- Motoneuron with motor axon
- Muscle fibers (extrafusal)
- Muscle spindle, including intrafusal muscle fibers
- Sensory neurons and axons that convey information from mechanoreceptors in the muscle to the spinal cord
- Spinal cord and higher centers

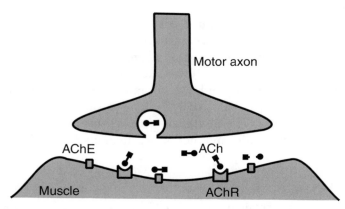

Figure 22.2 Normal neuromuscular junction. Diagrammatic representation of the neuromuscular junction, showing the motor axon, presynaptic terminal, postjunctional muscle membrane, and muscle fiber. (ACh = acetylcholine; AChE = acetylcholinesterase; AChR = acetylcholine receptor.)

Normal Neuromuscular Function

Motor Function

Input descending from the brain to the spinal cord activates the motoneurons. Action potentials that develop in the axon hillock of the motoneuron are transmitted to the nerve terminal by saltatory conduction. Calcium flows into the depolarized nerve terminal and promotes the release of acetylcholine (ACh) vesicles into the synaptic cleft (Figure 22.2). ACh binds to specific ACh receptors at the end-plate of the muscle fiber membrane and opens ionic channels that allow sodium and calcium into the cell and potassium and chloride out. The net effect of this ion flux is depolarization of the postsynaptic (muscle) membrane. Depolarization causes an action potential to be created in the muscle fiber membrane adjacent to the end-plate. This action potential is propagated throughout the muscle fiber. The propagated potential releases calcium from the sarcoplasmic reticulum, which, in turn, causes the muscle to contract. Contraction ends when calcium is taken back by the sarcoplasmic reticulum. Activation of one motoneuron results in activation of every muscle fiber innervated by that neuron. The motor unit potential is the summation of the action potentials from the muscle fibers comprising that unit.

Most muscle fibers are extrafusal, or outside of the muscle spindle. Some motoneurons activate intrafusal muscle fibers, whose contraction maintains the mechanoreceptor in a state of readiness to perform. The spindle ensures that extrafusal muscle fibers generate a desired level of force. If the force required to shorten a muscle is greater than expected, then contraction of the intrafusal muscle fibers stretches the muscle spindle, which sends signals to the spinal cord that promote further contraction of the extrafusal muscle fibers. This feedback loop ensures that the muscle is appropriately shortened. The additional force is generated by recruitment of nonfunctioning motor units and increased rate of discharge of already functioning motor units.

Sensory Function

Nerve terminals are excited by the sensory stimulation and create afferent action potentials in sensory nerves. The impulses enter the dorsal horn where some information ascends the dorsal columns ipsilaterally, some ascends contralaterally, and some is used for segmental reflexes. Cell bodies of the afferent neurons are in the dorsal root ganglia.

Abnormal Neuromuscular Function

The possible sites of abnormal function of the peripheral nerves and muscle are

- Motor neuron cell body, sensory neuron cell body, or both
- Root
- Plexus nerve axons, peripheral nerve axons, or both
- Plexus nerve myelin, peripheral nerve myelin, or both
- Neuromuscular junction
- Muscle

Specific disorders characteristic of each lesion site are listed in Table 22.3. Degeneration of the motoneuron cell body results in axonal degeneration and loss of innervation of the muscle fibers. With time, some muscle fibers are reinnervated by surviving motor axons (Figure 22.3). Others are not innervated, because of a limited ability of surviving axons to innervate additional muscle fibers. The membranes of actively denervated muscle fibers are unstable, causing the resting potential to fluctuate. These fluctuations occasionally result in spontaneous muscle fiber action potentials. Axonal degeneration causes the same physiologic changes in distal nerve and muscle as neuronal degeneration.

Lesions of myelin cause impaired saltatory conduction in peripheral nerves. Damaged myelin causes slowed conduction and, if severe, conduction block.

Table 22.3 Sites of Damage in Nerve and Muscle

Site	Disorder
Neuron cell body	Amyotrophic lateral sclerosis
Root	Cervical or lumbar radiculopathy
Axonal neuropathy	Toxic neuropathy
Demyelinating neuropathy	Guillain-Barré syndrome
Neuromuscular junction	Myasthenia gravis
Muscle	Muscular dystrophy

Muscle lesions cause instability of the muscle fiber membrane. The unstable membrane discharges spontaneously and may fail to be activated by normal neuromuscular transmission. The tension generated by abnormal muscle fibers is reduced, so that more units must be recruited to generate the desired force. This correction is partly conscious but largely automatic and is part of the feedback control mechanisms.

Basics of Nerve Conduction Studies and Electromyography

Nerve Conduction Studies

The time required for nerve conduction is measured by stimulation of a peripheral nerve and recording potentials from nerve or muscle. Details of methodology are presented in Chapter 23. Normal values for nerve conduction velocity are established for all of the major nerves (Table 22.4). A nerve conduction velocity is abnormal if it is more than 2.5 or 3.0 standard deviations from the mean.

Disorders of the myelin sheath slow the motor and sensory nerve conduction velocities. Unraveling or fragmentation of the myelin reduces the impedance between spaces inside and outside the axon. This interferes with the electrotonic depolarization between nodes that is essential for saltatory conduction. Demyelinated axons do not have the capacity to conduct in the same way as unmyelinated fibers. Therefore, if severe enough, a demyelinating disorder can result in failure of transmission of impulses down the nerve.

Nerve conduction velocities are typically normal or near normal in disorders of neuronal or axonal degeneration, because surviving axons conduct

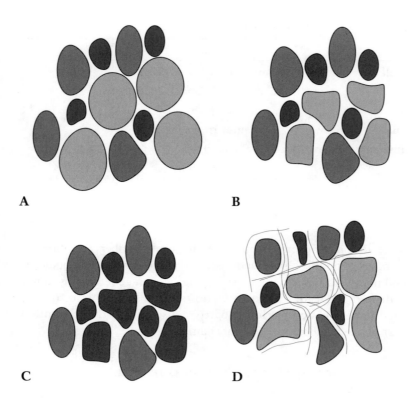

Figure 22.3 Neuromuscular disorders and muscle fiber composition. A. Normal cross-section of a skeletal muscle. Shades of gray indicate which motor axon innervates the muscle fibers. B. Same muscle after denervation by loss of axon innervating the fibers in light gray. Atrophy of muscle fibers innervated by this axon. C. Reinnervation of denervated muscle fibers by axons supplying surrounding muscle fibers. D. Myopathy with degeneration of selected muscle fibers and increase in connective tissue.

action potentials at a normal velocity. The amplitude of the compound action potential is often reduced, however, because the numbers of functioning axons is reduced. Disorders of the muscle usually have normal nerve conduction velocities.

Electromyography

EMG is the recording of motor unit potentials (MUPs). It can distinguish active from chronic denervation and myopathic from denervat-

Table 22.4   Normal Data for Nerve Conduction Studies[a]

Nerve	Distal Latency	Nerve Conduction Velocity	Amplitude
Motor nerve conduction studies			
Median	≤3.8 ms @ 7 cm	≥50 m/sec	≥5 mV
Ulnar, below elbow	≤3.1 ms @ 7 cm	≥50 m/sec	≥5 mV
Ulnar, across elbow[b]	—	≥50 m/sec	≥5 mV
Radial	≤3.4 ms @ 6 cm	≥50 m/sec	≥5 mV
Peroneal	≤6.0 ms @ 8 cm	≥40 m/sec	≥2.5 mV
Tibial	≤5.0 ms @ 10 cm	≥40 m/sec	≥2.6 mV
Sensory nerve conduction studies			
Median	≤3.5 ms @ 13 cm	≥55 m/sec	≥10 µV
Ulnar	≤3.2 ms @ 11 cm	≥54 m/sec	≥10 µV
Radial	≤2.8 ms @ 10 cm	—	≥18 µV
Sural	≤4.2 ms @ 14 cm	≥42 m/sec	≥4 µV

[a]Distal latency is in milliseconds at the specified distance between stimulating cathode and active recording electrode.
[b]Ulnar conduction across the elbow is usually compared to distal conduction and conduction on the contralateral side. Relative slowing of conduction velocity across the elbow of 10 m/sec or greater is considered significant.

ing disorders, as well as distinguishing among several different types of myopathic disorders.

The instability in muscle fiber membrane potential that characterizes neuropathies and myopathies may occasionally reach threshold, producing a single muscle fiber action potential. These spontaneous potentials never occur in normal muscle at rest and are called *fibrillation potentials* and *positive sharp waves*. These spontaneous potentials may not develop for 3–4 weeks after a nerve injury.

The MUPs are the summed action potentials of muscle fibers in proximity to the needle electrode. Since the fibers discharge almost synchronously in the individual muscle fibers, the appearance is biphasic or triphasic, but the exact phase characteristics depend on the orientation of the recording electrode surfaces to the muscle fibers. Some normal MUPs may have four or more phases, but units with more than four phases (*polyphasics*) comprise only approximately 10% of motor units in normal subjects. Normal MUPs are less than 15 ms in duration. In neuropathic conditions, new nerve sprouts reinnervate denervated muscle fibers. However, these nerves do not conduct as efficiently as the original connections, so potentials from these muscle fibers lag behind the potentials from the native muscle fibers—that is, they lack the synchrony of the normal MUPs. Therefore, the MUP has a polyphasic appearance with prolonged duration. The amplitude is also often increased because each motor axon innervates more and more muscle fibers.

Myopathic conditions produce MUPs of reduced amplitude because damaged muscle fibers may not respond to neuromuscular transmission. The MUPs are polyphasic in appearance but normal in duration.

A maximal voluntary contraction normally activates so many motor units that individual units cannot be identified. In neuropathic conditions, the number of motor axons is reduced, so there are fewer active motor units, but each is firing faster than normal. Myopathic conditions do not cause a loss of motor units but more motor units must be recruited to produce or maintain a given tension than in a normal muscle.

23 ⬜⬜⬜ ⬜⬜⬜ ⬜⬜⬜

Nerve Conduction Studies

Methods of Routine Nerve Conduction Studies

The stimulus for nerve conduction is a square-wave pulse that can vary in amplitude and duration. Standard durations are 0.1 ms and 0.2 ms, but longer and shorter durations are occasionally used. Longer durations can produce sufficient current density to activate the axons several millimeters from the active electrode, thereby introducing inaccuracy in identification of a normal response. Long duration stimuli should only be used when maximal voltage does not elicit a maximal response (e.g., in obese individuals). Even then, results should be interpreted with caution.

Stimulus voltage is varied continuously and can be set by controls on the instrument on the stimulator handset. The maximum voltage output varies between instruments but is usually 250 V. A brief direct current (DC) pulse of 250 V is not normally injurious to skin or neural tissues.

Motor Nerve Conduction Studies

Figure 23.1 shows a diagram of the techniques used to study motor nerve conduction velocity (NCV). The active recording electrode (G1) is placed over the midbelly of the muscle, and the reference (G2) is placed 2 cm distal to G1. Nerve stimulation evokes a compound motor action potential (CMAP) from the muscle. This is the summed potentials of multiple muscle fibers. The CMAP is sometimes called the M response (M for muscle), but CMAP is the preferred term. If the active recording electrode is not correctly placed, the major negative deflection of the CMAP may have an initial positive component. Determination of latency is then difficult because there is no initial negative deflection.

The stimulating electrodes are usually on a wand with two rigid poles comprising the active and reference electrodes. They are placed on the skin over the

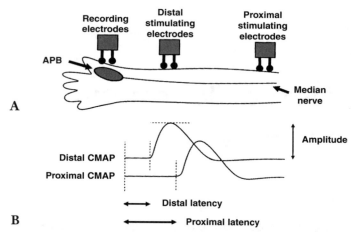

Figure 23.1 Motor nerve conduction velocity. A. Recording is made from a muscle with the active electrode on the skin overlying the end-plate region. The nerve is stimulated at two locations, proximally and distally. The stimulator is oriented so that the cathode is closer to the muscle. B. Simulated oscilloscope traces with proximal and distal stimulation. Dashed lines delineate the measurements made after data acquisition. (APB = abductor pollicis brevis; CMAP = compound motor action potential.)

nerve to be tested. Depolarization is greatest beneath the cathode, which is placed distally to the anode. The ground is attached on the same limb. All electrodes are coated with electrode gel and fastened to the limb with tape or Velcro straps. The stimulating electrode is usually held in position by hand.

For motor NCV, the setting of the low frequency filter is 10 Hz, and the setting of the high-frequency filter is 32 kHz (see Table 22.1). The oscilloscope is set for 2 ms per horizontal division and 2 mV per vertical division.

After all electrodes are in place, the instrument is set to deliver repetitive stimuli, usually at 1 Hz. The stimulus voltage is initially set to zero and then gradually increased with successive stimuli. A CMAP gradually appears and grows larger with the increasing stimulus voltage. Eventually, further increases in voltage do not cause any change in CMAP amplitude. A stable response is assured if the voltage is 25% greater than the voltage needed to produce the highest amplitude CMAP.

The following measurements are made of the CMAP:

- Latency from stimulation to takeoff of the CMAP
- Latency from stimulation to peak of the CMAP
- CMAP amplitude

After these measurements are made, the stimulating electrode is moved to a more proximal location on the nerve. It is not necessary to gradually increase the voltage for this second round of stimulation. If the waveform is the same as with distal stimulation, then only one or two stimuli are necessary. If the waveform is attenuated or has a different shape than the first CMAP, the examiner should increase the voltage to make sure that the changes are not due to incomplete activation. The same measurements are made on the CMAP with proximal stimulation as on the CMAP with distal stimulation. The distance between the two stimulation cathode positions is then measured along the course of the nerve.

When all the measurements have been made, the motor NCV is calculated from the following formula:

$$NCV = \frac{Dist}{PL - DL}$$

Where *PL* is the proximal latency, *DL* is the distal latency, and *Dist* is the distance between the stimulating cathodes. Latencies are measured in ms and distance in mm. Therefore, the final results are expressed as mm/ms, which is equivalent to meters per second (m/sec).

Sensory Nerve Conduction Studies

Sensory NCVs are measured more directly than motor NCVs (Figure 23.2). Only one stimulating site is needed, because sensory conduction studies do not encounter the delay of neuromuscular transmission seen with motor studies. The stimulation and recording are directly to and from the sensory nerve. However, sensory NCVs require that either the stimulating or recording electrode be over a purely sensory portion of the nerve. Nerves that have pure sensory segments include the superficial peroneal, sural, and radial nerves. Ring electrodes on the fingers are used for the median and ulnar nerves, since the motor axons of these nerves do not extend to the digits themselves (the nerves on the digits are purely sensory).

Sensory NCVs can be performed with activation in the normal direction of action potential propagation (*orthodromic stimulation*) or in the reverse direction (*antidromic stimulation*). The direction of stimulation should be consistent in an individual laboratory. Normative data are established for both directions of conduction. There is a slight discrepancy in the NCVs calculated with the two methods because of differences in geometry of volume conduction. In general, orthodromic stimulation is recommended, because there is less shock artifact and fewer nerve fibers are stimulated. Antidromic

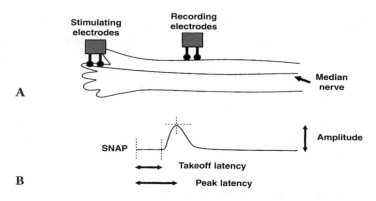

Figure 23.2 Sensory nerve conduction velocity. A. Electrode placement. B. Simulated oscilloscope traces of a sensory nerve action potential (SNAP). Dashed lines delineate the measurements made after data acquisition.

stimulation should be performed if no reproducible response is obtained from orthodromic stimulation.

The initial settings for sensory NCVs are as follows:

Stimulus frequency	1/sec
Stimulus intensity	0 V
Oscilloscope sweep speed	1 ms/div
Oscilloscope sensitivity	20 µV/div
Low-frequency filter	10 Hz
High-frequency filter	2 kHz

The stimulus voltage is gradually increased until a sensory neural action potential (SNAP) appears. When the potential no longer changes with increasing stimulus intensity, the trace is stored and the following measurements are made:

- Latency to takeoff of the potential
- Latency to peak potential
- Amplitude of the potential
- Distance between stimulating cathode and active recording electrode

Sensory NCV is calculated by the following formula:

$$NCV = \frac{Dist}{LT}$$

Where *Dist* is the distance between stimulating cathode and active recording electrode, and *LT* is the latency to takeoff of the potential. Unlike motor NCVs, both the takeoff and peak latencies of the SNAP can be used for interpretation. Takeoff latency more accurately represents conduction of the fastest fibers, so this is the preferred measurement. In our laboratory, we document both, but predominantly use takeoff for interpretation.

Sensory NCVs may be normal in patients with very proximal lesions of the nerve roots, especially avulsion, because the nerve fibers are damaged between the dorsal root ganglia and the spinal cord. The connection between the ganglia and the periphery is intact.

Sensory NCVs are occasionally irregular and of low amplitude, such that averaging is needed to clearly separate the signal from background electrical activity. This separation is especially important in older patients and in patients with peripheral neuropathy, in whom it may be almost impossible to define the SNAP without averaging.

Effect of Age and Temperature on Nerve Conduction Studies

The velocity of nerve conduction in the newborn is only half as fast as in adults. Velocity increases progressively and reaches adult speeds at approximately 3 years of age. After age 60 years, motor and sensory nerve conduction velocities slow slightly.

Normative data are defined for "normal" temperatures. Skin temperature of 34°C correlates with normal tissue and muscle temperature of 37°C. If the limb is cool, NCVs are slow. This is a common source of error when measuring NCVs. There are two methods for dealing with the effect of temperature: (1) warm the extremity with an infrared lamp or forced air heater, or (2) correct the NCV for temperature by adding 5% to the conduction velocity for each degree below 34°C. The latter is less desirable because of errors inherent in these calculations. The following guidelines should be followed when heating an extremity:

- Do not heat too rapidly or the patient may suffer skin burns.
- Ensure that sufficient time has elapsed for warming before performing the study. The skin temperature can reach a desirable temperature before deeper structures are warmed. (This is especially true in patients with peripheral vascular disease.)
- Turn the heat lamp off before performing the conduction study to eliminate artifacts created by the lamp.

Interpretation of Abnormalities

Reduced Conduction Velocity

If either motor or sensory conduction velocity is slower than three standard deviations below the mean, the study is interpreted as abnormal. This indicates an abnormality in the myelin component of the peripheral nerve. Axonal neuropathies may cause mild slowing of nerve conduction but usually not more than 5 m/sec below the lower limit of normal.

Polyneuropathies produce slowed conduction in several nerves, especially distally. Mononeuropathies produce slowing in conduction in isolated segments of individual nerves. *Conduction block* refers to the slowing or failure of conduction through selected segments of nerve. Multiple regions of conduction block are seen in patients with Guillain-Barré syndrome, chronic inflammatory demyelinating polyradiculoneuropathy, and multifocal motor neuropathy.

Increased Distal Motor Latency

The distal motor latency is the time for conduction through the distal nerve plus neuromuscular transmission plus propagation of the muscle fiber action potential to the region under the recording electrode. Distal latency is increased by demyelinating neuropathies, neuromuscular transmission defects, or dysfunction of the muscle fiber membrane. In practice, the most common cause for increased distal motor latency is demyelination or compression of the distal portion of the nerve.

Low-Amplitude Potentials

Low-amplitude CMAPs indicate a reduced number of functioning muscle fibers. This can be caused by motor units dropping out or by impaired excitation of muscle fibers. Decreased CMAP amplitude is seen in motor neuropathies, axonal degeneration, and myopathies.

Low-amplitude SNAPs indicate fewer functioning sensory axons. SNAP amplitude is more variable than CMAP amplitude in normal people. Caution is needed when interpreting a sensory conduction study on the basis of amplitude alone. Lesions that significantly affect SNAP amplitude usually slow conduction as well.

Dispersed Waveform

A dispersed waveform is usually caused by a demyelinating process. Demyelination does not slow the conduction velocity of each axon uniformly. The result is a poorly synchronized nerve volley that accentuates the normal dispersion pattern of the compound action potential. Axonal degeneration may also cause waveform dispersion when there is secondary demyelination.

Nerve Conduction Velocities for Specific Nerves

Median Nerve

Median motor NCV is calculated according to the formula given in the section on motor nerve conduction studies. The active recording electrode (G1) is placed over the belly of the abductor pollicis brevis (Figure 23.3). The reference (G2) is placed 2 cm distally. The cathode for proximal stimulation is placed over the median nerve proximal to the antecubital fossa. The anode is placed 2 cm proximal to this site. Normal distal latency is less than or equal to 3.8 ms. Normal motor NCV is greater than or equal to 50 m/sec.

Median sensory NCV is performed by using orthodromic stimulation. Stimuli are delivered to the fingers, and recordings are made from the median nerve at the wrist. Ring electrodes are placed on digits 2 or 3 for stimulation with the cathode as proximal as possible on the digit. The anode is 2 cm distal to the cathode. The active recording electrode (G1) is placed 13 cm proximal to the cathode and the reference (G2) is placed 2 cm proximal to the active electrode. The sensory NCV can also be measured by antidromic stimulation, however, the stimulus artifact is greater.

The median nerve is commonly studied for evaluation of suspected carpal tunnel syndrome. Absolute median motor distal latency and sensory NCV are usually abnormal. Some clinical neurophysiologists study incremental stimulation across the carpal tunnel to document the lesion. Compound motor action potentials are recorded in response to stimulation at 1-cm increments, beginning at the site of distal stimulation for median motor NCV and progressively moving onto the palm. Each successive CMAP will have a little shorter distal latency. A disproportionate change in latency between the two positions or a change in the waveform demonstrates evidence of median nerve compression in that segment. Normally, there is a latency change of 0.16–0.20 ms/cm distance across the tunnel. However, abnormalities of incremental stimulation in the presence of normal distal latency are not convincing evidence of compression.

The main pitfall to median NCV studies is the Martin-Gruber anomaly. See Chapter 31 for a review of nerve anomalies.

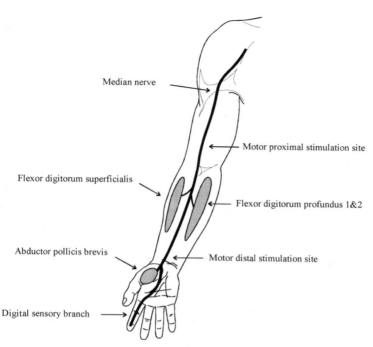

Figure 23.3 Median nerve anatomy. View of the medial aspect of the arm, showing innervation of the median-innervated muscles that are most important in neurophysiology. Xs refer to sites for stimulation, as labeled. Shaded areas represent approximate muscle positions. Sensory stimulation is delivered to the digital sensory branch. (NCV = nerve conduction velocity.)

Ulnar Nerve

For motor NCV, the ulnar CMAP is recorded from the abductor digiti minimi. G1 is placed over the belly of the abductor digiti minimi, approximately midway between the origin and insertion (Figure 23.4). G2 is placed 2 cm distal to G1. Distal stimulation is on the ulnar aspect of the wrist, 7 cm proximal to G1. Proximal stimulation is delivered so that the cathode is just below the ulnar groove at the elbow. More proximal stimulation is delivered at least 10 cm proximal to the ulnar groove. NCVs are calculated for the nerve segments between the wrist and groove and across the groove. An NCV across the elbow that is 10 m/sec less than that recorded distal to the elbow indicates an ulnar nerve lesion at the ulnar groove or cubital tunnel. If the NCV slows across the elbow, the contralateral side should be studied for comparison.

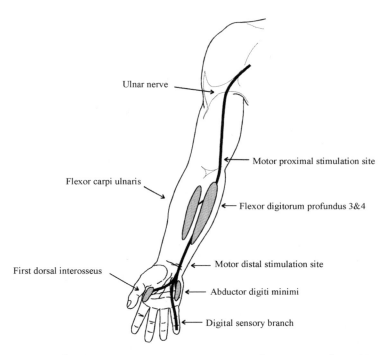

Ulnar nerve

Motor proximal stimulation site

Flexor carpi ulnaris

Flexor digitorum profundus 3&4

First dorsal interosseus

Motor distal stimulation site

Abductor digiti minimi

Digital sensory branch

Figure 23.4 Ulnar nerve anatomy. Format is similar view to that of Figure 23.3. (NCV = nerve conduction velocity.)

When measuring NCV across the elbow, a small error in measurement of distance or latency causes a large error in calculated NCV because of the short distance between stimulation sites. This error is exaggerated by the use of high-voltage, long-duration stimuli. High-voltage stimuli are volume-conducted through tissues and can depolarize the axonal membrane several millimeters from the cathode. Therefore, the distance measured on the skin may be longer than the distance between the site of activation and recording electrode. It is important to measure the distance with the elbow in the same position as it was during stimulation, usually flexed to 90 degrees.

Ulnar sensory NCV studies are performed by stimulating digit 5 (the little finger) using ring electrodes and recording from the ulnar nerve just above the wrist. Electrodes are placed as described for the median nerve, except that the distance between stimulating cathode and G1 is 11 cm. Antidromic stimulation can be performed if orthodromic stimulation fails to produce a measurable response or if this is the preference of the clinician.

Radial Nerve

Motor NCV is measured by recording from the extensor indicis. G1 is placed over the belly of the muscle. G2 is placed 2 cm distally. Needle electrodes can be used but are seldom required. The distal stimulation site is in the forearm, between the extensor carpi ulnaris and extensor digiti minimi, 10 cm proximal to the styloid process. Proximal stimulation is just proximal to the antecubital fossa, between the biceps tendon and brachioradialis. Sensory NCV is measured by recording from the superficial sensory branch on the dorsum of the hand after stimulating from a more proximal site (Figure 23.5).

Peroneal Nerve

The common peroneal nerve separates into superficial and deep peroneal branches. The superficial peroneal nerve innervates the peroneus longus and brevis and terminates in sensory branches that supply the lateral aspect of the lower leg and the dorsum of the foot and toes.

The deep peroneal nerve, also called the anterior tibial nerve, innervates the tibialis anterior, extensor digitorum longus, extensor hallucis longus, peroneus tertius, and extensor digitorum brevis. The terminal sensory branches supply the skin over the first two toes. The extensor digitorum brevis is occasionally innervated by the accessory peroneal nerve, a branch of the superficial peroneal nerve.

Peroneal motor NCV is usually determined by recording from the extensor digitorum brevis (Figure 23.6). Distal stimulation is in the lower leg, adjacent to the tendon of the tibialis anterior. Proximal stimulation is at the fibular neck. When the nerve is believed to be injured across the fibular neck, more proximal stimulation is then performed in the popliteal fossa. The NCV across the fibular neck is compared to the NCV distal to the neck. A difference of 10 m/sec or greater is abnormal.

Tibial Nerve

The tibial nerve innervates the medial and lateral gastrocnemius and soleus muscles and supplies sensation to those portions of the sole and dorsolateral foot that are not served by the sural and superficial peroneal nerves. The tibial nerve also innervates most of the intrinsic muscles of the foot via the medial and lateral plantar nerves. Tibial sensory NCVs are rarely performed and will not be discussed. Motor NCVs are performed by recording from the belly of the abductor hallucis muscle on the medial aspect of the foot (Figure 23.7). Distal stimulation is delivered to the nerve as it pass-

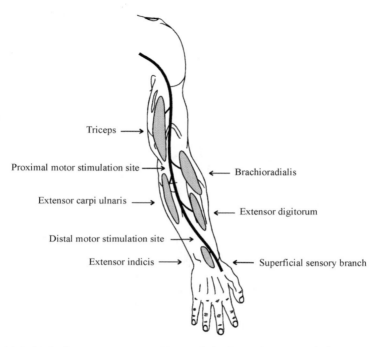

Triceps

Proximal motor stimulation site

Extensor carpi ulnaris

Distal motor stimulation site

Extensor indicis

Brachioradialis

Extensor digitorum

Superficial sensory branch

Figure 23.5 Radial nerve anatomy. View of the lateral aspect of the arm. Format is similar to that of Figure 23.3. (NCV = nerve conduction velocity.)

es behind the medial epicondyle, and proximal stimulation is delivered in the popliteal fossa.

Sural Nerve

The sural nerve is the only purely sensory nerve in the leg that is tested routinely. The sural is formed in the midcalf by the joining of branches from both the peroneal and tibial nerves. Sural sensory conduction is recorded from the nerve behind and slightly inferior to the lateral epicondyle. The stimulation site is on the posterior surface of the leg, 14 cm proximal to the recording site. There are no definite landmarks for the site of proximal stimulation, so some hunting may be needed. For most other NCV studies, the ground is placed proximal to the stimulating electrodes to minimize the potential for current to pass through the body. However, for sural sensory NCV, the ground is placed between the stimulating and recording electrodes.

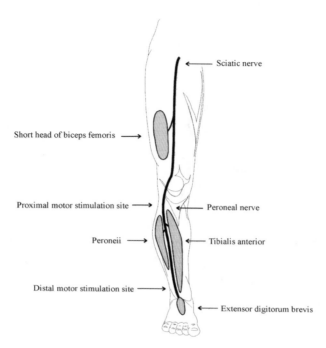

Figure 23.6 Peroneal nerve anatomy. View of the lateral aspect of the leg. Format is similar to that of Figure 23.3. The biceps femoris is not innervated by the peroneal nerve strictly; however, this muscle is most important for evaluation of peroneal nerve function. (NCV = nerve conduction velocity.)

In NCV, the ground is frequently placed between the stimulating and recording electrodes. This minimizes the stimulus artifact (sometimes called "shock artifact"), which can obscure the sural SNAP.

F-Wave Study

The F-wave study tests conduction of motor axons proximal to the stimulation site. When motor nerves are stimulated for routine NCV studies, the stimulation creates action potentials that travel not only orthodromically toward the muscle but also antidromically toward the motoneuron. The antidromic potential reaches the soma and depolarizes the dendrites. Depolarization is then conducted electrotonically back to the axon hillock, which is now repolarized. A new action potential is created and transmitted back to the muscle. The action potential activates

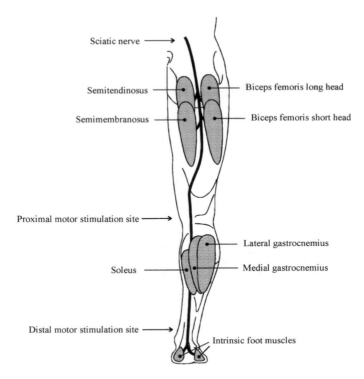

Figure 23.7 Tibial nerve anatomy. View of the posterior aspect of the left leg. The left side is lateral and right is medial. The format is similar to Figure 23.3. The terminal motor branches of the tibial nerve are the medial and lateral plantar nerves. (NCV = nerve conduction velocity.)

the motor end-plate, causing action potentials in muscle fibers. This late response is the F wave (Figure 23.8).

The recording electrodes for the F-wave study are placed in the same locations as for the motor NCV study. The stimulating electrode is over the nerve either proximally or distally. However, the stimulating electrodes are turned around, so that the cathode (negative pole) is toward the spine.

Normal values for F-wave conduction study are presented in Table 23.1. Interpretation is based on F-wave latency and the presence or absence of a response. Amplitudes are too variable to be of clinical use. Abnormalities of proximal conduction are unlikely to reduce amplitude without prolonging latency. Demyelinating peripheral neuropathies slow the F-wave response, since disorders that slow distal conduction also slow proximal conduction.

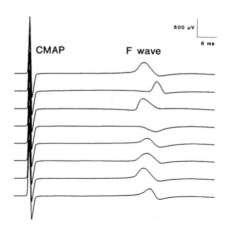

Figure 23.8 F-wave study of the median nerve. Stimuli are delivered to the distal median nerve. Recording is made from the abductor pollicis brevis. The responses to eight consecutive stimuli are shown in cascade format. (CMAP = compound motor action potential.)

An abnormal F-wave response is often the earliest electrophysiologic abnormality in Guillain-Barré syndrome.

The F wave and CMAP can be used to calculate a proximal motor conduction velocity. The F-wave latency is the sum of the time for conduction to the spinal cord and back down to the muscle. If the CMAP is recorded from the same stimulating electrode position, this latency can be subtracted from the F-wave latency to derive the time from conduction to the cord and then back to the stimulating electrode. Therefore, proximal NCV can be calculated according to the following formula:

$$NCV = \frac{2 \times Dist}{F - M}$$

Where *Dist* is the distance from stimulating electrode to spine, *F* is F-wave latency, and *M* is the CMAP latency. *Dist* is needed only for the calculation of proximal NCV. However, even if proximal conduction is not calculated, patient height should be measured since F-wave latency varies with limb and spine length.

Several disorders increase F-wave latency. F-wave studies are useful in most patients with suspected peripheral neuropathy to compare proximal

Table 23.1   Normal Data for F-Wave Studies*

Nerve	Maximum Latency (ms)
Median	31
Ulnar	31
Peroneal	51
Tibial	55

*During performance of the F-wave study, multiple trials are performed to a maximum of 10, or until one trial has a latency in the normal range. After 10 trials, the shortest latency is reported on the data sheet. If this latency exceeds the maximum latency listed on the table, the study is interpreted as abnormal, indicating slowing of proximal conduction in motor axons.

and distal conduction, but they are especially useful in proximal neuropathies such as the Guillain-Barré syndrome and chronic inflammatory demyelinating polyradiculoneuropathy. The F-wave latency is usually normal in patients with axonopathies, radiculopathies, and plexopathies. Severe axonopathies with secondary demyelination increase F-wave latency, but the delay is small as compared with the axonal changes seen on EMG. The F wave may be absent in demyelinating neuropathies, because the afferent and efferent compound action potentials are dispersed.

H-Reflex Study

The H reflex is the electrophysiologic counterpart of the tendon reflex. When the muscle is stretched by tapping the tendon, muscle spindles are activated and transmit afferent impulses to the spinal cord. Part of the reflex is generated by monosynaptic connections in the spinal cord, but much of the reflex is generated by polysynaptic pathways at both segmental and suprasegmental levels.

The H reflex is usually elicited from foot plantar flexors by stimulation of the tibial nerve. The patient lies prone with knees bent slightly. This is best done by placing a pillow under the feet. The stimulating electrode is in the popliteal fossa. The recording electrodes are over the soleus or medial gastrocnemius.

The oscilloscope time base is set at 10 ms/div and approximately 200 mV/div. The stimulator is set for repetitive stimulation at 1/sec or 0.5/sec,

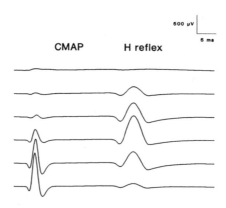

Figure 23.9 H-reflex study. Stimuli were delivered to the tibial nerve at the popliteal fossa, and recordings were made from the soleus. Each successive stimulus was of greater intensity. The first response is the H reflex because of the low threshold of afferent axons. At higher stimulus intensities, motor axons are directly stimulated, such that the compound motor action potential (CMAP) predominates and the H reflex disappears.

and the voltage is gradually increased until a response is obtained from the muscle (Figure 23.9). The first visible response, at approximately 30 ms, is the H reflex. As the stimulus voltage is increased further, a potential is recorded whose latency is much earlier than the H reflex. This early potential is the CMAP. The H reflex disappears as the CMAP amplitude increases with increments of stimulus voltage.

Normal H-reflex latency is 35 ms or less, and interside differences should not exceed 1.4 ms. H-reflex amplitude varies greatly between patients and between sides and cannot be used for clinical interpretation. A delayed or absent H reflex is associated with both demyelinating and axonal neuropathies, and may also be seen as an isolated finding in patients with S1 radiculopathy.

Blink Reflex

The blink reflex can be used to evaluate patients with lesions of the facial nerve, trigeminal nerve, or of the brain stem. However, neuroimaging is the preferred method to evaluate the brain stem, so the blink reflex is used predominantly to evaluate the cranial nerves.

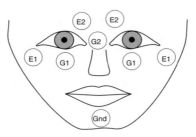

Figure 23.10 Blink reflex: electrode placement. G1 indicates the recording electrodes over the orbicularis oculi bilaterally. G2 is the reference for both electrodes. E1 is the site for direct stimulation of the facial nerve in front of the ear. E2 is the site of stimulation of the supraorbital nerve. (Gnd = ground.)

TECHNIQUES OF THE BLINK REFLEX

Surface electrodes are placed in the following positions (Figure 23.10):

- Active recording electrode (G1) is placed over the orbicularis oculi, usually below the eye.
- Reference electrode (G2) is placed on the nose.
- For direct response, stimulating electrodes are placed over the facial nerve anterior to the ear and slightly inferior to the external auditory canal, with the cathode distal (E1).
- For blink reflex, stimulating electrodes are placed over the supraorbital nerve with the cathode proximal (E2).
- Ground electrodes are placed below the chin.
- Electrodes are placed on the opposite side of the face corresponding to positions outlined above.

Stimulating and recording parameters are detailed in Table 23.2. Stimulus duration is 0.2 ms, and intensity is set high enough to establish a maximal direct response. This direct response is the CMAP produced in the orbicularis oculi.

NORMAL BLINK REFLEX

Before the blink reflex is performed, the facial nerve is stimulated and the CMAP recorded from the orbicularis oculi. This is termed the direct response and is a test of the integrity of the efferent system. The usual latency of the direct response is approximately 3 ms and should not exceed 4.1 ms.

Table 23.2 Blink Reflex Stimulus and Recording Parameters*

Parameter	Direct Response	Blink Reflex
Gain	1 mV/division	500 µV/division
Time base	1 ms/division	2 ms/division
Low-frequency filter	20 Hz	20 Hz
High-frequency filter	10 kHz	10 kHz
Stimulus duration	0.1 ms	0.1 ms

*Stimulus artifact may be further reduced by using an even shorter duration stimulus (e.g., 0.05 ms if the equipment allows this setting).

Then, the supraorbital nerve is stimulated to evoke the *blink reflex*. Stimulation of the supraorbital nerve results in a response composed of components R1 and R2 (Figure 23.11). R1 is a short loop reflex that is only projected ipsilateral to the stimulus. R2 is a longer loop reflex projected bilaterally.

Measurements are made of the latency of the direct response, R1, ipsilateral R2, and contralateral R2. R1 has a latency of about 10 ms and should not exceed 13 ms. R2 has a latency of about 30 ms and should not exceed 40 ms ipsilateral to the stimulus and 41 ms contralateral. Amplitudes are measured by some neurophysiologists. They are too variable to be used for clinical interpretation, however.

The blink reflex can be elicited not only by electrical stimulation but also by mechanical stimulation. A tap is delivered to the forehead by a hammer with a contact switch. The switch is connected to the EMG machine and triggers the sweep at the time of impact. The R1 with tap stimulation has an upper limit of normal of 16.7 ms. Mechanical stimulation usually offers no additional information over electrical stimulation, so this is not routinely performed.

INTERPRETATION OF THE BLINK REFLEX

Guides to the interpretation of the blink reflex are as follows:

- Prolonged direct response with otherwise normal latencies indicate a lesion of the facial nerve, such as Bell's palsy.
- Prolonged R1 indicates a lesion in the reflex pathway from trigeminal nerve to facial nerve. Facial nerve lesions also prolong R1 but are distinguished from brain stem or trigeminal nerve lesions because the

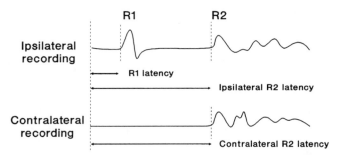

Figure 23.11 Blink reflex: normal response. R1 is seen only from the ipsilateral side. R2 is seen on both sides. The most important measurements are shown. Amplitude may be measured but is not routinely used in analysis.

direct response is prolonged as well. If the contralateral R2 is normal, then the afferent limb in the trigeminal nerve is normal, and a brain stem lesion is likely.

- If the latency of the direct response is normal, but the latencies of R1, ipsilateral R2, and contralateral R2 are prolonged, a lesion of the trigeminal nerve is likely, but brain stem lesions cannot be excluded.

Data on the interpretation of the blink reflex are presented in Table 23.3.

Sympathetic Skin Response

The sympathetic skin response is not strictly a nerve conduction. It is used to test the integrity of the sympathetic nervous system in patients with suspected autonomic neuropathy.

Electrodes are placed on the palm and dorsum of the hand or sole and dorsum of the foot, not overlying any particular muscles. The leads are fed to a machine capable of recording DC potentials. Gain is set to approximately 20 µV/div, with a sweep speed of 200 ms/div or, preferably, slower. The patient is asked to take a deep breath and then let it out. After a latency of a few seconds, there is a DC potential with the palm negative compared to the dorsum of the hand. The wave subsequently declines.

The study is interpreted as normal if the response is present, abnormal if the response is absent. No interpretation is made on the basis of amplitude or latency, although specific patterns have theoretical physiologic implications. In fact, the clinical utility of this technique is not universally accepted, and many laboratories do not offer this test.

Table 23.3   Interpretation of Blink Reflex Data

Direct	R1	R2 Ipsilateral	R2 Contralateral	Lesion Location
Normal	Normal	Normal	Normal	Normal response
Prolonged	Prolonged	Prolonged	Normal	Facial nerve
Normal	Prolonged	Normal	Normal	Brain stem pathways
Normal	Prolonged	Prolonged	Prolonged	Trigeminal nerve, but could be brain stem

Guidelines for Efficient Nerve Conduction Studies

Nerve conduction studies must be individually designed to answer clinical questions. Recommended studies for specific, common neuromuscular disorders are presented in Chapter 27. The following timesaving suggestions are applicable to virtually all conduction studies.

- If you do not know the patient prior to the examination, take a brief history and do a directed neurologic examination. Time invested in clinical evaluation saves time by directing the electrical studies and maximizing the information derived.
- Measure and mark the limbs for all anticipated nerve-conduction studies before starting.
- Gradually increase the stimulus voltage during the initial study so that the patient is not surprised by the shock. Once the optimal voltage is established, use this voltage for the initial stimulus for subsequent nerve conduction studies. There is no clinical value to sneaking up on the CMAP or SNAP.

Some neurophysiologists think that patients adjust to electrical stimuli over time. Studies in animals and humans suggest that each successive electrical shock is progressively less well tolerated, however. The nervous system would rather have one adequate shock than many incremental stimuli.

24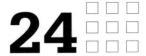

Electromyography

Technical Requirements

Electrodes

The three commonly used EMG electrodes are monopolar, coaxial, and single fiber (Figure 24.1). A monopolar electrode consists of a fine needle that is fully insulated with the exception of a very small region at the tip. The insulating material is usually a polymer plastic. The end of the wire opposite the needle point is soldered to multistrand wire that connects to the amplifier. The monopolar needle requires a reference, so a disk electrode is fixed on the skin overlying the study muscle using electrode gel and tape. A ground electrode is also placed on the skin proximal to the recording electrodes.

A coaxial electrode is composed of a fine wire inserted through the barrel of a hollow hypodermic needle. The wire is insulated, so that it does not touch the barrel of the needle. The recording surface is a small exposed portion of wire on the bevel of the needle that is held in place by epoxy or a similar cement. The opposite end of the wire is soldered to multistrand connector wire. The barrel of the needle is also soldered to another wire, so that the barrel can serve as a reference for the active recording surface. A ground electrode, but not a surface reference, is needed.

A single-fiber electrode is composed of a hollow needle with one or more insulated wires inserted through the barrel. The wires are turned and exposed on the side of the needle. This gives greater stability in longer-term recordings than when the electrode surface is on the bevel. The barrel serves as the reference for the single-fiber electrode.

Electromyography Machine Settings

The low-frequency filter is typically set to 10 Hz, and the high-frequency filter is set at 20 kHz. Most EMG instruments have a multiposi-

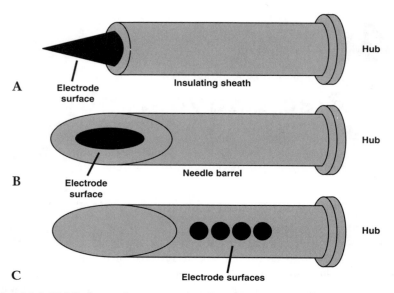

A

Hub

Electrode surface

Insulating sheath

B

Hub

Electrode surface

Needle barrel

C

Hub

Electrode surfaces

Figure 24.1 EMG electrodes. A. Monopolar electrode. B. Coaxial electrode. C. Single-fiber electrode.

tion switch or a software switch with several options for frequencies. Computerized EMG machines have filter settings preset, although the default settings are usually programmable by the user. The display is set for 10 ms/division. The ten horizontal divisions provide a total sweep time of 100 ms. The sweep rate of 10/sec is selected because it is the fastest sweep that is still below the flicker-fusion frequency of the human eye (i.e., approximately 16 frames per second). This is necessary for accurate visual analysis of the EMG. At faster frequencies, the traces appear fused, making it impossible to tell whether two potentials are on the same or subsequent traces.

Gain is first set at 50 μV/division to inspect resting activity, because the amplitude of fibrillation potentials may be only 50 μV. Analysis of single motor units requires a gain of 200 μV/division.

Electromyography Techniques

The EMG machine must be turned on before any electrodes are placed on the patient to avoid surges of current through the patient. The ground electrode is placed on the limb, proximal to the muscle to be studied. If a monopolar electrode is used, the reference is placed adjacent to the insertion point of the needle. Perotto (1994) is an excellent reference to the landmarks for needle insertion in specific muscles. The needle is inserted through the skin and into the muscle before the electrode junction box is switched on. If the box is switched on before insertion, the open loop between active and reference electrodes creates high voltage artifact.

EMG signals are usually analyzed by visual and auditory inspection. The clinical neurophysiologist watches as signals are displayed on the screen in real time and listens to the signals from the audio monitor. Experienced clinicians often hear abnormalities before they are seen. The pitch of the signals is a good indication of the rate of voltage change during a potential. It indicates the proximity of the electrode to the muscle fibers.

The four parameters that must be assessed are the following:

1. Insertional activity
2. Resting activity
3. Single motor unit analysis
4. Motor unit recruitment during maximal voluntary contraction

The patient is asked to completely relax the muscle to assess resting activity. A minimal muscle contraction is then requested to evaluate individual motor unit potentials (MUPs). The examiner's hand should be placed to oppose the action of the muscle. This shows the patient how to contract the muscle and helps to prevent dislodging the electrode by limb movement. Next, a maximal voluntary contraction is requested to evaluate motor unit recruitment. The limb must be held firmly to minimize movement.

Normal Electromyographic Activity

Insertional Activity

Normal insertional activity consists of a brief discharge of multiple muscle fiber action potentials. The duration is usually less than 500 ms, with abrupt onset and termination. An example of normal insertional activity is illustrated in Figure 24.2.

Insertion may provoke potentials that look like fibrillation potentials and positive sharp waves. These are the potentials of single muscle fibers and are not abnormal unless the discharge continues after needle movement has stopped.

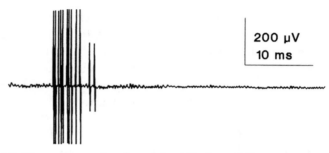

Figure 24.2 Normal insertional activity. The burst of activity was due to advancement of the needle electrode.

Spontaneous Activity

Normal muscles do not have spontaneous activity at rest. Persistent MUPs may occasionally be mistaken for abnormal spontaneous activity. Ensure that the patient has completely relaxed the muscle before interpreting abnormal spontaneous activity. Silencing of the muscle can occasionally be facilitated by contraction of an antagonist muscle.

Motor Unit Potentials

The patient is asked to contract the muscle enough to activate a few motor units. Each discharge is a MUP. (Sample MUPs are shown in Figure 24.3.) The amplitude of the MUP depends on the number of muscle fibers innervated by the motor axon and the proximity of the recording electrode to these muscle fibers. A typical MUP amplitude is 200 mV or greater. Amplitude is not as important as morphology in diagnosis. Most normal motor units are biphasic or triphasic. Up to 15% of motor units may be polyphasic before the muscle is classified as abnormal. The duration of most MUPs is usually less than 10 ms and should not exceed 15 ms.

Recruitment Pattern

With increasing volitional muscle contraction, motor units discharge faster and more units are recruited. With maximal contraction, so many units are activated that the baseline is obliterated. This is called a *full interference pattern*.

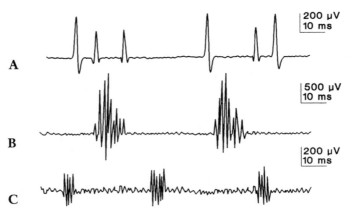

Figure 24.3 Motor unit potentials. A. Normal motor unit potentials. B. Neuropathic motor unit potentials. C. Myopathic motor unit potentials.

Abnormal Electromyographic Activity

Table 24.1 shows most of the common EMG findings, their origin, and their interpretation. Table 24.2 shows the expected EMG findings with neuropathic and myopathic disorders.

Abnormalities of Insertion

Increased Insertional Activity

Increased insertional activity indicates an exaggerated discharge, often with increased duration, such that the firing continues substantially after the end of electrode movement. None of the individual potentials is inherently abnormal. It is the repetitive and prolonged discharge that is abnormal.

Decreased Insertional Activity

Decreased insertional activity indicates a reduction in total activity with electrode movement. It is most common when there are few functioning muscle fibers, such as in long-standing denervation. An attack of periodic paralysis can result in abolition of insertional activity, since the muscle fibers are relatively inexcitable. Complete absence of insertional activity is more commonly caused by a faulty electrode than by absence of functioning muscle fibers.

Table 24.1   Common Electromyogram Findings

Potential	Physiologic Origin	Interpretation
Resting activity		
Fibrillation potential	Single muscle fiber action potential Due to membrane potential instability	Acute denervation or myopathy
Positive sharp wave	Same as for fibrillation potential The difference in electromyogram appearance is probably due to the orientation of the electrode to the muscle fiber	Acute denervation or myopathy May appear sooner than fibrillation potentials after denervation
Fasciculation potential	Spontaneous discharge of a motor unit	Denervation or motoneuron disease
Myotonia	Repetitive discharge of muscle fibers	Myotonic dystrophy, myotonia congenita, and some patients with periodic paralysis
Complex repetitive discharge	Repetitive discharge of muscle fibers	Denervation or myopathy
Motor unit activity		
Brief small-amplitude polyphasic potentials	Reduced number of functioning muscle fibers and dispersal of time of activation	Myopathy
Long-duration polyphasic motor unit potentials	Increased number of muscle fibers innervated by an axon Dispersed activation	Chronic denervation with motor unit reorganization
Maximal contraction		
Reduced recruitment	Reduced number of functioning motor units, requiring rapid discharge of single motor units	Denervation
Early recruitment	Reduced tension produced by each motor unit, so more units have to be recruited at faster rates even at relatively low effort level	Myopathy

Table 24.2   Electromyogram Abnormalities

Abnormality	Fibril-lations	Fascicu-lations	Polyphasic Motor Unit Potentials	Brief Small-Amplitude Polyphasic Potentials
Acute denervation	+	−	−	−
Chronic denervation	±	±	+	−
Myopathy	+	−	+	+
Neuromuscular junction transmission defect	±	−	−	±

Abnormal Spontaneous Activity

Fibrillation Potentials

Fibrillation potentials are single muscle fiber action potentials generated by abnormal spontaneous fluctuations in membrane potential that occasionally reach threshold (Figure 24.4). The potentials occur with a (more or less) random frequency, so that on the audio monitor they sound like raindrops. Fibrillation potentials occur at rest in patients with active denervation and with myopathies. Basic mechanisms of the membrane potential fluctuations were discussed in the Chapter 22.

Fibrillation potentials are brief biphasic waves with an initial negative component followed by a positive component. Amplitude is 20–200 µV with a duration of 1–5 ms. Fibrillation potentials occur at rest but may not be present at all recording locations within a given muscle. Multiple places in each muscle must be examined. Fibrillation potentials may not appear for 3–4 weeks after a nerve injury.

Positive Sharp Waves

Positive sharp waves are single muscle fiber action potentials that look different than fibrillation potentials. Unlike fibrillation potentials, the initial deflection is positive, followed by a return to baseline. There may be a small negative wave after the positive component, but the positive deflection is predominant. The frequency is random, as are fibrillation potentials.

Positive sharp waves, like fibrillation potentials, are prominent in active denervation and in myopathies. The different appearance of the two wave-

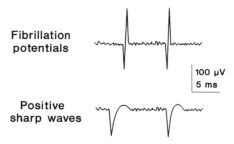

Fibrillation
potentials

100 μV
5 ms

Positive
sharp waves

Figure 24.4 Abnormal spontaneous activity. Fibrillation potentials and positive sharp waves.

forms may be explained by the location of the recording electrode. The fibrillation potential is biphasic because of the passing extracellular negativity created by propagation of the muscle fiber action potential. The membrane adjacent to the positive sharp waves may not be able to sustain an action potential, either due to focal damage from the underlying condition or to membrane deformation due to the electrode. Therefore, the action potential approaches the injured area but cannot excite it. The electrode sees the electrotonic potential that is trying to depolarize the membrane. This potential is an outward current, producing a positive extracellular field potential.

Fasciculations

Fasciculations are due to the spontaneous discharge of single motor units. The conformation of the MUP may be normal or may have a neuropathic appearance. Fasciculations are differentiated from voluntary MUPs by their pseudo-random frequency. The morphology and amplitude of fasciculation potentials may fluctuate, probably due to a shifting generator of the discharge.

Fasciculations are seen in normal individuals and in those with chronic denervation (most commonly motor neuron disease). They should not be interpreted as abnormal without other EMG evidence of chronic denervation. Pathologic fasciculations often have a polyphasic appearance and discharge irregularly at an average interval of 3.5 seconds. Nonpathologic fasciculations discharge at a mean interval of 0.8 seconds.

Myokymia

Myokymia is an involuntary repetitive discharge of a single motor unit at a frequency of 30–40/sec. The muscle moves under the skin, giving a rippling or quivering appearance on examination.

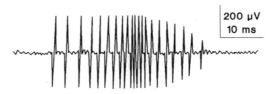

Figure 24.5 Myotonic discharges.

Myokymia occurs in several denervating disorders but is most common in the following: (1) multiple sclerosis, (2) brain stem glioma, (3) radiation plexopathy, (4) Guillain-Barré syndrome, and (5) gold neuropathy. The myokymia is localized to the face in multiple sclerosis and brain stem glioma. Myokymia occurs in radiation plexopathy but not in neoplastic infiltration of the brachial plexus, and its presence can be used as a distinguishing feature between the two. Syndromes of continuous muscle fiber activity may show a pattern of activation that suggests myokymia. It is likely that various lesions of the motor unit can produce myokymia, but the exact physiologic substrate of this pattern is not identified.

Myotonic Discharges

Myotonic discharges are repetitive muscle fiber action potentials. Needle movement evokes the discharges, probably by membrane deformation and resultant depolarization (Figure 24.5). The frequency waxes and wanes and has been described as having a "dive bomber" sound on the audio monitor.

The repetitive discharge is probably due to an abnormality in chloride conductance. Chloride is localized predominantly in the extracellular space. At the end of an action potential, the membrane is repolarized by closure of sodium channels and opening of potassium channels. The potassium efflux is responsible for the transient hyperpolarization that follows an action potential. As the potassium conductance falls to baseline, the membrane potential depolarizes toward normal. Normally, chloride conductance serves to keep the membrane from reaching threshold. If the chloride conductance is reduced, then the depolarization due to inactivation of potassium channels can result in another action potential. This cyclic depolarization, action potential, and repolarization occurs until the depolarization fails to reach threshold.

Myotonic discharges are seen in patients with myotonic dystrophy, myotonia congenita, paramyotonia congenita, and hyperkalemic periodic

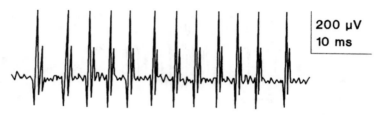

Figure 24.6 Complex repetitive discharges. Polyphasic potentials discharge repetitively. The frequency does not wax and wane as do myotonic discharges.

paralysis. Patients with inflammatory myopathies or acid maltase deficiency may have EMG evidence of myotonic discharges without clinical myotonia.

Complex Repetitive Discharges

Complex repetitive discharges are waxing and waning high-frequency synchronous discharges of several muscle fibers (Figure 24.6). Amplitudes range from 50 µV to 1 mV, and discharge rates range from 5–100/sec. Total discharge duration may be a few seconds. Older terms, which should not be used, are *pseudomyotonia* and *bizarre high-frequency discharge*. Complex repetitive discharges are seen commonly in chronic denervation and in some patients with myopathies. They can rarely occur in otherwise normal individuals and should not be interpreted as abnormal in the absence of other EMG abnormalities.

Complex repetitive discharges are thought to arise from discharge of a single muscle fiber that acts as a pacemaker, subsequently activating adjacent muscle fibers. The connection is direct electrical continuity, which accounts for the near synchrony of the discharge. Sudden changes in potential conformation likely are due to drop out of a group of fibers from the spread of electrical activation.

Abnormal Motor Unit Potentials

Neuropathic Motor Unit Potentials

Acute denervation, before reinnervation has occurred, results in loss of motor units. Surviving motor units have essentially normal function. Therefore, MUP analysis is usually normal, unless denervation is complete and there are no MUP.

Denervated muscle fibers are eventually reinnervated by sprouts of nearby surviving axons. Since the number of muscle fibers innervated by each surviving motor axon is increased, the amplitude of the reconstituted MUP is often greater than normal. The new connections are often not activated synchronously with the original connections, so the MUP is usually polyphasic and of increased duration (see Figure 24.3). High-amplitude, long-duration polyphasia is the hallmark of chronic denervation.

Myopathic Motor Unit Potentials

The instability of muscle fiber membrane potentials with myopathy results in alteration in the appearance of the MUP. Some muscle fibers are irreversibly depolarized and fail to be activated by neuromuscular transmission. This failure results in MUPs of low amplitude (see Figure 24.3). In addition, the loss of some muscle fibers and the asynchronous activation of remaining damaged fibers results in polyphasic MUPs whose duration is not prolonged, as it is for neuropathic units.

Myopathic MUPs are sometimes called *brief small-amplitude polyphasic potentials*. Although this term is discouraged by some neurophysiologists, it is a descriptive term. Unfortunately, the association of brief small-amplitude polyphasic potentials with myopathies is so strong in some minds that alternative interpretations are not considered. MUPs of similar appearance can be seen in some patients with denervation, especially early, due to desynchronization of terminal nerve conduction.

Abnormal Recruitment

Reduced Recruitment

Reduced recruitment indicates a decrease in functioning units. Single units can be identified and are often firing more rapidly to make up for the lack of recruitable units (Figure 24.7). Reduced recruitment is seen predominantly in axonal neuropathies but may also occur in demyelinating neuropathies, if some motor axons fail to transmit.

Early Recruitment

Early recruitment means that many units are recruited at an abnormally low level of effort (see Figure 24.7). This is typical of myopathies. The muscle contractions are ineffectual, so that additional units are recruited to generate the desired force. These units are often decreased in amplitude and produce an interference pattern that is reduced in amplitude but still able to obliterate the baseline.

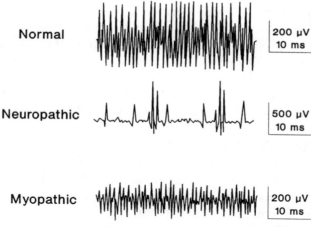

Figure 24.7 Recruitment patterns. **Normal** recruitment shows a mixture of motor unit potentials discharging at a high rate. Recruitment in **neuropathic** conditions is characterized by a reduced number of units. Units are polyphasic. Recruitment in **myopathic** disorders is characterized by low-amplitude potentials with a high frequency of discharge. A full recruitment pattern is developed with relatively weak contraction.

Electromyographic Testing of Specific Muscles

The most commonly tested muscles are listed in Table 24.3. The selection of muscles for examination is based on the clinical question and is discussed further in the Chapter 27.

Table 24.3   Muscles Commonly Studied in Electromyography

Muscle	Nerve	Plexus	Root
Upper extremity			
Abductor pollicis brevis	Median	MC	C8, T1
Biceps	Musculocutaneous	LC, UT	C5, C6
Deltoid	Axillary	PC, UT	C5, C6
Extensor digitorum communis	Radial	PC, MT, LT	C7, C8
First dorsal interosseus	Ulnar	MC, LT	C8, T1
Infraspinatus	Suprascapular	UT	C5, C6
Pronator teres	Median	LC, UT, MT	C6, C7
Serratus anterior	Long thoracic	—	C5, C6, C7
Supraspinatus	Suprascapular	UT	C5, C6
Triceps	Radial	PC, MT, LT	C7
Lower extremity			
Extensor digitorum brevis	Peroneal	SP	L5–S1
Gluteus medius	Superior gluteal	—	L4–S1
Medial gastrocnemius	Tibial	SP	S1–2
Peroneus longus	Peroneal	SP	L5–S2
Rectus femoris	Femoral	LP	L2–4
Short head of biceps femoris	Peroneal	SP	S1–2
Tibialis anterior	Peroneal	SP	L4–5
Vastus medialis	Femoral	LP	L2–4

MC = medial cord; LC = lateral cord; PC = posterior cord; UT = upper trunk; MT = middle trunk; LT = lower trunk; SP = sacral plexus; LP = lumbar plexus.

25

Special Tests of Neuromuscular Transmission

Repetitive Stimulation

Repetitive stimulation is a test of neuromuscular transmission and is indicated for patients with progressive weakness without sensory loss, patients with easy fatigability, and patients who have activity-dependent weakness.

Physiology

Normal neuromuscular transmission is one to one—that is, every motor axon action potential results in an action potential in each muscle fiber of the motor unit. This relationship fails at high rates of stimulation because some muscle fibers become refractory. The amplitude of the compound motor action potential (CMAP) then declines progressively. This is called the *decremental response*.

Normal individuals do not show a decremental response at stimulus rates less than 20/sec, but people with myasthenia gravis fail to fire repetitively even at low rates of stimulation. This is because there is an insufficient number of receptors available for binding with acetylcholine.

Unlike myasthenia gravis, botulism and the myasthenic syndrome are presynaptic defects in neuromuscular transmission caused by impaired mobilization or release of acetylcholine. The amount of transmitter released can be increased by repetitive stimulation at a fast rate, which is probably due to facilitated transmitter mobilization by the "priming" action potential.

Repetitive Stimulation at Slow Rates

Methods

Repetitive stimulation at slow rates is usually performed at 3/sec. Several different protocols have been suggested; I prefer the following:

1. Tape electrodes over the muscle under study with the active electrode (G1) on the belly and the reference (G2) distal.
2. Deliver a train of nine or ten pulses at a rate of 3/sec. Photograph or print the display.
3. Maximally exercise the muscle for 1 minute.
4. Repeat the trains of repetitive stimuli at 1-minute intervals until 5 minutes after the exercise.

Analysis of the responses can be performed in several ways. The most accurate method is to determine the area under the curve of the CMAP, essentially integrating the potential. The CMAP is produced by a bipolar recording. The negative deflection indicates depolarization, and the positive deflection indicates repolarization of the same muscle fibers. Therefore, only the negative portion of the CMAP is integrated. The negative area under the curve is thought to better correlate with the number of muscle fibers being activated than the measurements of the peak amplitudes. Most modem EMG machines perform this calculation automatically. The largest decrement is usually between the first and fourth or fifth responses.

The abductor digiti minimi, innervated by the ulnar nerve, is usually selected for repetitive stimulation studies, but the trapezius may be more sensitive to transmission defects. The spinal accessory nerve is stimulated at the base of the sternocleidomastoid muscle. G1 is placed on the belly of the upper portion of the trapezius, and G2 can be placed near the acromion. The patient exercises by holding onto the bottom of the chair with both hands and pulling the shoulders upward.

Interpretation

The repetitive stimulation study is considered abnormal if there is more than a 10% decrement from the first to fourth stimuli (Figure 25.1). After the fifth stimulus, the CMAP amplitude may increase, with the responses to the ninth stimulus being near the level of the first.

Repetitive stimulation is used mainly for the diagnosis of myasthenia gravis. In myasthenia gravis, the decremental response is usually greater than 10% but is not necessarily seen in all muscles. There are two reasons

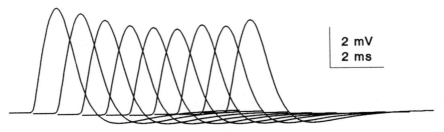

Figure 25.1 Repetitive stimulation at low rates. Responses to stimuli delivered at 3/sec are shown in overlapping format. This patient has a decay between responses 1 and 4.

that spinal accessory nerve stimulation of the trapezius is more sensitive than ulnar nerve stimulation of the abductor digiti minimi: (1) Distal muscles are less often affected than proximal muscles, and (2) distal muscles are more likely to be cool, and cooling of nerve and muscle can reduce the decrement to normal range.

Decremental responses occur in other disorders of neuromuscular transmission (e.g., partial denervation, myasthenic syndrome, botulism) and have been reported in multiple sclerosis. Repetitive stimulation is not used for the diagnosis of multiple sclerosis, however.

Repetitive Stimulation at Fast Rates

Methods

Repetitive stimulation at fast rates is too painful to be used routinely in clinical testing. Its greatest use is in the diagnosis of botulism and myasthenic syndrome, although paired stimuli may provide similar information. Electrode placement is the same as described above for repetitive stimulation at slow rates. The stimulus rate is 20–30/sec, and the responses are recorded and analyzed for decrement or increment.

Interpretation

Normal muscles show no significant increment or decrement in response to nerve stimulation at 20–30/sec. Faster frequencies are not used because a decremental response may appear when muscle fibers are no longer able to keep up with the rate of nerve activation. Patients with botulism, myasthenic syndrome, hypocalcemia, and hypomagnesemia have defects in transmitter release. The first response is often of very low amplitude, but successive stimuli evoke progressively larger responses. The response is not only facilitated by repetitive stimulation but also by sustained exercise. The incremental response is somewhat greater with myasthenic syndrome than with botulism. Myasthenia gravis may produce an incremental response with repetitive stimulation at fast rates; however, the magnitude of the increment is usually limited.

Paired Stimulation

The response to paired stimuli can be abnormal in any disorder of neuromuscular transmission. The technique is predominantly used for diagnosis of presynaptic defects such as botulism and myasthenic syndrome, however.

Physiology

A single stimulus gives a reproducible CMAP. If a second stimulus is given after the first, the CMAP is usually smaller if the interval between stimuli is short. This is because the second stimulus arrives within the refractory period of some of the muscle fibers (Figure 25.2). The second response usually disappears when the interval falls below 5 ms.

In presynaptic disorders, the second stimulus may produce a larger CMAP than the first for two reasons. First, release mechanisms are "primed," probably due to the increased availability of calcium. Since more transmitter is released, the second stimulus may activate some muscle fibers that the first did not. Second, if a muscle fiber did not reach threshold, the end-plate potential (EPP) likely has not completely decayed when the second arrives. Summation of the EPPs can bring the muscle fiber membrane to threshold. The result is that the second CMAP is greater than the first.

Methods

For paired stimulation, electrodes are placed as described for repetitive stimulation. Stimuli are given with variable interstimulus intervals. There is no uniformly agreed-on protocol, but it is reasonable to start at an interstimulus interval of 15 ms and gradually reduce the interval. The most helpful data are obtained with interstimulus intervals of 5–10 ms.

The amplitude of the CMAP obtained in response to the first and second stimuli of each pair is measured. The ratio of the two responses is used for interpretation.

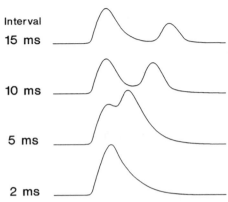

Figure 25.2 Paired stimulation. Paired stimuli are delivered at variable inter-stimulus intervals. The responses are recorded, and the amplitude to the first and second responses measured. No facilitation is normal. Facilitation of the second response is a positive result.

Interpretation

It is normal for the second CMAP to be smaller than the first. With shorter interstimulus intervals, the second response becomes smaller and eventually disappears, usually at or below 5 ms. An abnormal response results in a larger second response at interstimulus intervals of 5–10 ms. Normal paired stimulation is consistent with a diagnosis of botulism or myasthenic syndrome; however, it is not diagnostic.

Single-Fiber Electromyography

Single-fiber EMG is a time-consuming study used predominantly for the diagnosis of myasthenia gravis. False positives occur. Many clinicians do not routinely perform single-fiber EMG because of the time required and the relative rarity of cases to be studied. The two main studies performed during single-fiber EMG are jitter analysis and fiber density determination.

Jitter Analysis

Physiology

Single muscle fibers do not discharge exactly synchronously in creating a motor unit potential. There may be several milliseconds differ-

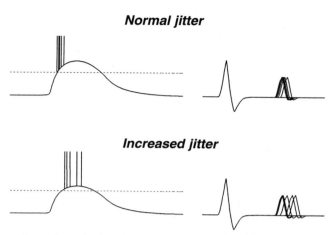

Figure 25.3 Physiologic basis for jitter on single-fiber EMG. Left side is an intracellular recording after nerve stimulation.

ence in the time of activation. This is termed the *interpotential interval* (IPI). The IPI for two muscle fibers (normally less than 4 ms) is reproducible from discharge to discharge. The normal variation is less than 50 µs. Disorders of neuromuscular transmission may increase the variation because synaptic transmission is less secure, that is, the EPP is smaller, so that the muscle fiber action potential is higher on the hump of the EPP (Figure 25.3). The time to threshold after the EPP is more variable.

The term *jitter* is derived from the appearance of the potentials on the oscilloscope display. The display is set so that the sweep is triggered by the first muscle fiber action potential. The second muscle fiber action potential appears a few milliseconds after the first. Since the first action potential is fixed in position on the display by the triggering apparatus, the second "jitters" back and forth as the IPI varies slightly.

Blocking is failure of discharge of either the first or second muscle fiber action potential. This is due to the muscle fiber's EPP not reaching threshold. Disorders of neuromuscular transmission may not only result in increased jitter but also in blocking.

Methods

The electrode is inserted into the muscle in the region of highest end-plate density. The extensor digitorum communis (EDC) is the most commonly studied muscle. After insertion of the electrode, the patient is asked to make a mild contraction (in the case of the EDC, extension of the middle finger [digit 3]). The examiner wants to record potentials from two muscle fibers of one motor unit. The action potentials can be defined as being from one unit if there is an almost perfect time lock between activation of the two fibers. A pair is accepted if the following criteria are met:

- Muscle fibers are clearly of the same motor unit
- Rise time is less than 300 ms
- Amplitude is greater than 200 µV
- IPI is greater than 150 µs

Measurements are made from the beginning of the upstroke of the potentials. This is best accomplished by using a computer to make direct measurement of the mean consecutive differences (MCDs) of the IPIs. The IPIs of consecutive discharges are subtracted, and the absolute values stored. The sum of these absolute values is divided by the number of trials to give the MCD. The MCD is more accurate than the standard deviation of the IPI, since the MCD is a more direct index of discharge-to-discharge variation.

A second method of jitter determination is possible without a computer. Ten consecutive discharge pairs are superimposed on the oscilloscope screen or on photographic paper. Because of the triggering, the first potential of each pair should be exactly superimposed. The second potentials will occur within an expected range. The range of IPI variation is the time from takeoff of the earliest of the second potentials to the takeoff of the last of the second potentials. This is termed the R_{10} (for range of 10 pairs). The R_{10} is determined for five electrode positions in the muscle, and the mean R_{10} range is calculated (MR_{10}).

An estimated MCD is calculated for the tested muscle from the following formula (Ekstedt et al., 1974):

$$MCD = MR_{10} \times 0.37$$

This formula results in an accurate estimation of the true MCD, which could have been calculated directly. In practice, jitter analysis is now usually performed on digital machines that analyze the pairs automatically.

Jitter analysis involves not only calculation of variation of IPI, but also the number of failures of conduction (termed *blocking*). Normal individuals have no blocking.

Interpretation
The mean consecutive difference should be less than 55 µs for EDC. Normative data are also available for other muscles. A normal muscle

may have increased jitter in one of twenty muscle fiber pairs, but increased jitter or blocking in two or more of twenty pairs is abnormal. The findings are not subtle. Most patients with generalized myasthenia have greatly increased jitter in a large proportion of pairs. Patients with ocular myasthenia may have increased jitter only in facial muscles.

Jitter analysis is a more sensitive test than repetitive stimulation to detect disorders of neuromuscular transmission. For example, patients with myasthenia gravis often have increased jitter in clinically unaffected muscles. Normal jitter in a clinically weak muscle is strong evidence against the diagnosis of myasthenia.

Increased jitter can be seen in partially denervated muscles as well as in disorders of neuromuscular transmission. Chronic heavy exercise may also increase jitter in otherwise normal individuals, probably due to mild denervation and reinnervation.

Blocking is a more specific sign of neuromuscular transmission disorders and is seldom seen in normal individuals. Some individuals 50 years or older may have blocking due to motor unit reorganization. Jitter is not significantly increased with age. In myasthenia gravis, blocking always occurs in the setting of increased jitter.

Fiber Density Determination

Fiber density is used to document chronic denervation. Increased fiber density is a sign of local reinnervation of denervated muscle fibers.

Physiology

Muscle fibers innervated by a single motor axon are scattered widely through a muscle; often only one muscle fiber is innervated by a single motor unit within a 300-μm radius. Fiber density is increased in patients with axonal neuropathies because denervated muscle fibers are reinnervated by sprouts from nearby surviving motor axons.

Methods

As was described for jitter analysis, a single-fiber EMG electrode is also used for fiber density determination. The needle is inserted into the muscle, the patient is asked to make a mild contraction, and a single muscle fiber action potential is recorded. A potential meets criteria for study if it has an amplitude of at least 200 μV and a rise time of less than 300 μs. When a potential is isolated, the clinical neurophysiologist looks for other muscle fiber action potentials that are part of the same motor unit. A muscle fiber action potential is classified as being part of the same motor unit if

Table 25.1   Normal Data for Fiber Density Determinations*

	Age (years)			
	10–25	26–50	51–75	>75
Extensor digitorum communis	1.87 ms	1.89 ms	2.00 ms	3.155 ms
First dorsal interosseous	1.66 ms	1.79 ms	ID	ID
Tibialis anterior	2.12 ms	2.11 ms	2.07 ms	ID

ID = insufficient data.
*Upper limits of normal, calculated as mean ±2.5 standard deviations from the mean.

it occurs reproducibly in the same time relation to the first muscle fiber action potential. The secondary potential must also be at least 200 μV in amplitude with a rise time of less than 300 μs. This ensures that the potentials are within a 300-μm radius.

   If the index potential is the only one identified in that motor unit, that electrode position has a fiber density of 1.0. If three muscle fiber potentials meet the criteria, the fiber density is 3.0. The fiber density is determined for at least twenty locations within the muscle and averaged across all examined locations. The muscle fiber density is expressed as a grand mean.

Interpretation

   Normal values for fiber density are shown in Table 25.1. Increased fiber density indicates partial denervation and local reinnervation. Young children may have increased fiber density in the absence of neuromuscular disease.

26

Quantitative Electromyogram Analysis

Routine EMG analysis is visual, with the neurophysiologist determining on the basis of training and experience whether a particular pattern is normal or abnormal. The neurophysiologist depends on the appearance of the trace and the sound from the audio monitor. Quantitative EMG analysis has capitalized on the same advances in computer hardware and software as digital EEG analysis. The purpose of quantitative EMG analysis is to provide more consistent and sensitive analysis.

Motor Unit Analysis

For digital motor unit analysis, the neurophysiologist must be especially careful about technique. Skin temperature must be at least 34°C in order for muscle temperature to be 37°C. The computer is able to identify motor unit potentials on the basis of a clear waveform that is separate from the background with defined amplitude and upstroke parameters. The upstroke velocity is an indicator of proximity of the motor unit fibers to the recording electrode. After a motor unit potential is selected, the duration and number of phases are calculated. Motor unit statistics are tabulated and can be compared with normative data for the particular muscle and patient age. Because the results of the analysis can differ between specific machines and in different laboratories, each laboratory should establish normal values for its population and equipment.

In practice, modern EMG machines are able to identify discrete motor unit potentials and perform motor unit analysis with relative ease and accuracy. This is far from the tedious process of manual unit selection and analysis, a process that should now be abandoned.

By quantitative motor unit analysis, diagnostic sensitivity to subtle myopathic or neuropathic conditions can be improved.

Recruitment Analysis

Motor unit recruitment with increasing effort allows for analysis of the discharge properties of individual motor units. Measured parameters may include recruitment frequency and average discharge rate per unit. Recruitment frequency is the frequency of motor unit discharge at which additional units are recruited. Average discharge rate is a function of the number of active units. The average discharge rate increases with enhanced effort. Overall, these measures show overlap between patients with and without neuropathic and myopathic disorders, so digital recruitment analysis is less important than single motor unit analysis.

With maximal muscle contraction, the interference pattern can show a characteristic appearance, ranging from a full pattern in normal conditions to the rapid firing of single units in neuropathic conditions, to low-amplitude units with early recruitment in myopathic conditions. Digital analysis lends itself well to this evaluation, although the computer is impaired by its inability to take into account patient effort.

Some laboratories have the ability to measure muscle tension and correlate this with electrical activity during recruitment. Complex calculations can be performed using digitized recruitment data as a function of force. There is considerable overlap between normal patients and patients with neuromuscular disorders, however. This technique is of interest but should be considered a research tool until methods and interpretations become more standardized.

Electromyogram Monitoring

EMG monitoring has recently been used during surgery on the spine. Dorsal rhizotomy is used for treatment of spasticity. Electrical stimulation is used to activate dorsal rootlets. Repetitive stimulation produces a pattern of activation of the muscles innervated by corresponding ventral roots that indicates whether the selected dorsal root subserves muscle spindle input or cutaneous and proprioceptive input.

Surgery for a tethered spinal cord involves dissection of tissue, some of which may include neural elements. Selective stimulation of tissue while recording from leg muscles and the anal sphincter can help to determine whether the patient will have increased deficit after surgery. These monitoring methods should be performed only by neurophysiologists trained in their use.

Monitoring of facial nerve function can be performed during surgery in the region of the nerve (e.g., cerebellopontine angle, acoustic nerve, vestibular nerve, and mastoid). Stimulation of the facial nerve and monitoring of contraction of facial muscles can help to ensure the integrity of the facial nerve during dissection.

27

Evaluation of Common Neuromuscular Problems

Electrophysiologic testing is designed to answer specific clinical questions. The first task is to localize the site of the lesion. For this, Table 27.1 shows the expected nerve conduction study (NCS) and EMG findings with different lesion sites in the nerve-muscle axis. Table 27.2 presents a suggested evaluation of patients with specific complaints. Table 27.3 shows the NCS and EMG findings in common specific disorders. The following are recommendations on studies to choose for several common clinical questions.

General Questions

Peripheral Neuropathy

Peripheral neuropathies have a predominantly distal distribution, and the longest nerves are the ones most likely affected. The following conduction studies are recommended as an initial screen:

- Tibial motor conduction
- Sural sensory conduction
- Tibial F wave

If these studies are normal, the patient does not have a generalized demyelinating neuropathy.

EMG should be performed in distal muscles. Myopathies are occasionally mistaken for neuropathies, so proximal muscles should be studied as

Table 27.1   Clinical Correlations of Nerve Conduction Velocities and Electromyogram Findings

Disorder	Nerve Conduction Velocities	Electromyogram Finding
Axonal neuropathy	Reduced CMAP amplitude Otherwise normal NCVs	Acute denervation, chronic denervation, or both
Demyelinating neuropathy	Slow motor and sensory NCVs Delayed F waves	Reduced recruitment
Motor neuron degeneration	Normal NCVs except possibly reduced CMAP amplitude	Acute and chronic denervation
Sensory neuron degeneration	Normal except possibly low sensory neural action potential amplitude	Normal
Myopathy	Normal Low CMAP amplitude (occasionally)	Myopathic findings
Neuromuscular transmission defect	Normal or reduced CMAP amplitude Abnormal repetitive stimulation Abnormal response to paired stimulation	Normal or mild denervation

NCVs = nerve conduction velocities; CMAP = compound motor action potential.

well, especially if the NCS is normal. Ask the patient which movements are most impaired, and study the muscles that perform those movements. If there are no localizing symptoms and the request does not specify an area to study, the tibialis anterior and rectus femoris should be examined. Some clinical neurophysiologists prefer to study the extensor digitorum brevis because of its distal location. I disagree. The muscle belly is small, and it is easy to insert the needle into a tendon or through the muscle into connective tissue.

Myopathy

Some clinical neurophysiologists perform EMG without NCSs when evaluating patients for myopathy. The observation of typical myopathic features on EMG does not exclude the existence of a concurrent neuro-

Table 27.2   Recommended Evaluation of Common Neuromuscular Problems*

Problem	Nerve Conduction Velocities	Electromyogram Finding
Brachial plexopathy	Median motor NCV Median sensory NCV Median F wave	First dorsal interosseous Pronator teres Biceps Triceps
Carpal tunnel syndrome	Median motor NCV Median sensory NCV	Abductor pollicis brevis
Cervical radiculopathy	Median motor NCV Median sensory NCV Median F wave	Abductor pollicis brevis First dorsal interosseous Extensor digitorum communis Biceps Triceps Deltoid Cervical paraspinal muscles
Fatigue or weakness that is not localized	Peroneal NCV (Consider repetitive and paired stimulation)	Tibialis anterior Quadriceps First dorsal interosseous Deltoid (Consider single-fiber EMG)
Footdrop	Peroneal motor NCV Peroneal F wave	Tibialis anterior Peroneus longus Short head of biceps femoris
Hand pain, weakness, or both	Median NCV Ulnar NCV	Abductor pollicis brevis First dorsal interosseous
Lumbar plexopathy	Tibial motor NCV Peroneal motor NCV Sural sensory NCV Tibial F wave Peroneal F wave	Tibialis anterior Medial gastrocnemius Vastus medialis
Lumbar radiculopathy	Tibial motor NCV Sural sensory NCV Tibial F wave H reflex	Tibialis anterior Medial gastrocnemius Vastus medialis Lumbar paraspinal muscles
Meralgia paresthetica	Tibial motor NCV Sural sensory NCV Femoral distal latency Lateral femoral cutaneous nerve condition	Rectus femoris Vastus medialis Tibialis anterior Medial gastrocnemius
Motoneuron disease	Tibial motor NCV Sural sensory NCV	Muscles in three nerve distributions in three extremities
Peripheral neuropathy	Tibial motor NCV Sural sensory NCV Tibial F wave	Tibialis anterior Medial gastrocnemius

Table 27.2 *(continued)*

Problem	Nerve Conduction Velocities	Electromyogram Finding
Peroneal palsy	Peroneal motor NCV Superficial peroneal sensory NCV Peroneal F wave	Tibialis anterior Peroneus longus Short head of biceps femoris
Radial neuropathy	Radial motor NCV Radial sensory NCV	Extensor digitorum communis
Sciatic neuropathy	Tibial motor NCV Peroneal motor NCV Sural sensory NCV Tibial F wave Peroneal F wave	Tibialis anterior Medial gastrocnemius Vastus medialis Gluteus medius

Spinal stenosis	See Lumbar radiculo-
	  pathy, above
		See Lumbar radiculopathy,
		  above

Ulnar neuropathy	Ulnar motor NCV
	  below elbow
	Ulnar motor NCV
	  across elbow
	Ulnar sensory NCV
		First dorsal interosseous

Tarsal tunnel
  syndrome
	Medial plantar motor
	  NCV
	Lateral plantar motor
	  NCV
		Abductor hallucis

Thoracic outlet syndrome	Median motor NCV Median sensory NCV Ulnar motor NCV Ulnar F wave Ulnar sensory NCV	Abductor pollicis brevis First dorsal interosseous Extensor digitorum communis

NCV = nerve conduction velocity.

*These studies are recommended as a minimum evaluation to look for the indicated disorder. In many cases, additional studies have to be done to localize the lesion. For example, if the recommended studies for carpal tunnel syndrome are abnormal, the ulnar and radial nerves should also be examined to differentiate between an isolated mononeuropathy and a polyneuropathy or plexopathy. Also, the study should not be guided only by the requisition.

Table 27.3 Nerve Conduction Velocity and Electromyogram Findings in Common Neuromuscular Disorders

Disorder	Nerve Conduction Velocities	Electromyogram Findings
Amyotrophic lateral sclerosis	Decreased CMAP amplitude or Nl NCVs	Widespread denervation
Carpal tunnel syndrome	Increased median motor DL Decreased median sensory NCV	Denervation of APB
Guillain-Barré syndrome	Increased F-wave latency Decreased motor and sensory NCV	Usually Nl Reduced recruitment Occasional mild denervation
Muscular dystrophy	Decreased CMAP amplitude Otherwise Nl NCV	Myopathic features primarily in proximal muscles
Myasthenia gravis	Abnormal response to repetitive stimulation	± Fibs
Peroneal palsy	Decreased peroneal motor NCV Decreased peroneal CMAP amplitude	Denervation of TA and EDC Short head of biceps femoris is normal
Polymyositis	± Decreased CMAP amplitude Otherwise Nl NCV	Myopathic features mainly in proximal muscles
Pronator teres syndrome	Decreased median motor NCV Nl pronator teres	Denervation of APB Denervation of FDS
Radiculopathy	Usually Nl NCVs Nl F waves	Denervation in dermatomal distribution
Thoracic outlet syndrome	Decreased ulnar SNAP amplitude Increased ulnar F wave latency	Denervation hand intrinsics, including APB
Tarsal tunnel syndrome	Increased tibial motor DL Decreased NCV of medial or lateral plantar nerve	Denervation of AHB
Ulnar neuropathy: Guyon's canal	Increased ulnar motor DL Decreased ulnar sensory NCV	Denervation of FDI
Ulnar neuropathy: cubital tunnel	Slow conduction across cubital tunnel	Denervation of FDI, ADM, and ulnar-innervated portion of FDP

NCV = nerve conduction velocity; CMAP = compound motor action potential; DL = distal latency; Fibs = fibrillation potentials and positive sharp waves; Nl = normal; SNAP = sensory nerve action potential; ± = may or may not be present but not a prominent feature; ADM = abductor digiti minimi (quinti); AHB = abductor hallucis brevis; APB = abductor pollicis brevis; EDC = extensor digitorum communis; FDI = first dorsal interosseous; TA = tibialis anterior; FDP = flexor digitorum profundus; FDS = flexor digitorum superficialis.

*Not all findings are diagnostic in individuals with a particular disorder. Also, findings may not be specific, so alternative diagnoses should be considered.

pathy, however. At least one motor and sensory nerve conduction should be performed. For motor conduction studies, I prefer to study the tibial nerve because the peroneal nerve is more susceptible to pressure palsies, especially when mobility is impaired by weakness. The sural nerve is preferred for sensory conduction studies because it is technically easier to study than the superficial peroneal.

The EMG should be directed at weak muscles. If these show no abnormalities, additional muscles need not be examined. If they show myopathic changes, clinically unaffected muscles should be studied to determine the extent of disease. Alternatively, if the muscles show neuropathic changes, the EMG study must be expanded to determine whether the denervation is from mononeuropathy, polyneuropathy, or motor neuron disease. Additional NCSs may be needed.

Vague Questions

Neurophysiologic studies should not be a substitute for neurologic consultation, but this is sometimes the case. Some patients have poorly defined reasons for the requested study due to poorly defined clinical data. If the clinical neurophysiologist cannot develop a sense of the problem by a brief history and physical examination, the following screening tests should be performed:

Nerve conduction velocity (NCV)
  Tibial motor NCV
  Tibial F wave
  Sural sensory NCV
EMG
  Tibialis anterior
  Medial gastrocnemius
  Rectus femoris

If all test results are normal, it is unlikely that the patient has any of the common neuromuscular diseases. The only generalized neuromuscular disorders that these studies might miss are neuromuscular transmission defects and rare motor neuronopathies. The impression may read as follows: "Normal study. No evidence of generalized myopathy or neuropathy. If a specific disorder is suspected, additional studies may be helpful and will be performed on request."

Specific Questions

Recommended minimum NCS and EMG studies for specific clinical questions are presented in Table 27.2. If all of the recommended studies are normal, further examination is not indicated. If abnormalities support the diagnosis, other investigations may be needed. Refer to the chapters on specific disease processes for guidelines on additional studies to diagnose the disorders.

28

Disorders of
Peripheral Nerve

The essentials of differential diagnosis of neuromuscular disorders is described in detail in Chapter 22. The most important types of information obtained from nerve conduction studies (NCSs) and EMG are the location of the lesion and the classification of the lesion type. This chapter discusses electrophysiologic features of some of the more important neuropathies. Clinical characteristics are not presented in detail. Refer either to standard neurology texts or especially *Peripheral Neuropathy* by Dyck et al. (1993) for an excellent discussion of peripheral neuropathies.

Mononeuropathies

The hallmark of mononeuropathies is slowed conduction in an isolated nerve; reduced compound motor action potential (CMAP) amplitude, sensory neural action potential (SNAP) amplitude, or both; and EMG signs of denervation in innervated muscles. Signs of denervation may not be seen if the lesion is minor or due to neurapraxia. Signs of acute denervation may not be present for 3–4 weeks. Therefore, a repeat study is indicated if the initial study was within 4 weeks of the onset of a mononeuropathy. Some studies must be done immediately, especially after trauma, to determine if the nerve is in continuity. The presence of even a few motor unit potentials often reassures the clinician that reinnervation and restoration of function is possible.

Median Nerve

Carpal Tunnel Syndrome

Carpal tunnel syndrome (CTS) is the most common entrapment neuropathy. Motor and sensory conduction of the median nerve through the wrist is usually slowed—that is, motor distal latency is prolonged and sensory nerve conduction velocity (NCV) is slow. At least one of these measures is abnormal in at least 90% of patients with clinically diagnosed CTS. Median motor NCV between the arm and wrist is normal. F waves are normal. Additional conduction studies are often performed because merely measuring sensory and motor conduction may miss 17–19% of patients with CTS; SNAP latency is prolonged in 85% of patients, and motor distal latency is prolonged in 66% of patients. The two most common methods of evaluating patients with mild CTS are palmar stimulation and median-radial SNAP comparisons.

Palmar stimulation is performed by stimulating the median nerve at 1 cm increments on either side of the palmar crease while recording the median SNAP. Patients with CTS will have slowed conduction of sensory axons across one or more segments.

Median-radial SNAP comparisons are used in our laboratory to evaluate patients with mild CTS. A difference in SNAP latency of 0.5 seconds or more is considered abnormal and indicative of mild slowing of conduction. Comparison with ulnar nerve conduction can also be done.

Motor comparisons can also increase diagnostic sensitivity for CTS. The difference in motor distal latency between the median and ulnar nerves should not exceed 1.8 ms, a greater difference suggests CTS. Likewise, a difference in the median motor distal latencies of greater than 1.0 ms suggests CTS on the side of longer latency.

The EMG of median-innervated muscles in CTS is often normal; however, there may be signs of acute denervation when injury is severe. If acute denervation is present in the abductor pollicis brevis, at least one ulnar-innervated muscle should be examined (e.g., first dorsal interosseous) to ensure that the lesion is not in the lower plexus (roots C8–T1). Also, more proximal median-innervated muscles should be examined to localize the lesion at the carpal tunnel rather than pronator teres or elsewhere. The most convenient muscles to examine are the flexor digitorum superficialis and the radial half of the flexor digitorum profundus. These should be normal.

Pronator Teres Syndrome

In pronator teres syndrome, the median nerve is compressed as it passes through the pronator teres muscle in the proximal forearm. Median motor NCV through the forearm is slow, but the distal latency is normal. Sensory NCV is normal because the segment tested is distal to the pronator teres.

The EMG usually shows acute and chronic denervation of the abductor pollicis brevis, flexor digitorum superficialis, and median-innervated portion of the flexor digitorum profundus. The pronator teres is not denervated because it is innervated proximal to the site of compression. This is an important feature that distinguishes the pronator teres syndrome from compression of the median nerve by the ligament of Struthers.

Compression by the Ligament of Struthers
The ligament of Struthers is a fibrous band above the medial epicondyle. The clinical syndrome of median nerve compression by the ligament of Struthers resembles the pronator teres syndrome. Most median-innervated muscles of the forearm are weak. The differentiating feature is involvement of the pronator teres. In pronator teres syndrome, the pronator teres is tender but its strength is normal, and there is no denervation on EMG. When median nerve compression occurs at the ligament of Struthers, the pronator teres is weak and shows acute and chronic denervation on EMG. Other neurophysiologic findings are as described for the pronator teres syndrome.

Anterior Interosseous Syndrome
The anterior interosseous nerve is a branch of the median nerve that innervates several muscles in the forearm, including the flexor digitorum profundus of the first two digits, flexor pollicis longus, and pronator quadratus. This syndrome is caused by injury of the nerve after it leaves the main trunk of the median nerve. NCVs are usually normal. Stimulation of the anterior interosseous nerve at the elbow may reveal increased distal latency of the CMAP recorded from the pronator quadratus. The EMG shows denervation in the flexor pollicis longus, median-innervated portion of the flexor digitorum profundus, and pronator quadratus.

Ulnar Nerve
The most common locations for lesions of the ulnar nerve are Guyon's canal and near the elbow. Many diabetics show wasting and denervation in the ulnar-innervated intrinsic muscles of the hands. These patients have a prominent ulnar neuropathy superimposed on a more generalized polyneuropathy.

Entrapment at Guyon's Canal
The ulnar nerve passes from the forearm into the hand through Guyon's canal. Ulnar compression at the wrist is analogous to CTS. Unlike compression of the ulnar nerve at the elbow, the ulnar-inner-

vated flexors in the forearm are unaffected, and the sensory loss is confined to the ulnar side of the hand, sparing the forearm.

Ulnar NCVs are slowed across the wrist, and the distal latency is increased when recording from the abductor digiti minimi. The EMG shows denervation of the abductor digiti minimi and first dorsal interosseous but a normal pattern in the flexor digitorum profundus and flexor carpi ulnaris.

Entrapment Near the Elbow

The ulnar nerve is especially susceptible to injury as it crosses under the medial epicondyle of the humerus. Ulnar motor NCV is slow across the elbow but usually normal in the forearm. The difference in NCV should exceed 10 m/sec to be significant. The CMAP is small in amplitude if the nerve damage is severe. SNAPs are often absent or very small in amplitude. Stimulation can be performed at measured intervals across the cubital tunnel for precise localization.

With entrapment near the elbow, the EMG shows acute and chronic denervation of the ulnar-innervated intrinsic muscles of the hand and the ulnar-innervated portion of the flexor digitorum profundus. The flexor carpi ulnaris is not denervated because its innervation leaves the main ulnar nerve proximal to the elbow.

Lesion of the Palmar Branch of the Ulnar Nerve

Pressure on the palmar branch of the ulnar nerve can produce damage distal to nerve branches innervating the abductor digiti minimi and digit 5. Therefore, routine motor and sensory NCVs are normal, including motor distal latency. Distal latency to the first dorsal interosseous is prolonged, and denervation is seen in this muscle. The superficial sensory branch of the ulnar nerve may be damaged, especially in bicycle riders.

Radial Nerve

The most common sites of injury to the radial nerve are at the spiral groove and in the forearm as the nerve penetrates the supinator muscle. Less common sites are the elbow with radius dislocation, the wrist from handcuffs, and damage to the recurrent epicondylar branch (a form of tennis elbow).

Compression at the Spiral Groove

NCV across the spiral groove is slow. The CMAPs and SNAPs are absent if the lesion is complete. With severe but incomplete lesions, the distal latency of the CMAP may be prolonged and distal conduction studies slowed.

The EMG shows acute and chronic denervation of all radial-innervated finger and wrist extensors. Proximal lesions cause denervation of the triceps as well. It is important to determine if any motor units can be activated by attempted voluntary contraction. The presence of motor units indicates that the nerve is in continuity, and there is a better prognosis for recovery.

Posterior Interosseous Syndrome

As the radial nerve enters the forearm, it divides into the posterior interosseous nerve and a superficial sensory branch. The posterior interosseous nerve supplies the finger and wrist extensors. Injuries to the nerve cause weakness without sensory loss.

In posterior interosseus syndrome, nerve conduction is slowed through the involved segment. The EMG shows denervation in the wrist and finger extensors, with sparing of the extensor carpi radialis longus and the supinator. Both muscles are innervated by branches that arise proximal to the lesion.

Brachial Plexus Lesions

Upper Plexus Lesion (Erb's Palsy)

Proximal muscles are more severely affected than distal muscles, and intrinsic muscles of the hand are spared. The most prominent denervation is in the deltoid, biceps, supraspinatus, and infraspinatus. The serratus anterior and rhomboids are spared because their innervation is proximal to the lesion.

Lower Plexus Lesion

The lower brachial plexus is susceptible to trauma, but is especially sensitive to neoplastic infiltration. Tumors arising from the apex of the lung will produce infiltration, compression of the lower plexus, or both. Denervation is most prominent in muscles innervated by the median and ulnar nerves (roots C8–T1).

Neoplastic infiltration is differentiated from radiation plexopathy mainly on clinical grounds; however, NCS and EMG can be helpful. Tumor infiltration usually slows conduction through the plexus, whereas conduction is usually normal in radiation plexopathy. The EMG shows myokymia in many patients with radiation plexopathy but not in patients with neoplastic infiltration.

Idiopathic Brachial Plexitis

NCVs may be normal or show slowing through the plexus. Severe lesions may cause slowing of distal median and ulnar conduction. The EMG may show denervation not only in weak muscles but also in muscles that seem clinically unaffected. Sufficient time must elapse before the EMG is abnormal, however. In practice, EMG shows denervation at about the time that the patient has developed significant weakness. Therefore, if there is pain but no weakness, the initial EMG may be normal, and a later study may be more revealing.

Peroneal Neuropathy

Peroneal pressure palsy occurs most commonly at the fibular neck. Peroneal palsy is diagnosed by slowed NCV of the peroneal nerve across the fibular neck or reduced amplitude of the CMAP when stimulating above the lesion site. Denervation is seen in the tibialis anterior and peroneii; however, there is no denervation in the short head of the biceps femoris. This latter muscle is innervated by a branch of the peroneal division which takes off proximal to the fibular neck.

Slowing across the fibular neck is significant if it is at least 10 m/sec slower than distal conduction velocity. Amplitude difference is significant if the response to proximal stimulation is at least 25% less than the response to distal stimulation.

Occasionally, sciatic nerve lesions may be misdiagnosed as peroneal palsy. The peroneal division of the sciatic nerve is more susceptible to damage than the tibial division. Abnormalities in the tibial distribution may be subtle. Therefore, it is important to study some tibial-innervated muscles, even in cases that appear to be isolated peroneal palsy.

Tibial Neuropathy

Tibial nerve entrapment behind the medial malleolus is called *tarsal tunnel syndrome*. It is relatively uncommon. The motor distal latencies of the medial plantar nerves, the lateral plantar nerves, or both are often increased. To test the medial plantar nerve, a recording is made from the abductor hallucis; to test the lateral plantar nerve, a recording is made from the abductor digiti quinti. Sensory conduction through the tarsal tunnel is performed by stimulation in the medial or lateral plantar nerves and recording from the tibial nerve behind the medial malleolus. Because of the tremendous effect of foot temperature on nerve conduction, especially sensory, subtle differences in latency should be interpreted with caution, and the absence of a SNAP on the affected side should support the clinical diagnosis. Motor distal latencies are less dependent on temperature than sensory conduction. Differences in left-right and medial-lateral conductions are evidence for tarsal tunnel syndrome.

Some neurophysiologists use incremental stimulation through the tarsal tunnel, similar to that performed for carpal tunnel syndrome. This probably does not add anything to careful measurement of medial and lateral plantar nerve motor distal latency and sensory latency, however.

Sciatic Nerve Lesions

Piriformis Syndrome

Piriformis syndrome is compression of the sciatic nerve by the piriformis muscle. It is a clinical diagnosis with no unique electrophysiologic findings. Denervation in the distribution of the peroneal division of the sciatic nerve, with lesser or no involvement of muscles innervated by the tibial division, is the only EMG finding. Denervation of distal muscles with sparing of the gluteus medius is supportive of piriformis syndrome, since this muscle receives innervation from a branch of the sciatic that arises proximal to the lesion. Piriformis syndrome is differentiated from peroneal neuropathy at the fibula by involvement of the short head of the biceps femoris in the former but not in the latter. The innervation of this muscle is proximal to the popliteal fossa.

Sciatic Stretch

The lithotomy position (extension, abduction, and slight flexion of the legs) is used in many surgical procedures. This position stretches the sciatic nerve as it passes through the sciatic notch into the leg. The patient awakens from anesthesia with weakness of sciatic-innervated muscles. This syndrome is also seen in patients who sustained sudden forward flexion at the waist.

With the sciatic stretch, tibial motor and sural sensory NCVs are typically normal; however, there may be increased tibial F-wave latency. The EMG is normal or shows only a decreased number of motor units immediately after injury.

Multiple Mononeuropathies

Diabetes mellitus and polyarteritis nodosa are the most common disorders that cause multiple mononeuropathies in the United States. Leprosy is a common cause worldwide.

Polyarteritis Nodosa

Polyarteritis nodosa is an idiopathic connective tissue disorder characterized by multifocal vasculitis. This is a clinical diagnosis and can be supported but not confirmed by electrophysiologic studies.

Affected nerves show slowed or blocked conduction at the site of arteritis, and EMG shows acute and chronic denervation in affected areas. Complete denervation causes fibrillation potentials and positive sharp waves and absence of motor unit activation with attempted voluntary effort.

Leprosy

Leprosy is probably one of the most common causes of neuropathy worldwide. The neuropathy is caused by either primary nerve infiltration or by infarction of the vasa nervorum.

Nerve conduction in the involved regions of the nerves is blocked or slowed. The EMG shows acute and chronic denervation in muscles innervated by involved nerves. If the neuropathy is predominantly due to cutaneous vasculitis, only the distal sensory branches may be involved.

Polyneuropathies

Demyelinating Neuropathies

Guillain-Barré Syndrome

Motor and sensory NCV studies of the upper and lower limbs may be normal early in the course but later are slowed. The earliest changes are prolongation or absence of the F wave and dispersion of the CMAP. EMG evidence of denervation is unusual but may develop in severe cases. Reduced recruitment and conduction block are seen early in the course.

When demyelination is severe, permanent axonal loss may occur in distal muscles. The EMG and NCV usually return to normal, but conduction slowing may persist in severe cases.

Chronic Inflammatory Demyelinating Polyneuropathy

With chronic inflammatory demyelinating polyneuropathy, the first electrophysiologic abnormality is slowing of the F wave. Motor and sensory NCVs of the upper and lower extremities slow subsequently. EMG is normal in the first weeks of disease but later shows widespread denervation. The denervation is typically a mixture of acute and chronic findings: fibrillation potentials, positive sharp waves, and high-amplitude long-duration polyphasic motor unit potentials. Although patients often clinically improve, NCVs usually remain slow.

Some investigators have followed serial NCVs to assess response of chronic inflammatory demyelinating polyneuropathy to treatment. This is not routine practice now, but parameters for assessing progression versus improvement will likely become standard in the future.

Multifocal Motor Neuropathy

Patients who present with muscle weakness and wasting without sensory findings on clinical or neurophysiologic examination are evaluated for the possibility of amyotrophic lateral sclerosis (ALS) and progressive muscular atrophy. Patients with multifocal motor neuropathy have segmental conduction block of motor axons with sensory axons being unaffected, however.

F waves are absent or prolonged. Motor NCVs show conduction delay in isolated segments of the nerves. Sensory NCV is normal, even through segments of delayed motor conduction.

Axonal Neuropathies

Axonal neuropathies comprise a huge group; many of these are toxic-metabolic.

Most toxic neuropathies cause axonal degeneration, but demyelination is occasionally seen. The compounds that most often cause neuropathy are vincristine, cisplatin, lead, and ethanol. There are no specific findings on NCV and EMG to differentiate between toxic axonal neuropathies and other causes of axonal neuropathy.

Neuronal Degenerations

Amyotrophic Lateral Sclerosis

ALS is the most common neuronal degeneration affecting the peripheral nervous system. Both upper and lower motoneurons degenerate. Motor and sensory NCVs are normal, although CMAP may be of reduced amplitude. The EMG shows widespread denervation. A screening examination for motoneuron disease should include examination of at least three muscles in different nerve distributions in each of three limbs. The head may be substituted for one limb. Features of both acute and chronic denervation are typical, but acute changes may be mild as the disease progresses. Fasciculations are common in ALS, but fasciculations in the absence of other clinical or electrophysiologic abnormalities are not diagnostic. Fasciculations occur in other, less serious, disorders and in some normal individuals.

Spinal Muscular Atrophy

Motor NCVs in spinal muscular atrophies are normal or only mildly slowed. Sensory NCVs are normal. The EMG shows prominent denervation with fibrillation potentials and positive sharp waves. Recruitment may be incomplete, with rapid firing of single units. Long-duration polyphasic motor unit potentials (neuropathic motor units) are rare early in the disease but then become prominent with ongoing motor unit reorganization.

Poliomyelitis

Poliomyelitis is caused by a neurotropic enterovirus that destroys anterior horn cells. Motor NCVs are normal or near normal. EMG shows chronic denervation in patients who have had the disease. Since poliomyelitis is focal or multifocal, the EMG findings are most prominent in muscles that are clinically involved. It is my impression that when the polio afflicts a patient at a very young age, the motor unit potentials are less polyphasic than if the patient is affected later in life, probably because of improved reinnervation of the young muscle. Signs of motor unit reorganization are often seen in muscles that were clinically unaffected.

Lay and medical attention has focused on patients with a past history of polio who have a variety of complaints including increasing weakness, pain, and so on. This has been termed *postpolio syndrome.* EMG shows chronic signs of denervation with high-amplitude, long-duration polyphasic motor unit potentials, with occasionally some fibrillation potentials. The role of the clinician is to determine whether there are any signs of new disease responsible for the symptoms. The neurophysiologist can, in most cases, document the prior denervation but cannot specifically rule out many other neuromuscular diseases on the basis of EMG alone. Prominent signs of active denervation should suggest new axonal damage. Unfortunately, repetitive stimulation and single-fiber EMG often provide abnormal responses after polio.

Selected Neuropathies

Several major classes of neuropathy do not fall clearly within the above categories. The most important classes are reviewed here.

Diabetic Neuropathy

Diabetes mellitus is the cause of four different neuropathies:

- Small-fiber polyneuropathy
- Large-fiber polyneuropathy

- Autonomic neuropathy
- Mononeuropathy and mononeuropathy multiplex

The small-fiber neuropathy is a distal predominantly sensory neuropathy. C-fiber dysfunction predominates, although axonal degeneration also involves motor fibers. NCV studies may be normal because compound action potentials are mediated by large myelinated fibers. EMG is usually normal as well. The most sensitive test of small-fiber dysfunction is the sympathetic skin response.

The large-fiber neuropathy involves both motor and sensory axons, with particular loss of fibers serving motor function, vibration, joint perception, and two-point discrimination. Autonomic neuropathy is also a predominantly small fiber disorder and is a common feature of all diabetic neuropathies. Mononeuropathy can affect one or several nerves (mononeuropathy multiplex). Mononeuropathy multiplex is diagnosed by finding multifocal NCV changes, EMG changes, or both. The most commonly affected nerves are femoral, lumbosacral plexus, oculomotor, abducens, ulnar, and median, but any cranial nerves may be affected. Mononeuropathy of the femoral nerve or proximal lumbar plexus is often termed *diabetic amyotrophy*. Mononeuropathy affecting individual spinal roots is termed diabetic radiculopathy.

Nerve conduction is slowed in most patients with diabetic neuropathy, even though the demyelination is often secondary to axonal degeneration. The EMG usually shows denervation in clinically affected muscles. Patients with isolated mononeuropathies or radiculopathies superimposed on a polyneuropathy will often have fibrillation potentials and neuropathic motor unit potentials in clinically affected muscles.

Hereditary Neuropathies

Hereditary Motor-Sensory Neuropathy Type I

Hereditary motor-sensory neuropathy type I (HMSN-I) is the demyelinating or hypertrophic form of Charcot-Marie-Tooth disease. Motor and sensory NCVs are slow, often at 20–30 m/sec, and distal motor latencies are prolonged. F waves are absent or delayed. The EMG may suggest mild denervation, but the features of axonal degeneration are much less prominent than the features of demyelination. Slowing of nerve conduction may involve the facial nerve, causing an abnormal blink reflex.

Hereditary Motor-Sensory Neuropathy Type II

HMSN-II is the neuronal form of Charcot-Marie-Tooth disease. It is clinically similar to HMSN-I; however, the NCV and EMG findings are very different. Motor and sensory NCVs are either normal or mildly slow, indicating relative preservation of myelin. Motor distal latency may be increased, and CMAP and SNAP amplitudes may be reduced. The EMG shows signs of acute and chronic denervation, including prominent fibrillation potentials, fasciculations, and high-amplitude long-duration polyphasic motor unit potentials.

Hereditary Motor-Sensory Neuropathy Type III

HMSN-III, also known as Dejerine-Sottas disease, is a demyelinating condition clinically similar to HMSN-I but distinguished by inheritance and severity of disease. Motor and sensory conduction velocities are slow, and motor distal latencies are increased because of demyelination of distal nerve segments. Denervation changes on EMG are not as prominent as are the slowed NCVs.

A focal form of HMSN-III has been described. Only one nerve is affected. NCVs in other nerves are normal. The EMG is normal except in the distribution of the affected nerve, where there is prominent acute and chronic denervation.

Hereditary Motor-Sensory Neuropathy Type IV

HMSN-IV is Refsum's disease, with both central and peripheral nervous system involvement. In the peripheral nervous system, demyelination causes slowed NCVs. Degeneration of anterior horn cells causes EMG features of acute and chronic denervation.

Hereditary Motor-Sensory Neuropathy Type V

HMSN-V is the combination of peripheral neuropathy and upper motor neuron degeneration. The electrophysiologic changes are similar to HMSN-IV, and the two are distinguished by clinical features.

Friedreich's Ataxia

This is a hereditary ataxia transmitted by autosomal recessive inheritance. There are clinical and electrophysiologic features of peripheral neuropathy. Motor NCVs are usually normal, but SNAPs are absent or of low amplitude. If a SNAP is obtainable, sensory NCV is found to be normal or only mildly slowed because the sensory defect is due to sensory neuron degeneration.

29 Disorders of Muscle

The major categories of muscle disease are dystrophies, inflammatory myopathies, and metabolic myopathies (endocrine, genetic, and toxic). Table 29.1 summarizes the clinical and neurophysiologic findings in these disorders.

Motor and sensory conduction velocities are normal in most disorders, although selected metabolic disorders affect peripheral nerves in addition to muscles. Compound motor action potential (CMAP) amplitude may be reduced because muscle fibers fail to be activated. EMG is essential for diagnosis. Insertion may elicit complex repetitive discharges. At rest, there are fibrillation potentials and positive sharp waves. Motor unit potentials (MUPs) are reduced in amplitude and brief in duration. With increasing effort, units are recruited earlier than normal because of reduced tension output of the muscle fibers (termed *early recruitment*).

Muscular Dystrophies

Duchenne type and Becker's muscular dystrophy are characterized by normal nerve conduction velocities (NCVs). The EMG shows fibrillation potentials, complex repetitive discharges, and early recruitment. Fibrillation potentials are not as common as in inflammatory myopathies and denervation. Toward the end of the disease, muscle is replaced by fat and connective tissue, and insertional activity is reduced or absent.

Limb-girdle muscular dystrophy is the common phenotypic expression of several disorders. Many male patients diagnosed with limb-girdle dystrophy actually have Becker's dystrophy, a neuropathic disorder, or a metabolic myopathy. The EMG shows myopathic features in the majority of patients. Those with neuropathic features probably have a spinal muscular atrophy.

Table 29.1   Muscular Dystrophies

Disorder	Clinical Findings	Nerve Conduction Velocities and Electromyogram Findings
Duchenne type muscular dystrophy	Weakness Pseudohypertrophy of calves Gower's sign XR	Myopathic MUPs Early: increased insertional activity, fibs Late: reduced insertional activity, no fibs
Becker's muscular dystrophy	Features of Duchenne type muscular dystrophy with later onset and longer survival XR	Similar to Duchenne type muscular dystrophy with possibly more fibs CRDs
Scapuloperoneal dystrophy	Footdrop Shoulder weakness Onset in childhood AD or XR	Myopathic MUPs
Humeroperoneal dystrophy (Emery-Dreifuss)	Weakness of arms, shoulders, legs in peroneal distribution Contractures of neck, elbows Cardiac defects XR	Mixed myopathic and neuropathic patterns on EMG
Facioscapulohumeral dystrophy	Facial weakness followed by arm weakness and scapular winging AD	Early: mild changes Later: myopathic MUPs
Limb-girdle dystrophy	Progressive weakness of pelvic and shoulder girdle muscles in adults Sporadic, AR, or rarely AD	Usually myopathic MUPs Occasionally signs of denervation
Myotonic dystrophy	Muscle wasting and weakness with clinical myotonia Associated baldness, cataracts, endocrinopathies. AD	Myotonia in patients and some asymptomatic relatives May be myopathic MUPs, and mild slowing of nerve conduction velocity with reduced numbers of motor units

XR = X-linked recessive; MUP = motor unit potential; fibs = fibrillation potentials; CRD = complex repetitive discharge; AD = autosomal dominant; AR = autosomal recessive.

Myotonic dystrophy is characterized by myotonia on EMG. Myotonia is the repetitive discharge of muscle fibers with an initially high frequency that gradually declines. This produces a "dive bomber" sound in the audio monitor. Myopathic MUPs may also be seen. Occasional neuropathic features include slow motor conduction and a reduced number of functioning motor units.

Facioscapulohumeral muscular dystrophy is an autosomal dominant disorder characterized by progressive weakness of the face and shoulder girdle. Scapuloperoneal dystrophy is probably a variant phenotype of the same genetic disorder. The EMG may be normal in mild or early cases. Typical findings are myopathic MUPs and early recruitment. Fibrillation potentials are occasionally seen but are not prominent. Neuropathic changes are seen both by electrophysiologic and histologic studies in some patients, suggesting that this is a neuropathic disorder rather than a dystrophy.

Inflammatory Myopathies

The electrophysiologic changes in all inflammatory myopathies are essentially the same. NCVs are normal, although the CMAP amplitude may be reduced. The typical EMG findings are fibrillation potentials and positive sharp waves, myopathic MUPs, and complex repetitive discharges. Fibrillation potentials are more common in inflammatory myopathies than in muscular dystrophies. Abnormalities are more prominent in clinically weak muscles. The EMG is normal in approximately 10% of patients with typical polymyositis. This may be due to sampling error or to periods of relative inactivity during the course of the disease (Table 29.2).

Metabolic Myopathies

Mitochondrial disorders may present as neuropathy or myopathy. Therefore, NCV and EMG should both be done when a mitochondrial myopathy is suspected. Tibial motor conduction and sural sensory NCV are a sufficient screen. If the sural sensory neural action potential is absent with a normal tibial motor NCV, a sensory NCV in the arm or superficial peroneal sensory NCV should be performed.

Endocrine myopathies may be associated with the following disorders:

- Cushing's syndrome
- Addison's disease
- Thyrotoxicosis

Table 29.2 Inflammatory Myopathies

Disorder	Clinical Findings	Nerve Conduction Velocities and Electromyogram Findings
Polymyositis	Proximal weakness Increased CK Inflammatory infiltrate on muscle Bx	Myopathic MUPs Fibs PSWs CRDs May be inconsistent findings within and between muscles
Dermatomyositis	Symptoms of polymyositis with discoloration of eyelids Rash on dorsum of fingers, especially MCP and PIP joints	See polymyositis, above
Inclusion body myositis	Proximal and distal weakness in adults, commonly asymmetric CK concentration mildly increased Dx by Bx	See polymyositis, above May also have some neuropathic features
Viral myositis	Muscle pain and increased CK	See for inclusion body myositis, above

CK = creatine kinase; Bx = biopsy; MUP = motor unit potential; fib = fibrillation potential; PSW = positive sharp wave; CRD = complex repetitive discharge; Dx = diagnosis; PIP = proximal interphalangeal; MCP = metacarpal phalangeal.

- Hypothyroidism (rarely)
- Hyperparathyroidism (rarely)

NCVs are normal except in hypothyroidism, in which case they may be slowed. EMG may show minor myopathic features in all of these disorders (Table 29.3).

Steroid myopathy (Cushing's syndrome) is a clinical diagnosis. The EMG usually does not show myopathic features. The NCVs are also normal, although CMAP amplitude may be reduced.

Carnitine palmityl transferase deficiency usually manifests normal NCV and EMG findings. Patients with carnitine deficiency have myopathic findings with small-amplitude polyphasic MUPs. Fibrillation potentials are seen but are rare.

Table 29.3   Metabolic Myopathies

Disorder	Clinical Findings	Nerve Conduction Velocities and Electromyogram Findings
Mitochondrial myopathies	Muscle weakness with other manifestations (e.g., ptosis, ophthalmoplegia, cardiac abnormalities) Mild increase of CK concentration	Myopathic MUPs, but findings may be subtle or absent May have some neurogenic appearance as well.
Myotonia congenita	Myotonia with or without muscle cramps Onset in youth or young adults AD, AR, or sporadic	Myotonia Repetitive stimulation may reveal sustained decrement that is greater with increasing stimulus frequence Some patients have myopathic MUPs
Hypokalemic periodic paralysis	Episodic weakness provoked by rest after large carbohydrate meal	Normal between episodes Reduced MUPs during attack Reduced CMAP amplitude
Hyperkalemic periodic paralysis	Episodic weakness provoked by rest after exercise or cold	Between attacks: possible myopathic patterns During attack: myotonia, increased insertion, reduced MUPs to volition or stimulation

CK = creatine kinase; AD = autosomal dominant; AR = autosomal recessive; MUP = motor unit potential; CMAP = compound motor action potential.

Syndromes of Continuous Muscle Fiber Activity

Disorders of increased muscle fiber activity are classified into the following categories depending on the site of defect:

- Tetanus
- Stiff-man syndrome
- Schwartz-Jampel syndrome
- Neuromyotonia (Isaac's syndrome)

Tetanus is characterized by involuntary discharge of motor units. The toxin works at the spinal level, blocking postsynaptic inhibition, thereby increasing the excitability of motoneurons. The EMG shows repetitive MUPs that are abolished by peripheral nerve or neuromuscular block. The discharges are attenuated during sleep and with general or spinal anesthesia.

Stiff-man syndrome is not really a disorder of muscle; it is due to excessive motoneuron activation. The reason for the enhanced discharge is unknown. Excessive motor unit activity results in involuntary muscle contraction involving predominantly proximal muscles. Affected muscles show normal MUPs with coactivation of agonists and antagonists. Discharges are attenuated by sleep, general anesthesia, benzodiazepines, peripheral nerve block, or neuromuscular block.

Schwartz-Jampel syndrome is characterized by multiple congenital anomalies in association with increased muscle fiber activity. The defect is probably at the nerve terminal. Clinically, the muscle activity looks similar to that of myotonia, but on EMG the discharges have the appearance of complex repetitive discharges, lacking the frequency modulation of true myotonia. The discharges are abolished by neuromuscular block but not by nerve block.

The term *neuromyotonia* is designed to differentiate this type of continuous discharge from myotonia of primary muscle origin, as in myotonic dystrophy. Neuromyotonia differs from stiff-man syndrome in that the EMG shows continuous activity of single muscle fibers rather than complete motor units. The muscle fibers discharge repetitively at frequencies that are initially high and gradually decline. This is similar to true myotonia, but the discharges have an invariant decline in frequency rather than a waxing and waning frequency. Also, these discharges are apparent at rest, whereas myotonia is evoked primarily by needle insertion. The amplitude of MUPs may be reduced because of loss of functioning muscle fibers due to continuous activity. The defect is probably in the terminal motor axon. Therefore, the discharges are abolished by neuromuscular block but not by peripheral nerve block, spinal block, or general anesthesia (Table 29.4).

Miscellaneous Disorders of Muscle

Myotonia congenita is usually characterized by normal NCVs, but the EMG shows myotonia. Repetitive stimulation produces a decremental response. The decrement is greater with high frequencies of stimulation.

Paramyotonia congenita is characterized by myotonia that worsens with exercise or exposure to cold. The NCVs are normal. Repetitive stimulation often results in a decremental response.

Table 29.4 Syndromes of Continuous Muscle Fiber Activity

Disorder	Clinical Findings	Nerve Conduction Velocity and Electromyogram Findings
Stiff-man syndrome	Progressive stiffness of proximal muscles Pain	Increased motor unit potentials at rest Coactivation of antagonists, especially proximal muscles
Schwartz-Jampel syndrome	Multiple congenital anomalies with increased muscle activity	Repetitive motor unit potentials, but with a firing pattern like complex repetitive discharges
Neuromyotonia (Isaac's syndrome)	Progressive rigidity of trunk and limbs, present at rest but exacerbated by movement Persists during sleep	Continuous activity of single muscle fibers, look like complex repetitive discharges Present at rest Appearance of myokymia, at times
Tetanus	Muscle spasms starting in the face, and generalizing Often asymmetric	Continuous motor unit discharges, abate during sleep or sedation

The *periodic paralyses* are a family of disorders all characterized by abnormal loss of excitability of the muscle fiber membrane. Between attacks, NCVs are normal. The EMG is often normal but may show some myopathic features, indicating a myopathy. During an attack, motor nerve stimulation activates fewer muscle fibers. Therefore, the CMAP is smaller. Myotonia may be seen in hyperkalemic periodic paralysis, blurring the distinction between this entity and paramyotonia congenita.

30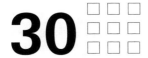

Disorders of Neuromuscular Transmission

Disorders of neuromuscular transmission typically produce abnormalities on repetitive stimulation, paired stimuli, and single-fiber EMG testing. Similar abnormalities are occasionally seen in peripheral neuropathies and motor neuronopathies, however.

Repetitive stimulation and single-fiber EMG are performed on patients who are being evaluated for the possibility of myasthenia gravis. Paired stimuli are performed mainly for botulism. Myasthenic syndrome is associated with abnormalities on both repetitive stimulation and single-fiber EMG testing.

Table 30.1 summarizes clinical and neurophysiologic features of these disorders of neuromuscular transmission.

Myasthenia Gravis

Myasthenia gravis is due to failure of neuromuscular transmission. Antibodies bind to the acetylcholine receptor on the postsynaptic membrane. This binding stimulates internalization and degradation of the receptor. Therefore, there are fewer receptors available for binding with acetylcholine. When an action potential depolarizes the presynaptic membrane, the transmitter cannot activate enough receptors to evoke an action potential in the muscle fiber. The sarcolemmal depolarization is insufficient.

Sensory conduction studies are normal as are motor nerve conduction velocities (NCVs), but the amplitude of the compound motor action potential (CMAP) may be reduced. Repetitive stimulation results in a decremental response.

The EMG is usually normal. The amplitudes of the motor unit potentials (MUPs) may fluctuate. Occasional myopathic MUPs may be seen but not fibrillation potentials and long-duration polyphasic potentials. Single-

Table 30.1   Disorders of the Neuromuscular Junction

Disorder	Clinical Findings	Nerve Conduction Velocities and Electromyogram Findings
Myasthenia gravis	Weakness that worsens with activity Ptosis Diplopia	Normal CMAP Repetitive stimulation elicits decremental response with low stimulus rates Abnormal single-fiber EMG with increased jitter and blocking
Myasthenic syndrome	Generalized or proximal weakness, often with dry mouth, impotence, and/or other signs of autonomic dysfunction	Decremental response at low rates of repetitive stimulation Incremental response at high rates of repetitive stimulation Facilitation with exercise
Botulism	Gastrointestinal distress with abdominal cramping, diarrhea, dry mouth, followed by weakness with bulbar involvement	Low CMAP amplitude, increases with exercise. Repetitive stimulation elicits little or no decrement with low rates, incremental response with high rates

CMAP = compound motor action potential.

fiber EMG shows increased jitter. The constellation of neurodiagnostic findings must be considered together.

Increased jitter and variable MUP amplitude can be observed with denervating diseases. Signs of active and chronic denervation should be notably absent for a diagnosis of myasthenia gravis.

Neonatal Myasthenic Syndromes

A new classification of neonatal myasthenic syndromes was presented by Misulis and Fenichel (1989). The classification is based on pathophysiology (Table 30.2). Diagnosis of these syndromes depends on techniques not readily available in most laboratories (e.g., muscle acetylcholinesterase assay, in vitro intracellular electrophysiology, and receptor-binding studies). Most laboratories can narrow the differential diagnosis by clinical examination. Repetitive stimulation is usually not helpful, because it is abnormal in virtually all patients with genetic myasthenia. Normal repetitive stimulation responses at 3 Hz have been reported in some patients with impaired acetylcholine receptor function.

Table 30.2   Neonatal Myasthenia*

Genetic

Presynaptic

Abnormal acetylcholine resynthesis or mobilization
Abnormal Ach release

Postsynaptic
End-plate acetylcholinesterase deficiency
Reduced number of acetylcholine receptors
Impaired function of acetylcholine receptors
Slow-channel syndrome

Acquired

Acetylcholine receptor antibody positive

Transitory neonatal
Juvenile myasthenia
Generalized
Mainly ocular

Acetylcholine receptor antibody negative
Juvenile myasthenia
Mainly ocular
Relapsing ocular

---

*Antibody-negative juvenile myasthenia may occur in individuals who are genetically predisposed.

Source: Adapted with permission from KE Misulis, GE Fenichel. Genetic forms of myasthenia gravis. Pediatr Neurol 1989;5:205.

Acetylcholinesterase deficiency and slow-channel syndrome are characterized by repetitive discharges of muscle fibers by a single neural stimulus. A motor nerve is stimulated in the usual manner. A needle electrode is placed into the muscle for recording motor unit activity. In these disorders, a single stimulus produces prolonged depolarization of the postsynaptic membrane. In the case of acetylcholinesterase deficiency, the prolonged depolarization is due to failure of breakdown of acetylcholine and resultant sustained activation of postsynaptic receptors. In slow-channel syndrome, the sustained depolarization is due to prolonged open time of the ion channel associated with the acetylcholine receptor.

Routine nerve conduction studies and EMG are performed in all patients to look for neuropathies or myopathies that could be confused with genetic myasthenia. Transitory neonatal myasthenia occurs in children of myasthenic mothers. Repetitive stimulation at 3 Hz produces a decremental response.

Botulism

Botulism is due to toxins isolated from one of several strains of *Clostridium botulinum*. Botulinum toxin interferes with release of acetylcholine from the presynaptic terminal. Miniature end-plate potential amplitude is usually normal, but the frequency is very low. End-plate potential amplitude is reduced.

Nerve conduction studies are normal except for reduced CMAP amplitude. Successive stimuli result in a further reduction in CMAP amplitude. The EMG shows small MUPs initially because of a reduced number of functioning neuromuscular junctions. Later, signs of acute denervation develop. Repetitive stimulation at slow rates produces a decremental response. Repetitive stimulation at fast rates produces a small initial decrement followed by a much more pronounced increment.

The diagnosis of botulism depends on the response to paired stimuli. At short interstimulus intervals (less than 15 ms) the response to the second pulse is greater than to that of the first. This is because the second impulse activates some terminals that were not activated by the first pulse due to summation of end-plate potentials.

Myasthenic Syndrome

Myasthenic (Eaton-Lambert) syndrome is characterized by progressive weakness without sensory loss, often in association with systemic malignancy. The etiology of the weakness is not completely known but is believed to be due to circulating factors that interfere with release of transmitter from the presynaptic terminal. The effect is similar to that of botulism, in that a bacterial toxin inhibits transmitter release.

The nerve conduction studies are normal except for marked reduction in CMAP amplitude. Repetitive stimulation at 3 Hz depresses the CMAP further, giving a marked decremental response. Repetitive stimulation at low rates produces a decremental response. Repetitive stimulation at high rates produces an incremental response, similar to that of botulism. Sensory conduction studies are normal. The EMG shows repetitive discharge of single motor units, due to incremental activation.

Paired stimulation at short interstimulus intervals results in facilitation of the second response. This is similar to the response seen in botulism. In contrast, however, paired stimuli with interstimulus intervals of greater than 15 ms also results in facilitation of the second response. The pathophysiology of the facilitation with short and long latency paired stimuli is different. Therefore, this represents an actual facilitation of transmitter release.

31

Troubleshooting in Nerve Conduction Studies and Electromyography

Common Errors Encountered in Nerve Conduction Studies

Early Positive Component to the Compound Motor Action Potential

A propagating action potential should produce a negative deflection in a surface electrode as it passes. The appearance of an initial small positive potential is usually caused by poor positioning of the surface electrodes. Either the active electrode is not centered over the end-plate zone, or the reference electrode is positioned over an excited membrane. These conditions can be corrected by placing the recording electrode squarely over the muscle belly and placing the reference distally on an area of skin overlying bone.

Unstable Waveform of the Compound Motor Action Potential or Sensory Neural Action Potential

Unstable waveform is usually due to poor fixation of the recording electrodes. Movement of the limb with stimulation dislodges the electrodes and changes the recording geometry. New gel should be used and the electrodes should be firmly reapplied. If this is not effective, consider changing the electrode leads, since breakage of the multistrand wires can produce the same artifact.

No Recordable Potentials

A completely flat baseline is not normal. Baseline activity should be present even if the nerve is completely degenerated. Tap the recording electrodes to produce artifact. If this does not produce a response, check that the electrode junction box is switched on, the cables are firmly in their sockets, and the gain is properly set. If this fails, look further to determine if an electrode lead is broken. This is best accomplished by using a completely different electrode set.

In most machines, a disconnected electrode results in high-amplitude 60-Hz artifact. Some amplifiers, however, block in response to high-amplitude potentials (i.e., they transiently fail to amplify anything and then gradually recover). During the recovery phase, the baseline activity slowly increases in amplitude.

Excessive 60-Hertz Interference

Excessive 60-Hz interference is usually due to one of the following problems: (1) poor grounding, (2) unequal electrode impedances, or (3) high-amplitude electronic noise in the vicinity. Poor grounding occurs if the ground electrode is old and has breaks in some strands of wire, if the ground electrode was moved several times during the study without replenishing gel or tape, or if the ground electrode has poor electrical continuity with the skin. Some electrode boxes have two sockets for ground to accommodate different size plugs. Only one should be used; using both may augment 60-Hz interference.

Unequal electrode impedances can degrade common mode rejection, causing increased 60-Hz artifact. High-amplitude electronic noise is prominent when there are power trunk lines or high-power equipment in the vicinity. Our laboratory has had special difficulty with interference from centrifuges, fluorescent lights, oscilloscopes, and computers.

An occasional cause of augmented 60-Hz interference is excessive length of electrode leads. Stray capacitance and inductance create noise that is dependent on the length of the electrode leads. This is more apt to be a problem during portable studies rather than during studies in the EMG laboratory. The noise can be minimized by keeping the leads short but lengthening the cable from the electrode box.

Mistaking F Wave for H Reflex

Mistaking F wave for H reflex is a common error. While performing an H reflex, it is important to ensure that the response appears at a lower stimulus intensity than the direct compound motor action potential (CMAP) and that the reflex response disappears with maximal stimulation of the nerve. At maximal stimulation, an F wave usually occurs at about the same latency as the H reflex response.

High-Voltage, Long-Duration Stimulus Required for Stable Wave

A high-voltage, long-duration stimulus is usually due to improper positioning of the stimulating electrode. If the probe is not positioned immediately overlying the nerve, more charge is required to depolarize the distant axons. When high-voltage stimuli are used, the nerve may be activated a considerable distance from the probe and the measures of distance are no longer accurate.

Common Errors Encountered in Electromyography

No recordable potentials and 60-Hz interference are encountered in EMG studies as well. The solutions are the same. A few potentials errors are unique to EMG.

Poor Motor Unit Potential Waveform

The normal morphology of motor unit potentials (MUPs) is degraded if the electrode is distant from the active muscle fibers, especially when the electrodes are inserted into superficial fascia. The electrode should be repositioned if the MUPs do not meet the criteria described in Chapter 24. Also, be sure that the patient is making the required contraction. If the patient does not perform the task correctly, the muscle being studied may not be activated, even though the electrode is properly positioned. The distant MUPs are from nearby muscles. If monopolar electrodes are used, poor MUP waveform can be helped by moving the surface reference closer to the needle electrode.

Fibrillation Potentials with Poor Motor Unit Potential Waveform

If the electrode is outside the muscle, MUPs will have poor waveform, and fibrillation potentials will not be seen. Insertion of the needle into a tendon may result in spontaneous discharges, which look like fibrillations, generated at the myotendinous junction, however. The morphology of the motor units is degraded. The needle should be repositioned.

Ultra-Short–Duration Spontaneous Potentials

Ultra-short–duration spontaneous potentials can resemble fibrillation potentials but are of much shorter duration. They tend to follow the electrode—that is, movement of the electrode often does not abolish the activity. This is the EMG equivalent of the electrode pop seen on EEG.

Mistaking Voluntary Activity for Spontaneous Activity

Voluntary activity may seem to be spontaneous activity in patients who cannot relax. This is especially true in the elderly. Distant motor unit activity can be mistaken for positive sharp waves. Avoid this problem by interpreting only potentials that have a fast upstroke.

Mistaking Phasic Activation for Polyphasic Potentials

Phasic activation can be mistaken for polyphasic potentials if there is excessive reliance on audio output rather than on visual analysis. During phasic muscle activation, multiple motor units may discharge almost simultaneously. The sound is raspy and suggests a polyphasic potential. Reproducible polyphasic potentials are not present on visual inspection. Phasic activation is most common in elderly individuals and in patients with upper motoneuron disorders.

Mistaking Complex Repetitive Discharge for Myotonia

Close analysis of the onset and offset of the discharge and of the change in frequency during the discharge should clearly distinguish complex repetitive discharges from myotonia.

Common Errors in Repetitive Stimulation

The most common reason for a false-positive decremental response is poor fixation of the stimulating and recording electrodes, which is especially prominent with testing of proximal muscles. The distance of the electrode from the nerve can be increased by contraction of surrounding muscle. Because of muscle and joint movement with repetitive stimulation, the instability of the stimulus may not be appreciated when only single shocks are used.

The most common error in repetitive stimulation is interpretation. A decremental response is supportive of myasthenia gravis but can also be seen in other disorders, especially with denervation.

Anatomic Variation

The most common anatomic anomalies are the Martin-Gruber anomaly and the accessory peroneal nerve.

Martin-Gruber Anomaly

The Martin-Gruber anastomosis is a connection between the median and ulnar nerves (Figure 31.1). Fibers from the brachial plexus descend into the arm in the median nerve. Distal to the elbow, the fibers cross to the ulnar nerve and descend through the forearm into the hand with the ulnar nerve. The fibers that were originally with the median nerve innervate muscles that are normally median innervated. The median fibers innervate any of several muscles that are normally ulnar innervated. These include the abductor digiti minimi, adductor pollicis, and first dorsal interosseous. The innervation may be derived from both the median and ulnar nerves. Conduction studies produce a CMAP that is larger after stimulation of the median nerve at the elbow than at the wrist. This is because stimulation at the wrist does not activate the thenar muscles innervated by the anomalous median nerve axons.

The collision technique can be used to diagnose this anomaly. Refer to Figure 31.1 during this discussion. A CMAP is recorded in response to stimulation of the median nerve at the wrist. Then, the stimulus is delivered to the median nerve at the elbow. Third, the stimulus is delivered to the ulnar nerve at the wrist. Fourth, stimuli are delivered to both the median nerve at the elbow and ulnar nerve at the wrist. The action potential from ulnar stimulation propagates antidromically until it collides with the orthodromic action potentials of nerves destined for the ulnar nerve. The action potentials in those nerves will not reach the hand.

Variations in Innervation of Hand Muscles

There are several potential variations in innervation of the intrinsic muscles of the hand, often involving the flexor pollicis brevis or

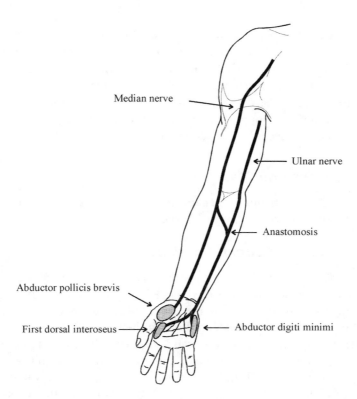

Figure 31.1 Martin-Gruber anomaly. Axons from the ulnar nerve cross over to the median nerve in the arm. They then cross again distally in the forearm to the ulnar nerve.

adductor pollicis. These muscles may be innervated exclusively by the median nerve, exclusively by the ulnar nerve, or by both.

Accessory Peroneal Nerve

The common peroneal nerve bifurcates into the deep and superficial peroneal nerves. The deep peroneal nerve innervates the tibialis anterior and extensor digitorum brevis. In approximately 25% of patients, a branch of the superficial peroneal nerve extends behind the lateral malleolus and turns to innervate the lateral aspect of the extensor digitorum brevis. The clue to presence of an accessory peroneal nerve is that the CMAP with stimulation at the knee is larger than with stimulation near the ankle. An accessory peroneal nerve should be mentioned in the comment section of the report but should be interpreted as normal.

Pathologic States

Patients with polyneuropathies may have superimposed mononeuropathies that are clinically significant. Some clinical neurophysiologists believe that in the setting of polyneuropathy, mononeuropathies should be diagnosed only rarely. Patients may benefit from treatment of the mononeuropathy, however, so every effort should be made to distinguish a mononeuropathy from an underlying polyneuropathy. Should a patient with diabetic neuropathy not be treated for his or her carpal tunnel syndrome?

There are no firm guidelines as to what constitutes significant slowing of conduction when generalized neuropathic changes are seen. Our laboratory uses a 10 m/sec discrepancy in conduction velocity. This is reasonable for most studies. Patients with peripheral neuropathies may have sufficient slowing of distal segments such that conduction across the elbow may not be slowed by 10 m/sec, however. Our laboratory does not interpret focal slowing unless it is at least 10 m/sec but in the presence of a polyneuropathy the impression might read as follows: "Abnormal study consistent with a peripheral polyneuropathy. Conduction in motor axons across the elbow was slowed in comparison to distal conduction, but the difference was less than 10 m/sec. Focal compression of the ulnar nerve at the elbow is possible but cannot be diagnosed by this study."

If the EMG portion of the study shows clear-cut denervation in an ulnar distribution, the impression can be stronger. An ulnar neuropathy can be diagnosed, but mention should be made of the peripheral polyneuropathy.

IV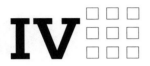
Evoked Potentials

32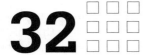

Evoked Potential Basics

Electrophysiologic Basis of Evoked Potentials

Sensory evoked potentials (EPs) are the responses of nervous tissue to stimulation. Motor EPs are the responses of muscles to stimulation of the motor cortex. Motor EPs are not commonly used in routine clinical practice and are not discussed in Part IV. This part concentrates on sensory EPs. The three clinically useful modalities of sensory stimulation are auditory, visual, and somatosensory.

The important role of sensory EPs in the diagnosis of multiple sclerosis, transverse myelitis, optic neuritis, acoustic neuromas, and other disorders has been modified by the development of magnetic resonance imaging. Sensory EP technology, however, continues to serve an important function in the evaluation of optic neuropathy and myelopathy, in screening for acoustic neuroma, and in intraoperative monitoring of central nervous system function. Somatosensory-evoked potentials (SEPs) are used to monitor both spinal cord function during corrective surgery for scoliosis and cerebral function during carotid surgery. Brain stem auditory-evoked potentials (BAEPs) are used to monitor some posterior fossa explorations. It is likely that intraoperative monitoring will be the predominant future role of sensory EPs.

EPs are very low-amplitude responses superimposed on normal EEG activity. The responses to many trials must be averaged to make the potentials stand out from background activity. The visual-evoked potential (VEP) is the only one that is seen without averaging. It can be observed on routine EEGs during low-frequency photic stimulation.

Neural Generators of Evoked Potentials

There are many generators of EPs, since responses are recorded from multiple sites along the afferent pathways. The VEP is most likely due to charge movement associated with conduction in the projections from the lateral geniculate to the visual cortex. Central SEP activity is due to thalamocortical projections, but impulses conducted in peripheral nerves and the dorsal columns are recorded as well. The BAEP is recorded from the nerve volley in the eighth cranial nerve and potentials generated by tracts and nuclei in the brain stem. Specific locations of generators are discussed in the individual sections on VEP, BAEP, and SEP.

The generators of EPs are of two basic types: nerve fiber bundles and nuclei. Nerve fiber bundles include both peripheral nerves and central tracts. The recorded potential is due to the advancing front of the compound action potential. The vector of this potential is determined by the direction of projection of the axons.

Potentials generated in nuclei are not easily described by vectors and axonal conduction. Movement of charge in nuclei is a combination of axonal action potentials and charge movement during synaptic transmission. Synapses are oriented in virtually all directions on a cell's dendrites and soma, such that it is impossible to predict the ultimate vector of positivity and negativity. Also, because of the complex orientation of the synapses, there is no guarantee that the field will conform to a simple dipole. Therefore, hypotheses of the sources of individual EP waves are developed on the basis of human pathology and animal studies in addition to a knowledge of basic neuroanatomy.

Theory of Averaging

The EPs are of very small amplitude and in most instances cannot be seen without averaging. The EP is superimposed on higher-amplitude EEG activity unrelated to the stimulus and other potentials, such as movement artifact and EMG. Averaging brings out the EP by the assumption that most potentials not caused by the stimulus occur in a random fashion and will not produce a potential of substantial amplitude after averaging many trials. This assumption is generally true but has two possible sources of error. First, the stimulus may cause a slight movement of the patient that is sufficiently reproducible from trial to trial to be detectable in the average. An experienced neurophysiologist can usually identify such abnormal waveforms. Second, 60-Hz interference can appear to be a high-amplitude sinusoidal wave on averaging. To prevent this latter error, the stimulus rate should not be an even harmonic of 60 Hz. The electronics of averaging and analog-to-digital (A/D) conversion are discussed in detail in Part I.

Artifact Rejection and Analysis Time

Artifact rejection is an important part of noise reduction. An electronic window is created within specified times and voltages. Potentials larger than the set voltage window are rejected from the average. If a trial contains a potential outside of the window, the entire trial is considered unreliable and therefore is rejected. When a trial is rejected, an indicator usually shows this on the screen. Also, at the end of the averaging period, most EP machines will display the percent of trials that were rejected.

The time window serves several purposes. Acquisition of data is delayed by a short interval, in part to prevent stimulus artifact from affecting the input amplifier. This is most important for SEPs; however, there can be an element of stimulus artifact with BAEPs due to current movement in the earphone leads. Pattern reversal VEPs have virtually no stimulus artifact. Limiting the duration of recording is important for resolution of the waves, since each point must be converted into digital format for averaging. The number of points that can be remembered is limited by computer memory and governed by the number of channels being recorded, the total time to be sampled, and the time between samples. See Chapter 5 for details. The following formula shows this relationship:

$$\text{Number of samples} = \frac{\text{Channels} \times \text{duration}}{\text{Sample interval}}$$

where *channels* is the number of channels being recorded, *duration* is the time being averaged, and *sample interval* is the time between samples. For most EPs, at least 256 and preferably 512 samples per trial are needed. If four channels are recorded, there are 2,048 samples for each run, and if two trials are recorded, 4,096 data points must be stored in memory. Although an EP machine remembers only the running averages and not each trial, available memory can be quickly depleted by recording several averages of several channels each.

General Principles of Evoked Potentials

This section discusses the general principles of performance and interpretation of EPs. Much of this also applies to other neurodiagnostic tests but is specifically directed toward the applications of EPs.

The three major modalities of EPs are discussed individually later in this section. The recommended parameters for stimulation and recording are derived in part from the *Guidelines* (American Electroencephalographic Society, 1994).

Table 32.1   Minimal Technical Requirements for Evoked Potential Machines

Parameter	Acceptable Range
Input amplitude range	5 µV–50 mV
Input impedance of differential amplifier	10 MΩ
Common mode rejection ratio	10,000:1 (80 dB)
Time resolution	20 µs/data point
Amplitude resolution	8 bit converter, 500 data points/trial
Averaging capacity	4,000 trials
Number of channels	For BAEP = 2 channels
	For SEP and PS-VEP = 4 channels
Noise level of amplifier	2 µV root-mean-square
Chassis leak current	<100 µA

BAEP = brain stem auditory-evoked potential; SEP = somatosensory-evoked potential; PS-VEP = pattern-shift visual-evoked potential.

Evoked Potential Equipment

The equipment used to record EPs is similar to that used for routine EEG and EMG studies and should fulfill the guidelines for electrical safety outlined in Part I. In general, modern and well-maintained machines meet the required limitations on allowable leakage current. Unsafe practices can endanger a patient even with the best equipment, however. The greatest risk is with SEPs, since the stimulus is an electrical pulse. The patient must be adequately grounded so that the path of current cannot traverse the heart or spinal cord. Normally, the path of current is between the two electrodes of the stimulator; however, current can flow from stimulating electrode to ground if one lead has poor skin contact or high impedance. Minimal technical requirements for EP machines are tabulated in Table 32.1.

Evoked potential equipment should be calibrated before each recording session by recording and averaging electronically generated calibration pulses. This procedure ensures that there is no problem with data acquisition and manipulation.

The calibration pulses may have one of two sources. Most EP machines have calibration outputs—that is, the output of a signal generator of defined frequency and amplitude. Such waveform generators are technically much simpler than the amplifiers and analog-to-digital converters that make up the essentials of the EP machine, so failure of the calibration pulse generator is very unusual. Alternatively, external calibration pulse generators are available at low cost. When triggered by the stimulator, these produce potentials of defined amplitude. Realistically, careful amplitude calibration is not as important as time calibration, since latency is a more important measure than amplitude. (Amplitude abnormalities are much less clinically important than latency abnormalities.)

Replications

Two replications of each waveform are recommended for each EP. Consistency of waveforms is best visualized if the traces are superimposed on the hard copy. Four replications may be necessary when recording SEPs to provide convincing identification of individual waves.

Normative Data

Normative data from Vanderbilt University Hospital Neurodiagnostic Laboratory are presented in the respective chapters on BAEP, VEP, and SEP. Testing equipment and environment differ between laboratories, however, and each laboratory should establish its own set of normative data. There are significant maturational effects on the latency of EPs, and the *Guidelines* recommends that normative data be established for each week of the perinatal period, for each month of infancy, and for each decade thereafter. At least 20 subjects from each age group should be tested for each evoked response. Responses from the left and right sides of the same subject cannot be treated as two subjects. Such data are used to establish normative data on interside differences in latency and amplitude.

Normative data are expressed as mean plus or minus standard deviation. A latency is considered abnormal if it exceeds 2.5 or 3.0 standard deviations from the mean. Some laboratories use two standard deviations; however, this allows an unacceptable percentage of false-positive interpretations. When normative data are displayed, it is evident that it does not subserve a normal distribution. Transformation of the data can result in a more normal distribution from which standard deviations can be calculated. Possible transformations include logarithm, square root, reciprocal, and so on. The neurophysiologist is encouraged to use a statistician to assist with these calculations.

Linear regression analysis allows a more precise evaluation of waveform latencies as a function of increasing age. The relationship between age and latency is not strictly linear, however, and such a level of precision is not needed.

Interpretation

When recordings are made from bipolar linkages, up or down is determined by which electrode is considered active and which is considered the reference. For routine EEG recording, a negative potential delivered to the active electrode is shown as an upward deflection of the pen. Polarity conventions have recently become fairly consistent. For SEPs and VEPs, traces are displayed so that a negative event at the active electrode (G1) produce an upward deflection. In contrast, for BAEPs, a positive event at the active electrode (G1) produces an upward deflection. The reason for this discrepancy is that with this polarity convention, most of the waves of interest are upward deflections.

Reports should be concise but thorough. A sample report is shown in Figure 32.1. It is most helpful to put the data in tabular form. Highlighting abnormal values is also helpful. The interpretation can have two sections. The first describes what is abnormal, and the second gives the implications of the abnormalities. Interpretation of the data in light of the clinical history is essential, since many physicians ordering EPs are not experts in this field.

Hard copies of the waveforms should be kept with the patient's record in the laboratory. Some equipment allows for selected waves to be printed on the report along with the tabular data. This is helpful for other neurophysiologists but is not of interest to most clinicians.

St. Nowhere's Hospital
Neurodiagnostic Laboratory

Patient: Jane Q. Doe
Hospital number: 12345
Study: Visual-evoked study
Requested by: Jim Public, M.D.
Date: 2/1/97
Clinical: 32F with transient visual obscurations
Medications: None
Notes: Visual acuity 20/20 OU

Technical: Pattern reversal visual-evoked potential study was performed using unilateral full-field stimulation. No deviation from standard laboratory procedures.

Data:

	Left	Right	Interside comparison
P100 latency (ms)	97.6	134.0	36.4 difference
P100 amplitude (µV)	10.2	12.4	1.22 ratio

Interpretation: The absolute latency of the P100 from stimulation of the right eye is prolonged. The interside difference in P100 latency is prolonged. Interside amplitude ratio is normal.

Impression: Abnormal visual-evoked potential study, consistent with a lesion in the right optic nerve

                            Mel Practice, M.D.   *2/1/97*
                                  Practice   **Date**

Figure 32.1 Sample visual-evoked potential report. Interpretation section states the abnormalities. Impression section presents the clinical implication of the findings. The visual-evoked potential traces are shown on a separate sheet.

33 Brain Stem Auditory-Evoked Potentials

The brain stem auditory-evoked potential (BAEP) is the complex of potentials produced by the brain and acoustic nerve in response to auditory stimulation. Most of the waves originate in the brain stem. The main use of BAEPs is for evaluation of patients with reduced hearing or with suspected disorders of the brain stem. A particularly sensitive and inexpensive method to screen for acoustic neuromas, measuring BAEPs is also used for intraoperative monitoring during surgery for posterior fossa lesions. The BAEP has less use with demyelinating disease than visual-evoked potentials (VEPs) and somatosensory-evoked potentials (SEPs).

Methods

Stimulus

Headphones are placed on the subject for delivery of the auditory stimulus. For older children and adults, the headphones are similar to those used for conventional stereo equipment. They completely envelope the ear, thereby reducing ambient noise. For infants and younger children, special earphones are placed in the external auditory canal because regular headphones can collapse the external canals of infants. Both sets of headphones should be provided with evoked potential (EP) machines.

The EP apparatus delivers electronic signals to the headphones, producing movement of the diaphragm. Three types of sounds are produced by the phones: clicks, pure tones, and white noise.

Type of Stimulus

Clicks, most commonly used for routine BAEP testing, are produced by a square-wave pulse delivered to the headphone. The rising phase of the pulse moves the diaphragm in one direction; the fall of the pulse returns the diaphragm to its original position. An initial movement of the diaphragm toward the eardrum is termed *condensation*; an initial movement away from the eardrum is termed *rarefaction*. These terms are derived from the roots *condense* ("to make more dense") and *rarefy* ("to make less dense"). EP machines can deliver both types of movement, but rarefaction is predominantly used for interpretation of routine studies. The duration of the electrical pulse driving the speaker membrane is 100 μs, which produces a sound complex of approximately 2 ms duration.

Pure tones are generated by some, but not all, EP machines. The stimulator delivers exact frequencies to the headphones. The most common use for this type of stimulus is pure tone audiometry. Pure tones are not used for routine BAEP testing but are useful for testing hearing at different frequencies. Some disorders, such as the hearing loss associated with ototoxic drugs, produce a predominant high-frequency hearing loss that is less well detected by BAEP testing using clicks than by pure-tone audiometry.

White noise is sound composed of all audible frequencies in equal proportions. It is similar to the sound made by a radio that is not tuned to an active station. During BAEP testing, a similar sound is delivered into the ear not being stimulated with clicks. This is called *masking*. Without masking the ear not being tested could be stimulated by bone conduction of the click delivered to the opposite ear.

Stimulus Rate

Clicks are delivered at 8–10/sec. This allows for reproducible identification of all waves. Waves I, II, VI, and VII are reduced in amplitude at faster frequencies.

Stimulus Intensity

Terminology for stimulus intensity is potentially confusing. The *Guidelines* (American Electroencephalographic Society, 1994) recommends that intensity be indicated in units of decibels peak equivalent sound pressure level, or dB pe SPL. This is measured directly by a sound meter using a constant stimulus of the same frequency and amplitude as the test stimulus to be measured. The dB scale is a log scale, so 0 dB is defined as a pressure of 20 micropascals. An alternative scale occasionally used is in reference to normal hearing threshold, or dB HL (for hearing level). Zero dB HL is the threshold for hearing for a population of normal people. This is approximately equivalent to 30 dB pe SPL. Sensation level, or dB SL, is in reference to the ear being tested. Zero dB SL is the threshold for that ear.

The *Guidelines* recommends stimulus intensities between 40 and 120 dB pe SPL. Many EP machines do not give stimuli louder than that recommended. For routine BAEP testing, intensity is set at approximately 65 dB SL or HL. Reducing stimulus intensity is necessary only if waveform identification is difficult. With decreasing stimulus intensity, waves II and VI are reduced more than the other waves, allowing for more accurate identification of waves I, III, and V.

Electrode Placement and Recording Parameters

Electrodes are placed in the following positions: (1) A1 (behind the left ear), (2) A2 (behind the right ear), and (3) Cz (at the vertex). These surface electrodes are identical in composition to those used for routine EEG recording. Detailed guidelines for placement of surface electrodes are included in Part II.

Recommended montages for recording of BAEP are Cz-Ai for channel 1 and Cz-Ac for channel 2 (where Cz is at the vertex, Ai is behind the ipsilateral ear, and Ac is behind the contralateral ear). Positions Ai and Ac are identical to A1 and A2 in the 10–20 Electrode Placement System for EEG surface electrode placement, which is described in Part II. Cz is identical to the position Cz in the 10–20 system.

Therefore, for stimulation of each ear, the first channel records the difference in potential between the ipsilateral ear and the vertex, and the second channel records the difference between the contralateral ear and vertex. Recording from the contralateral ear aids in identification of waves I, IV, and V.

Stimulus and recording parameters are summarized in Table 33.1.

Interpretation

Waveform Identification and Origin

The waves routinely analyzed in BAEP testing are numbered I through V. Waves VI and VII are also identified but not used in interpretation. Waves I and V should be identified first. Wave I is generated by the distal portion of the acoustic nerve and is approximately 2 ms after the stimulus. Wave I identification is aided by recording from a contralateral electrode derivation; it is the only wave present on ipsilateral but not contralateral recording.

Wave V may be generated by projections from the pons to the midbrain. There are several criteria for identifying wave V. It normally appears at approximately 6 ms and is often combined with wave IV into a single com-

Table 33.1   Brain Stem Auditory-Evoked Potential Stimulus and Recording*

Parameters	Values
Stimulus parameters	
Rate	8–10/sec
Intensity	115–120 dB pe SPL
Duration of electrical pulse	100 μs
Stimulus character	Monaural
	Contralateral masking with a 60 dB pe SPL white noise
Stimulus polarity	Rarefaction or condensation, summed independently
Number of trials	1,000–4,000
Recommended montages	
Channel 1	Cz-Ai
Channel 2	Cz-Ac
Recording parameters	
Low-frequency filter	10–30 Hz (–3 dB)
High-frequency filter	2,500–3,000 Hz (–3 dB)
Analysis time	10–15 ms
Number of trials	1,000–4,000
Measurements	Wave I peak latency
	Wave III peak latency
	Wave V peak latency
	I–III interpeak interval
	III–V interpeak interval
	I–V interpeak interval
	Wave I amplitude
	Wave V amplitude
	Wave V: wave I amplitude ratio

dB pe SPL = decibels peak equivalent sound pressure level.
*Special circumstances may occasionally dictate changes in these standard parameters.
The amplitude of wave III is often decreased on contralateral recording. Waves I, III, and
IV are the major peaks used in interpretation. Waves II and IV are between I and III, and
III and V, respectively. Their latency and amplitude is variable.
Source: Modified with permission from American Electroencephalographic Society.
Guidelines in EEG, evoked potentials, and polysomnography. J Clin Neurophysiol
1986;11:60.

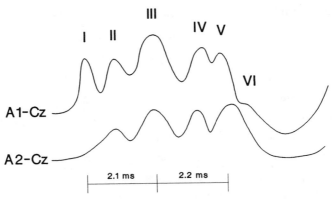

Figure 33.1 Normal brain stem auditory-evoked potential. Waves are numbered according to conventions described in the text. The top trace was recorded from the ipsilateral side, and the bottom trace was recorded from the contralateral side.

plex waveform. Wave V is also the first waveform whose falling edge dips below the baseline.

The wave III–V complex has a wider separation with recording from the contralateral ear than recording from the ipsilateral ear. This means that the contralateral wave IV is of slightly shorter latency and wave V is of slightly longer latency. Wave V is the last to disappear as stimulus intensity is decreased.

Wave III is thought to be generated by the projections from the superior olive through the lateral lemniscus. It is the major peak between waves I and V.

Data Analysis

Latency is a more important measure than amplitude in the interpretation of BAEP data. The most important measurements are wave I latency, wave I–III interpeak latency, and wave III–V interpeak latency. A sample normal BAEP test is shown in Figure 33.1. Normative data are shown in Table 33.2. Interpretation of abnormalities is detailed in Table 33.3.

Increased wave I latency is seen if the most distal portion of the acoustic nerve is affected. Most acoustic neuromas do not affect wave I.
Increased wave I–III interpeak latency indicates a defect in the pathway from the proximal eighth nerve into the inferior pons. The lesion may

Table 33.2   Brain Stem Auditory-Evoked Potential Normal Data

Waveform	Male[a]	Female[a]
Wave I latency	2.10	2.10
I–III interpeak interval	2.55	2.40
III–V interpeak interval	2.35	2.20
I–V interpeak interval	4.60	4.45
Interside I–V difference	0.50	0.50
Wave V: wave I amplitude ratio[b]	0.50	0.50

[a]All latencies are given in milliseconds (ms) and represent the upper limit of normal.
[b]The V:I amplitude ratio is a simple ratio, without units.
Source: Data used at Vanderbilt University Hospital, Nashville, Tennessee.

Table 33.3   Interpretation of Brain Stem Auditory-Evoked Potential Abnormalities

Finding	Interpretation
Increased wave I latency	Lesion of distal portion of acoustic nerve
Increased I–III interpeak latency	Lesion of pathway from proximal cranial nerve VIII to pons, either in the nerve or in the brain stem (e.g., acoustic neuromas)
Increased III–V interpeak latency	Lesion between caudal pons and midbrain
Increased I–III and III–V interpeak latencies	Lesion affecting brain stem above caudal pons plus either the caudal pons or acoustic nerve
Absence of wave I with normal III and V	Peripheral hearing disorder Conduction in the caudal pons cannot be evaluated
Absence of wave III with normal I and V	Normal
Absence of wave V with normal I and III	Lesion above the caudal pons, considered an extreme of wave III–V interpeak interval prolongation
Absence of all waves	Severe hearing loss

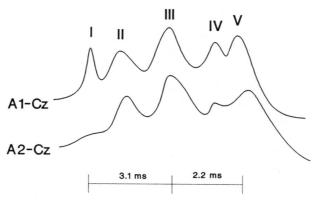

Figure 33.2 Increased I–III interpeak interval of the brain stem auditory-evoked potential. This is due to a lesion between the intracranial portion of the eighth nerve and caudal pons.

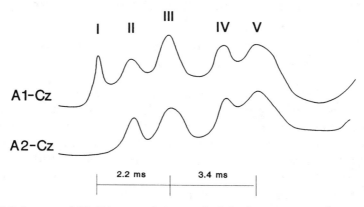

Figure 33.3 Increased III–V interpeak interval of the brain stem auditory-evoked potential. This is due to a lesion above the caudal pons.

be either in the nerve or in the brain stem. This is the most common abnormality found in patients with acoustic neuromas (Figure 33.2).

Increased wave III–V interpeak latency indicates a defect in conduction between the caudal pons and midbrain (Figure 33.3).

Increased wave I–III and wave III–V interpeak latencies indicate that the lesion is affecting both the brain stem above the caudal pons and either the caudal pons or the acoustic nerve. In most instances, the prominent lesion is in the pons.

Absence of wave I with normal III and V may indicate a peripheral hearing disorder, with the caveat that conduction in the caudal pons cannot be evaluated. Absence of wave I with prolonged latency or absence of wave III, wave V, or both usually indicates a defect of conduction in the eighth nerve along with a lesion in the caudal pons; however, this is difficult to evaluate without a recordable wave I–III interpeak interval.

Absence of wave III with normal waves I and V is normal, but if the wave I–V interval is prolonged, then a lesion affecting conduction somewhere from the eighth nerve to the midbrain is suspected.

Absence of wave V with normal waves I and III is uncommon, but when present, it indicates a lesion affecting the auditory pathways above the caudal pons. This is considered an extreme prolongation of the wave III–V interval.

Pediatric Brain Stem Auditory-Evoked Potentials

Brain Stem Auditory-Evoked Potentials for Disorders of Childhood

Often, BAEPs are used to evaluate children with suspected hearing loss, especially infants and children who cannot cooperate with conventional audiometry. An abnormal BAEP test result is usually associated with abnormalities on behavioral testing of hearing; however, a normal BAEP test result does not guarantee normal hearing. If the lesion is of the peripheral auditory structures, threshold may be increased, but there may not be a change in wave I–V interpeak interval.

Abnormal BAEPs are recorded in children with several metabolic disorders: phenylketonuria, maple syrup urine disease, nonketotic hyperglycinemia, and Leigh's disease. Wave I–V interpeak interval is typically increased. BAEP testing is not important in the diagnosis of these disorders, however, because BAEP abnormalities are not disease-specific.

Neonatal Brain Stem Auditory-Evoked Potentials

Special care is needed in recording BAEPs in the newborn. Ordinary headphones may produce sufficient pressure to close off the external auditory canal. The result is absent or poor waveforms. Special earphones that do not deform the canal are routinely provided with EP machines.

Sedation is usually required to record EPs in neonates. This is best accomplished by the use of chloral hydrate, meperidine plus secobarbital, or meperidine plus promethazine plus chlorpromazine (DPT). Sedation does not affect short-latency EPs such as the BAEP.

BAEP testing is performed on infants to evaluate respiratory and feeding dysfunction, particularly with suspected perinatal asphyxia and in premature infants. The wave I–V interpeak latency is prolonged in premature infants and may be related to delayed maturity of brain stem nuclei and pathways. There is an almost linear relationship between the decline in wave I–V interpeak latency and the reduction in apnea frequency.

The wave I–V interpeak interval is increased in term newborns who have experienced episodes of total asphyxia with subsequent damage to brain stem nuclei. The mortality and neurologic morbidity in such newborns is high. Newborns who have experienced prolonged partial asphyxia sustain mainly hemispheric damage, and the wave I–V interval may be normal despite a poor neurologic outcome.

Brain Stem Auditory-Evoked Potential in Specific Disorders

Acoustic Neuromas

Prolongation of the wave I–III interpeak interval is the most sensitive finding in the diagnosis of acoustic neuroma. If there is difficulty in obtaining wave I, the technician should place an electrode in the external auditory canal for better recording. Alternatively, electrocochleography can aid with identification of wave I. In patients with very large tumors, there may be such severe damage that there are no reproducible waves after I. In early cases, the BAEP has been abnormal, when imaging revealed an acoustic neuroma. A sample finding with acoustic neuroma is shown in Figure 33.2.

Brain Stem Tumors and Stroke

BAEP test results are abnormal in most patients with intrinsic tumors of the brain stem. This is especially true in patients with pontine involvement. The usual abnormality is delay or loss of waves III and V and increased wave I–III and wave III–V interpeak intervals.

BAEP test results are also abnormal in most patients with brain stem stroke. A few patients with extensive brain stem infarctions have been reported to have normal BAEPs, however. In some of these patients the amplitudes of the waveforms were low; however, amplitude abnormalities are not emphasized in the interpretation of BAEPs.

Approximately 50% of patients with transient ischemic attacks affecting the posterior circulation have latency abnormalities, and 50% of patients who recover from definite brain stem strokes have normal BAEPs. A sample recording from a patient with a brain stem lesion is shown in Figure 33.3.

Multiple Sclerosis

BAEP testing is less sensitive than VEPs and SEPs for detection of clinically unsuspected lesions in patients being evaluated for multiple sclerosis. The usual abnormalities are reduction in wave V amplitude and increased wave III–V interpeak latency.

Most abnormalities are asymmetric, affecting the response from only one ear. Caution in the interpretation of amplitude abnormalities is recommended. BAEP testing cannot distinguish a demyelinating disease from tumors or infarction.

Coma and Brain Death

The Medical Consultants on the Diagnosis of Death (1981) cited BAEP testing as a confirmatory test, along with EEG and radionucleotide brain scan. The commission criteria are enumerated in Chapter 17.

BAEP test results are consistent with brain death if there are no reproducible waves after wave I. Wave II may be intact in less than 10% of brain-dead patients, reinforcing the hypothesis that wave II is generated by the intracranial portion of the eighth nerve. The presence of wave II is consistent with cerebral death in a patient who otherwise fulfills all other clinical criteria and has no subsequent waves on the BAEP potential.

Miscellaneous Disorders

Abnormal interpeak latencies are reported in patients with meningitis, B_{12} deficiency, epilepsy, alcoholism, and diabetes mellitus. The abnormalities associated with diabetes and meningitis (i.e., increased wave I–III interpeak intervals) are consistent with a lesion of the acoustic nerve.

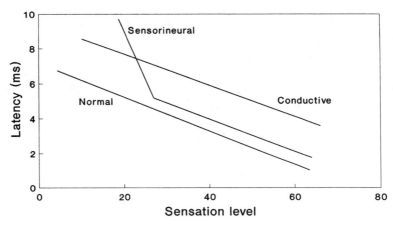

Figure 33.4 Relationship between sensation level and latency of wave V. This is essentially a semilog plot, since sensation level is an exponential parameter. Conductive hearing loss results in an increased latency at all intensities. Sensorineural hearing loss results in recruitment at low intensities but a normal slope at higher intensities.

Audiometry

Audiometry is a variation of evoked responses that evaluates dysfunction of the ear and proximal eighth nerve. The BAEP technique is the same as described previously, except that special attention is given to the latency of wave V at different stimulus intensities. The wave V latency is plotted against the stimulus intensity at 20, 40, 60, and 80 dB greater than threshold (Figure 33.4). Because of the nature of the decibel scale, this is essentially a semilog plot.

The relationship between wave V latency and stimulus intensity is linear in normal individuals, with higher intensities producing shorter latencies. Conductive hearing loss does not change the slope of this relationship but prolongs the latency at each intensity. Therefore, the curve is shifted up. The response looks as if the intensities are turned down at every point, which is in effect what occurs with conductive loss. Sensorineural hearing loss produces a curve with two slopes. At low intensities, there is decreased responsiveness of the end-organ, so that for a given intensity the wave V latency is prolonged. With increases in intensity, there is more recruitment of nerves than normal, so that the slope of the curve is steeper. At high intensities, sufficient recruitment has occurred such that the latency may be normal. At this point, the slope reverts to normal. This L-shaped curve is typical for sensorineural hearing loss.

Audiometry is useful for evaluating patients for hearing loss when the localization of the lesion is in doubt. Audiometry can also be used to follow patients receiving chemotherapeutic agents that cause ototoxicity.

34 Visual-Evoked Potentials

The visual-evoked potential (VEP) is the potential recorded from the occipital region in response to visual stimuli. The VEP differs from other evoked responses in that the response is a long-latency response. (Brain stem auditory-evoked potentials and somatosensory-evoked potentials [SEPs] are short-latency responses.) There are long-latency components to the brain stem auditory-evoked potential and SEP, but these are not routinely used for interpretation because they are too variable for clinical usefulness.

The VEP is the only evoked response that is visible without averaging. During routine EEG, photic stimulation is used to activate epileptiform discharges in patients suspected of having seizures. The photic stimulation is a bright flash delivered to subjects with their eyes closed. At flash frequencies of less than 5–7/sec, an evoked response is recorded from the occipital leads. A driving response is recorded at faster flash frequencies. The VEP is highly reproducible as long as the patient maintains fixation and has no change in visual acuity.

Stimulus

The VEP stimulus may be flash, full-field pattern reversal, or half-field pattern reversal. Flash is used in patients who cannot cooperate with the level of fixation required for pattern-reversal stimulation. The latencies of flash stimulation are more variable than pattern-reversal stimulation, so that the flash VEP is only useful to test continuity of the visual pathways. Full-field pattern reversal is the usual stimulus for the VEP. Since each eye is examined separately, this tests the anterior visual pathways especially well. Half-field pattern-reversal stimulation is used for localization of lesions behind the optic chiasm. Although many laboratories still perform

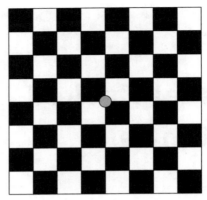

Figure 34.1 Pattern-reversal stimulus for the visual-evoked potential. The black-and-white checkerboard pattern is generated on a cathode ray tube or light-emitting diode array. The black squares become white, and the white become black at a rate of 2/sec.

half-field testing, modern imaging procedures have reduced the clinical application of this technique.

Flash Stimulus

The flash stimulus is delivered by a strobe light placed in front of the patient. The device is similar to that used for photic stimulation during routine EEG. Typically, the eyes are closed. Sufficient light passes through the lids to activate the retina.

An intact flash VEP indicates continuity of the pathways from the retina to the lateral geniculate. Flash VEPs have been recorded in the absence of a functioning cortex. Therefore, flash stimuli are not used if reproducible waveforms can be obtained with pattern-reversal stimuli.

Pattern-Reversal Stimulus

Pattern-reversal stimulation is generated by a video display attached to a pattern generator or video card connected to a computer. The patient, in a sitting position, fixates on a small target in the middle of the display. On the display is a checkerboard pattern (Figure 34.1). At regular intervals, the pattern is electronically reversed so that the white squares become black and the black squares become white; thus, there is pattern reversal. The response is recorded from occipital leads and averaged over many trials.

Several parameters influence the response, including the following:

- Size of the checks
- Size of the visual field stimulated
- Frequency of pattern reversal
- Luminance of the display
- Contrast between background and foreground
- Fixation of the patient

Table 34.1 summarizes the stimulus and recording parameters for the VEPs.

Check size affects the amplitude and latency of the VEP. Size is measured in minutes of visual field arc, where there are 60 minutes (60′) per degree of arc. The maximal response is elicited by a check size between 15′ and 60′. The wide range of check size is made possible by differences in other variables, notably size of the stimulus field. With smaller checks, the latency of the response is increased and the amplitude is reduced. With larger field sizes, the amplitude is reduced. The fovea is stimulated better by smaller checks, and the periphery is stimulated better by larger checks. The recommended check size is 28′ to 32′ of the visual field arc, which is a compromise between the two extremes.

Stimulus field size should be at least 8 degrees (8°) of the visual field arc, since approximately 80% of the response is generated by the central 8° of vision.

A smaller field size has been recommended to increase sensitivity to subtle defects, but the false-positive rate is unacceptable. Visual acuity is the limiting factor in the presence of reduced stimulus field and reduced check size.

Reversal rate should be 2/sec, which is an interstimulus interval of 500 ms. Faster reversal rates cause an increase in the latency of the major wave, P100. Rates faster than 5–7/sec produce the entrained driving response seen on routine EEG during photic stimulation.

Low luminance is known to cause an increase in P100 latency and a decrease in amplitude. Standard video monitors used for routine VEP testing produce sufficient luminance, but this should be checked periodically. Note that pupillary diameter can greatly affect retinal illumination, so marked interside differences in pupil diameter must be considered in interpretation of the VEP. Although there are no specific recommendations for luminance levels, it is recommended that luminance levels remain consistent during and between studies.

Table 34.1   Visual-Evoked Potential Stimulus and Recording Parameters*

Stimulus Parameters	Values
Reversal rate	2/sec (500 ms interval)
Contrast	>50%
Check size	28–32 min of arc
Field size	8° of arc
Number of trials	100–200
Recommended electrodes	
MO	5 cm above inion
RO	5 cm right of MO
LO	5 cm left of MO
MF	12 cm above nasion
A1	Left ear or mastoid
Recommended montages	
Channel 1	LO-MF
Channel 2	MO-MF
Channel 3	RO-MF
Channel 4	MF-A1
Recording parameters	
Low-frequency filter	1.0 Hz (–3 dB)
High-frequency filter	100 Hz (–3 dB)
Analysis time	250 ms
Measurements	N75 latency from each eye
	P100 latency from each eye
	Interocular latency difference
	Amplitude (baseline to P100 or N75 to P100)
	Interocular amplitude ratio (larger: smaller)

MO = midline occipital; RO = right occipital; LO = left occipital; MF = midline frontal.
*Special circumstances may occasionally dictate changes in these standard parameters.
Source: Modified with permission from American Electroencephalographic Society. Guidelines in EEG, evoked potentials, and polysomnography. J Clin Neurophysiol 1994;11:48.

Contrast between the light and dark squares must be greater than 50%. In practice, the contrast is much greater than this. Lower contrast results in a delayed and lower amplitude P100.

Fixation on the target is helpful, but not essential, for a good reproducible response. Intentionally poor fixation does not affect the P100 latencies in most individuals but can cause a reduction of amplitude. Some individuals may be able to voluntarily reduce the amplitude sufficiently to make the P100 not identifiable.

Half-Field Pattern Reversal

Half-field stimulation is given to one eye at a time and only to one half-field, either right or left. The pattern-reversal technique is the same as that used for full-field stimulation, with the checkerboard on one side of the screen blocked out. Comparing the responses with stimulation of the two half-fields tests the visual pathways behind the optic chiasm.

Magnetic resonance imaging and computerized tomography provide excellent visualization of the retrochiasmatic visual pathways and are superior to VEP for detection of lesions in these regions. Therefore, half-field stimulation is not commonly used for evaluation of patients with suspected brain pathology.

Half-field stimulation is typically performed by having the patient fixate on a spot that is not directly adjacent to a luminant box with either half-field stimulation. The left and right half-fields are alternately stimulated with the stimulated area at least one check-width from the fixation point. Only one eye is stimulated at a time. Montage is shown in Table 34.2.

Significant findings should be prolonged P100 latency from any half-field or increased interocular difference for any half-field.

Electrode Placement and Recording Parameters

Although there are significant variations between laboratories, the *Guidelines* (American Electroencephalographic Society, 1994) recommends electrode positions as detailed in Table 34.1. Most interpretation is performed using the midline occipital (MO) electrode. Electrodes on both sides of the midline (RO and LO) can be helpful for interpretation of abnormal studies. Some laboratories use a Cz-Oz derivation, having not converted to conformity with the new guidelines. This table also outlines the montages recommended.

The laterally placed electrodes facilitate accurate waveform identification, especially for half-field stimulation. For routine pattern-reversal stimulation, placement of electrodes is dictated by findings. If the waveforms are poor or unusual, use of lateral electrodes, use of more anterior electrodes, or both is recommended to look for an unusual potential distribution.

Table 34.2   Half-Field Visual-Evoked Potential Stimulation and
Recording Parameters

Parameter	Values
Electrodes	
LO	Left occipital
RO	Right occipital
MF	Midfrontal
RT	Right posterior temporal
LT	Left posterior temporal
Montage for left half-field stimulation	
Channel 1	LO-MF
Channel 2	MO-MF
Channel 3	RO-MF
Channel 4	RT-MF
Montage for right half-field stimulation	
Channel 1	LT-MF
Channel 2	LO-MF
Channel 3	MO-MF
Channel 4	RO-MF
Measurements	P100 latency
	P100 amplitude
Derivations	Left half-field interocular latency difference
	Right half-field interocular latency difference
	Left eye half-field latency difference
	Right eye half-field latency difference
	Left half-field interocular amplitude ratio
	Right half-field interocular amplitude ratio
	Left eye half-field amplitude ratio
	Right eye half-field amplitude ratio

MO = midline occipital; MF = midline frontal.

Waveform Identification

Normal Waveforms

Inspection of the normal VEP reveals three identifiable waveforms, N75, P100, and N145 (Figure 34.2). The positive potential at approx-

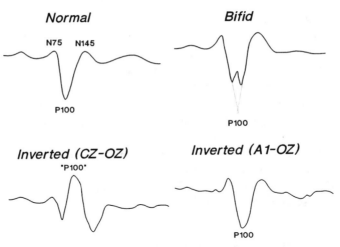

Figure 34.2 Normal visual-evoked potentials. The top left wave is the most common observed. The other waveforms are variants of normal, as described in the text.

imately 100 ms (P100) is used for interpretation. The negative N75 and N145 that precede and follow the P100 are helpful for identification but not for routine interpretation.

Variant Waveforms

There are two common variations in the VEP waveform: bifid and inverted (see Figure 34.2). Both are due to variation in the anatomic orientation of the visual cortex and optic radiations. The main clinical concern regarding the bifid pattern is where to call the P100. If the split in the P100 is fairly narrow, it is reasonable to use a point that is extrapolated from the ascending and descending slopes. If the derived P100 latency is normal, the VEP is interpreted as normal. Some patients will exhibit a widely split P100, not amenable to extrapolation. This may be due to defects in the projection to the upper and lower segments of the calcarine cortex, possibly from visual field defects. Stimulation of only the lower half of the visual field may improve the bifid waveform, but the latency is often abnormal anyway. There is controversy as to whether or not a bifid waveform should be considered abnormal on its own. The most conservative approach is to simplify the waveform by lower-half stimulation and localize the P100 by recording from Pz and Cz in addition to midline occipital derivations. Using these techniques, the test is abnormal if the latency of the resultant waveform is increased.

The inverted waveform is an artifact of a montage commonly used in recording the VEP. In some patients, the positivity of the VEP is shifted superiorly and anteriorly. Using a Cz-Oz montage, the Cz electrode is more positive than the Oz electrode, causing a reversed direction of the deflection. N75 and N145 are reversed as well, and one of these could be misinterpreted as the P100. If the waveform is not typical of the normal VEP, recordings should be made from channels other than Cz-Oz, such as A1-Oz, A1-Pz, and A1-Cz. These will allow for mapping of the topography of the VEP and aid greatly in the identification of the P100.

Interpretation of Data

The main indication for VEP is a suspected disorder of the anterior visual pathways. The most common abnormality is an increase in the latency of the P100 from one eye. This indicates a lesion in the optic tract anterior to the chiasm.

If the P100 is prolonged from both eyes, one would suspect bilateral optic nerve lesions, but the same recording could be obtained from a lesion in the region of the chiasm or from extensive retrochiasmal damage. To distinguish between these possibilities, VEP with half-field stimulation may be helpful. A lesion in the right optic tract will result in a prolonged P100 with stimulation of the left half-field.

The absolute latency of the P100 is considered prolonged if it exceeds 117 ms. Interside latency difference is even more sensitive than absolute latency, however. For example, if the P100 from full-field stimulation of the left eye is 110 ms, and that from stimulation of the right eye is 97 ms, the study would be interpreted as abnormal. The 13-ms interside difference is excessive, even though the absolute latencies are both within normal limits. Normal values are shown in Table 34.3.

Optic Neuritis

Optic neuritis typically increases the latency of the P100 using the pattern-reversal VEP. If the optic neuritis is unilateral, the increase is purely unilateral. A prolonged latency of the P100 from an asymptomatic eye suggests a previous subclinical episode of optic neuritis. A sample VEP from a patient with optic neuritis is shown in Figure 34.3.

Table 34.3   Visual-Evoked Potential Normal Data*

Measurement	Values
Pattern-reversal VEP	
Latency	117 ms
Interocular latency difference	6 ms
Amplitude	3 µV
Interocular amplitude difference	5.5 µV
Flash VEP	
Latency	132 ms
Interocular latency difference	6 ms

VEP = visual-evoked potential.

*Most laboratories do not interpret a study as being abnormal solely on the basis of low or unequal amplitudes. These data are used at Vanderbilt University Hospital, Nashville, Tennessee.

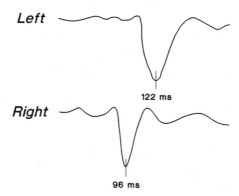

Figure 34.3 Visual-evoked potential with left optic neuritis. The response from stimulation of the left eye is prolonged. Upper limit of normal is 117 ms. The response from the right is normal.

After the acute phase of the optic neuritis, very few VEPs return to normal. Therefore, if a patient is being evaluated for previous optic neuritis, the VEP should be abnormal.

Multiple Sclerosis

Approximately 15% of patients with optic neuritis will later develop other signs of multiple sclerosis. In patients with optic neuritis, SEP testing is often performed to look for clinically silent lesions in the spinal cord. Conversely, when multiple sclerosis is suspected because of lesions in other parts of the central nervous system, VEP testing may be useful to show previous asymptomatic optic neuritis. Abnormal VEP latency is present in approximately 40% of patients with multiple sclerosis who do not have a history of optic neuritis. Virtually all patients with a history of optic neuritis have either an absolute increase in the latency of the P100 from the affected eye or an abnormal interside difference in latency, if the absolute latencies are normal.

Tumors

Tumors affecting the anterior visual pathways commonly produce compression of the optic nerve and chiasm. This results in visual field defects that affect each eye differently. The VEP is almost always abnormal, but the correlation between visual acuity and degree of VEP abnormality is poor. Reported abnormalities are alterations in absolute or interside latencies of the P100 and changes in wave morphology and amplitude. Latency changes are more reliable than morphology or amplitude changes.

Tumors affecting the posterior visual pathways are less likely to affect the VEP. Full-field pattern-reversal VEP testing is usually normal in patients with dense hemianopia. The use of electrodes lateral to MO may reveal an amplitude asymmetry with the higher amplitude ipsilateral to the side of the lesion, but amplitude asymmetries may be present in normal individuals. Half-field stimulation reveals abnormalities in some individuals; however, the sensitivity and specificity is not good enough to justify using this technique to screen for posterior lesions. Imaging techniques should be used.

Pseudotumor Cerebri

Patients with pseudotumor cerebri have increased intracranial pressure not associated with a structural defect, such as mass or obstruction in cerebrospinal fluid flow. If the increased pressure is untreated, patients may develop visual loss. If treatment is effective, the visual loss can improve; however, permanent deficits result if there has been long-standing increased pressure.

Most patients with pseudotumor cerebri have normal VEPs. A few patients are described with abnormalities in association with incipient visual loss; however, VEPs should not be used as screening procedures for increased intracranial pressure.

Functional Disorders

The pattern-reversal VEP is frequently used to evaluate patients with suspected functional visual loss. Few individuals can voluntarily suppress the VEP. An intact VEP usually suggests continuity of the visual pathways but does not fully exclude cortical blindness. Caution is needed in using pattern-shift VEP for the diagnosis of functional visual loss.

A normal flash VEP indicates continuity of the visual pathways only to the lateral geniculate. An intact flash response is expected with lesions of the optic radiations and visual cortex. Great care should be exercised in interpretation of latency abnormalities of the flash VEP.

Ocular and Retinal Disorders

Many ocular and retinal disorders cause abnormalities in the pattern-shift VEP. The effect of impaired visual acuity and effective retinal illumination on the VEP have been discussed previously in the section on Pattern-Reversal Stimulus. The VEP is not ordinarily used for the diagnosis of these disorders. Although some patients with glaucoma have an increased latency and reduced amplitude of the P100, a normal VEP cannot be interpreted as indicating normal intraocular pressure. The effects of ocular and retinal disorders on the VEP are of interest only in the interpretation of VEPs used to evaluate disorders at and behind the optic nerve.

Cortical Blindness

Some patients with documented cortical blindness have normal pattern-reversal VEPs. The use of smaller check size may help to bring out abnormalities; however, this is not routinely done in most neurodiagnostic laboratories.

Table 34.4   Visual-Evoked Potential Interpretation

Finding	Interpretation
Unilateral prolonged P100	Lesion of optic tract anterior to chiasm
Bilateral prolonged P100	Bilateral optic tract lesions or chiasmal lesion or extensive retrobulbar lesions
Normal P100 but increased interside difference	Lesion of the optic tract on the side of the longer latency
Absence of waves from one eye	Lesion of optic tract, retina, or of optics of light transmission to the retina Need to rule-out technical factors, such as stimulator failure
Binocular single-half-field defect	Lesion of the contralateral optic tract

Intraoperative Monitoring of Visual-Evoked Potential

The flash VEP has been used for intraoperative monitoring during surgery in the region of the optic nerve and chiasm with mixed results. An absence of change in VEP waveform or latency is correlated with no postoperative deterioration in vision. The main indications for VEP monitoring are surgery of optic glioma, meningioma in the region of the optic nerve or chiasm, pituitary adenoma, craniopharyngioma, and hypothalamic tumor (Table 34.4).

35

Somatosensory-Evoked Potentials

The somatosensory-evoked potential (SEP) is the response to electrical stimulation of peripheral nerves. Stimulation of almost any nerve is possible, but the most commonly studied are median, ulnar, peroneal, and posterior tibial. Recording is made of the afferent nerve volley, the potentials generated in the spinal cord and relay nuclei, and the potentials generated over the motor-sensory cortex. Short-latency responses are used in clinical practice; long-latency responses are too variable to be helpful.

The SEPs are helpful in the diagnosis of spinal cord disease that is not displayed by imaging studies (especially multiple sclerosis) and are used routinely for intraoperative monitoring of some surgical procedures, such as Harrington rod placement for scoliosis. SEP can be helpful for objective evidence of myelopathy in patients with negative imaging studies.

Overview of Stimulus and Waveform Generation

The stimulus for SEPs is a brief electric pulse delivered to the distal portion of the nerve. The electrical stimulus cannot selectively activate sensory nerves, so a small muscle twitch is associated. There are no effects of the retrograde volley in motor nerves on central projections of the sensory fibers.

Intensity of the stimulus is adjusted so that there is slight twitching of the innervated muscles. This intensity is sufficient to activate low-threshold myelinated nerve fibers. The compound action potential is conducted through the dorsal roots and into the dorsal columns. The impulses ascend in the dorsal columns to the gracile and cuneate nuclei, where the primary afferent fibers synapse on the second order neurons, which ascend through the brain stem to the thalamus. Thalamocortical projections are extensive, as are secondary intracortical associative projections.

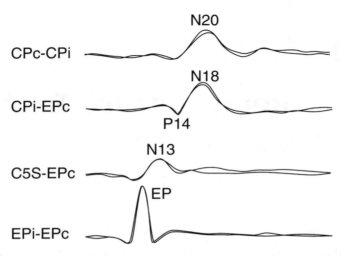

Figure 35.1 Normal median nerve somatosensory-evoked potentials. The potentials used for routine analysis are evoked potential (EP), P14, and N20.

Median Nerve Somatosensory-Evoked Potential

Median nerve SEPs are useful to assess conduction in the upper cervical cord and brain and to assess spinal cord disease when performed in conjunction with leg SEPs. A delay in conduction from the leg with a normal median response localizes the lesion to the region between the cauda equina and the cervical spinal cord. A sample median SEP is shown in Figure 35.1.

Stimulus and Recording Parameters

A summary of SEP stimulus and recording parameters is presented in Table 35.1. Specific recommendations for median nerve SEPs are presented in Table 35.2. For median-nerve SEPs, electrodes are placed as follows: (1) Erb's point on each side, (2) over the fifth or second cervical spine process (C5S or C2S), (3) at contralateral cortex (CPc) and ipsilateral cortex (CPi), and (4) a noncephalic reference (Ref).

Erb's point is 2–3 cm above the clavicle, just lateral to the attachment of the sternocleidomastoid muscle. Stimulation at Erb's point produces abduction of the arm and flexion of the elbow. The second and fifth spinous processes are identified by counting up from the seventh, notable by its prominence at the base of the neck. CPc and CPi are scalp electrodes halfway

Table 35.1 Somatosensory-Evoked Potential Common
Stimulus and Recording Parameters*

Stimulus parameters	
Stimulus rate	4–7/sec
Recording parameters	
Low-frequency filter	5–30 Hz (–3 dB)
High-frequency filter	2,500–4,000 Hz (–3 dB)

*See Tables 35.2–35.5 for specific recommendations for individual nerves.
Source: Modified with permission from American Electroencephalographic Society.
Guidelines in EEG, evoked potentials, and polysomnography. J Clin Neurophysiol
1994;11:48–73.

Table 35.2 Median Nerve Somatosensory-Evoked Potential Stimulus and
Recording Parameters

Parameter	Value
Number of trials	500–2,000
Analysis time	40 ms
Bandpass	30–3,000 Hz (–6 dB)
Simulating electrodes	
Cathode	Median nerve 2 cm proximal to wrist crease
Anode	2 cm distal to cathode
Recording electrodes	
CPc	Contralateral scalp, between C3/4 and P3/4
CPi	Ipsilateral scalp, between C3/4 and P3/4
C5S	Over C5 spinous process
EPi	Erb's point ipsilateral to the stimulus
Ref	Noncephalic reference, such as distal arm
Montage	
Channel 1	CPc-CPi
Channel 2	CPi-Ref
Channel 3	C5S-Ref
Channel 4	EPi-Ref
Measurements	Peak latency of EP potential
	Peak latency of P14 in neck-scalp derivation
	Peak latency of N20 in scalp-scalp or scalp-ear derivation

between C3 and P3 or C4 and P4, where CPc is contralateral to the stimulus and CPi is ipsilateral to the stimulus. These electrodes are over the motor-sensory cortex. Fz is in the midline frontal region. This is identical to the Fz electrode position of the 10–20 system used for routine EEG. EPi is Erb's point ipsilateral to the stimulus. The recommended channels are shown in Table 35.2

The *Guidelines* (American Electroencephalographic Society, 1994) suggests a recording time of 40 ms, beginning at the onset of the stimulus. Frequently, the first 1–5 ms are not recorded to reduce stimulus artifact. Longer recording times should be used only if there are no reproducible potentials. For adequate waveform identification, 500–2,000 trials should be averaged.

The recommended filter settings are the same for all of the SEPs: (1) low-frequency filter at 5–30 Hz (–3 dB) and high-frequency filter at 2,500–4,000 Hz (–3 dB), and (2) filter slope not exceeding 12 dB/octave for low frequencies and 24 dB/octave for high frequencies. The *Guidelines* cites an optimal bandpass as 30–3,000 Hz.

Waveform Identification

With stimulation of the median nerve, the recorded potentials are from Erb's point, the neck, and the scalp. The potential at Erb's point is labelled EP; the same potential in neck-scalp derivation is called N9. N13 and P14 are recorded, but only P14 is now the recommended spinal potential to be used for interpretation. N18 and N20 are recorded over the scalp, but only N20 is used for interpretation. Normative data for all SEPs are presented in Table 35.3.

Interpretation

The median SEP is used for thoracic outlet syndrome, cervical myelopathy, and intraoperative monitoring during carotid endarterectomy. Increased latency or loss of a waveform during surgery suggests ischemia.

Table 35.4 shows the postulated sites of origin of the waves comprising the median and peroneal SEP. Interpretation of abnormalities is as follows:

- *A delayed EP with normal EP-P14 and P14-N20 intervals* indicates a lesion in the somatosensory nerves at or distal to the brachial plexus.
- *An increased EP-P14 interval with a normal P14-N20 interval* suggests a lesion between Erb's point and the lower medulla.

Table 35.3 Somatosensory-Evoked Potential Normal Data[a]

Wave	Latency[b]	Interside Difference
Median nerve somatosensory-evoked potential		
N9/EP	11.80	0.87
P14	16.10	0.70
N20	21.50	1.20
N13-N20 interval	7.10	1.20
Peroneal nerve somatosensory-evoked potential		
LP	13.50	0.50
P27	31.80	2.24
N33	40.70	5.96
LP-N27 interval	19.38	2.30
Tibial nerve somatosensory-evoked potential		
LP	22.10	1.20
P37	41.70	1.40
LP-P37 interval	20.50	1.50

[a]These data are used at Vanderbilt University Hospital, Nashville, Tennessee.
[b]All latencies are presented in milliseconds (ms).

Table 35.4 Somatosensory-Evoked Potential Waveform Origins*

Waveform	Origins
Median	
EP	Afferent volley in plexus
N13	Dorsal horn neurons
P14	Caudal medial lemniscus
N18	? Brain stem and thalamus
N20	Thalamocortical radiations
Tibial	
LP	Dorsal roots and entry zone
N34	? Brain stem and thalamus
P37	Primary sensory cortex

*These origins are based on currently available evidence and are not backed by extensive clinical-anatomic correlation. Therefore, they are subject to change.

- *An increased P14-N20 interval with a normal EP-P14 interval* indicates a lesion between the lower medulla and the cerebral cortex.

Amplitude abnormalities should be interpreted with caution. A marked asymmetry can be caused by a lesion affecting some but not all of the afferent fibers. If the lesion is not sufficiently severe to produce a latency change, however, the study is probably normal. An absent N20 is abnormal when EP and N13 are present. If N13 is absent but EP and N20 are normal and the EP-N20 interval is normal, the study indicates a lesion between the brachial plexus and medulla, but no statement can be made of brain conduction.

Ulnar Somatosensory-Evoked Potential

For the ulnar SEP, the stimulating electrode is placed over the ulnar nerve in the lateral distal forearm, just before entry into the wrist. Recording electrodes, montages, machine settings, and analysis of results are identical to those described for the median nerve. Normal values should be established for individual laboratories.

Tibial Somatosensory-Evoked Potential

Lower extremity SEPs have included study of the peroneal and tibial nerves. In current practice, tibial studies are performed more commonly and are discussed here. The tibial nerve supplies the gastrocnemius and soleus muscles in the leg, as well as the small muscles of the foot. The sural nerve wraps around the lateral malleolus, and the terminus of the tibial nerve wraps around the medial malleolus. At the medial malleolus, the tibial nerve is superficial and can be stimulated for the SEP.

Stimulus and Recording Parameters

Stimulus and recording settings are similar to those outlined for peroneal SEP. Specific recommendations are presented in Table 35.5. The proximal stimulus electrode (cathode) is placed at the ankle between the medial malleolus and the Achilles tendon. The anode is placed 3 cm distal to the cathode. A ground is placed proximal to the stimulus electrodes, usually on the calf. Stimulus intensity is set so that each stimulus produces a small amount of plantar flexion of the toes. Recording electrodes are placed

Table 35.5 Tibial Nerve Somatosensory-Evoked Potential Stimulus and Recording Parameters*

Parameter	Value
Number of trials	1,000–4,000
Stimulating electrodes	Behind medial malleolus
Analysis time	60 ms
Bandpass	30–3,000 Hz (–6 dB)
Recording electrodes	
CPi	Ipsilateral cortex between C3/4 and P3/4
CPz	Midline between Cz and Pz
Fpz	Fpz position of 10–20 system
C5S	Over the C5 spinous process
T12S	Over the T12 spinous process
Ref	Noncephalic reference
Montage	
Channel 1	CPi-Fpz
Channel 2	CPz-Fpz
Channel 3	Fpz-C5S
Channel 4	T12S-Ref
Measurements	LP latency
	P37 latency
	LP-P37 interpeak interval

*Special circumstances may dictate changes in these standard parameters.
Source: Modified with permission from American Electroencephalographic Society. Guidelines in EEG, evoked potentials, and polysomnography. J Clin Neurophysiol 1994;11:2–127.

as listed in Table 35.5. Although the *Guidelines* recommends measuring potentials from T12S, measurements of these latencies are not normally used for routine SEP interpretation.

Analysis time is routinely 60 ms; however, if the cerebral potentials are not identifiable, recording times of 100 ms or more should be used.

Waveform Identification

The recorded waveforms with tibial stimulation include a potential recorded from the afferent nerve volley in the popliteal fossa,

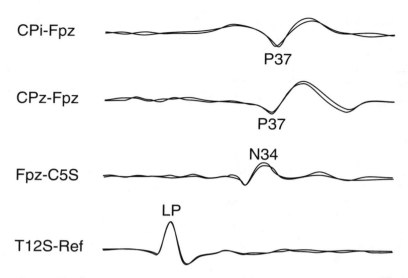

CPi-Fpz

P37

CPz-Fpz

P37

N34

Fpz-C5S

LP

T12S-Ref

Figure 35.2 Tibial nerve somatosensory-evoked potentials. Only LP and P37 are routinely used for interpretation.

potentials recorded over the lumbar spine (LP), and two potentials, N34 and P37, recorded over the cortex. A sample recording is shown in Figure 35.2.

Identification of the LP wave is usually easy. Patients with peripheral neuropathy may have desynchronization of the afferent volley, such that the amplitude of the nerve potentials may be low or inconsistent.

Identification of N34 and P37 is facilitated by overlapping averaged traces, which is currently recommended to aid visual interpretation of EPs in general. N34 is the main negative wave in the Fpz-C5S derivation and is preceded by a small positive wave that is not used for interpretation (P31). The P37 is the major positive wave in the CPi-Fpz and CPz-Fpz derivations. The amplitude may be very different between these channels, reflecting an anatomic variance in waveform distribution. Abnormalities of tibial SEPs are interpreted as follows:

Interpretation

Interpretation of tibial SEPs parallels interpretation of median SEPs. Absence of waveforms and increased interpeak latencies are the most important interpretive data. Abnormalities of tibial SEPs are interpreted as follows:

- *A prolonged LP with a normal LP-P37 interval* indicates a peripheral lesion. The lesion may be in the cauda equina but is more likely in the peripheral nerve.
- *A normal LP latency and a prolonged LP-P37 interval* indicate abnormal conduction between the cauda equina and the brain. Median SEP is required to localize the abnormality to the spinal cord. Normal median SEP indicates a lesion below the mid-cervical cord; prolonged median SEP indicates a lesion above the mid-cervical cord. A second lesion below the cervical cord cannot be excluded, however, since the P37 latency is already prolonged by the higher lesion.
- *A prolonged LP and an increased LP-P37 interval* suggest two lesions affecting the peripheral nerve and central conduction. A single lesion in the cauda equina is also possible.

36 ⬚⬚⬚
⬚⬚⬚
⬚⬚⬚

Evoked Potential
Monitoring

Evoked potential (EP) monitoring has become much more prevalent in the past decade, so much so that EP monitoring during surgery is a major part of the business of many laboratories. Orthopedic surgeons and neurosurgeons now consider somatosensory-evoked potential (SEP) monitoring a requirement for certain spinal surgeries. The need for adequate physiologic monitoring is clear, but there is less certainty as to what to do with the data that are acquired. The neurophysiologist needs to be knowledgeable not only in how to conduct and interpret EP monitoring, but he or she must also be ready to advise the surgeon of different possible outcomes dependent on the surgeon's reaction to the changes in the EP. This role has, unfortunately, opened up a new avenue of medicolegal liability for the neurophysiologist. This exposure is often increased by technically poor recordings, inadequate supervision of staff, and inaccurate interpretation of the data at the time of the surgery.

SEP is the most commonly monitored modality, with brain stem auditory-evoked potentials (BAEPs) used predominantly for posterior fossa surgery. Visual-evoked potential (VEP) is used in some institutions for dissection in the region of the optic nerve, chiasm, and pituitary gland; however, it is not in widespread use because of technical difficulties in delivering a high-resolution patterned stimulus to a positioned anesthetized patient. SEPs and BAEPs are less affected by anesthetics and involve techniques almost identical to those used for diagnostic evoked potentials.

Brain Stem Auditory-Evoked Potentials

The BAEP is often used to monitor brain stem integrity during posterior fossa surgery. It is recorded at intervals and compared not only with the previous intraoperative recordings, but also to a recording made before surgery. Anesthesia has virtually no effect on the BAEP, so reproducible waveforms are easily recorded in most patients. Monitoring of BAEPs is not useful during surgery for acoustic neuroma, since most patients are left with total loss of hearing in the affected ear.

Intraoperative BAEP monitoring methods for electrode position, stimulation, and recording are similar to those for routine diagnostic BAEP recordings. Headphones that completely cover the ear cannot be used, however, and earphones are used instead. Most equipment manufacturers supply earphones along with headphones. Since the surgery is being performed in an area that pathology might already have affected the BAEP, a preoperative study is desirable to ensure that reproducible waveforms can be obtained. The only other change from routine studies involves the use of longer than standard leads, to allow the EP machinery to be a workable distance from the head. With averaging and electronic noise reduction technology, this does not introduce excessive error in the recordings.

There is concern over incipient damage to the brain stem if any of the following occur:

- Loss of normal waveforms after wave I
- Decrease in amplitude of a major wave (III, V)
- Increase interpeak interval (I–III or III–V)

If all of the waves, including wave I, are lost, there could be failure to generate the click in the earphone or other technical problems, and caution must be exercised before suggesting brain stem dysfunction. If wave I (and usually also wave II) is present and later waves are not, this indicates severe abnormality in conduction in auditory pathways through the brain stem. Deterioration of the BAEP after surgery correlates with poor auditory function.

Anesthesia has a minimal effect on BAEP, making it an almost ideal monitoring modality. With anesthesia, all waves are delayed, but by no more than 0.2 ms. Cooling of the brain can result in prolonged interpeak latencies with prolonged surgery, but this should not be interpreted as indicative of brain stem or acoustic nerve damage if it occurs in a gradual, predictable, and bilateral fashion.

Somatosensory-Evoked Potentials

SEP monitoring is used mostly for surgery of the spine, but it is also used during carotid endarterectomy. Spine surgery uses either tibial or peroneal leg SEPs. The patient is tested before surgery to determine which type of response is obtainable.

Intraoperative monitoring of SEPs is performed chiefly for surgery on the spine but recently has been used for cerebrovascular surgery. The waveform is not significantly altered by anesthetic agents. In fact, the waves are frequently much easier to record in an anesthetized, paralyzed patient.

Corrective surgery for scoliosis typically includes vertebral fusion and Harrington rod insertion. If there is no change in waveform or latency of the SEP, there should be no deterioration in neurologic function after the surgery. Clearly, this statement needs validation by careful study, since, theoretically, there could be damage to the motor systems of the spinal cord, which is not tested with SEPs. A typical recording shows normal or prolonged waves of constant amplitude and latency throughout the surgery. The preoperative SEP may be abnormal because of compressive myelopathy from the scoliosis. If excessive stretch of the spinal cord occurs during insertion of the rods, there is either loss of amplitude or increase central conduction time of the SEP. Relieving tension on the spinal column causes the SEPs to return to the preoperative appearance.

Upper-extremity SEPs have been used during carotid endarterectomy to assess changes in the cerebral blood flow. If the cerebral waveform is lost, reduced in amplitude, or increased in latency, impaired conduction exists between the cervicomedullary junction and the cortex. One notable case from our experience is an elderly woman who was undergoing endarterectomy for right carotid stenosis with an ulcerated plaque. Preoperative evaluation found moderate atherosclerotic disease on the left as well. Throughout the surgery, the median SEP from the operated (right) side was stable; however, there was loss of the response from the unoperated (left) side. When the patient awoke, deficits from a left hemisphere infarction were evident. In this case, attention was focused predominantly on the operated side, but the loss of waves from the unoperated side correctly predicted the subsequent deficit.

At Vanderbilt University Hospital, we stimulate the median or tibial nerve continuously at a rate of 4.3/sec. Averages are continuously made, with 1,000–2,000 stimuli per average. The waveforms are continuously monitored by a technician, who prints a recording every 5 minutes. If there is any change in waveform or latency, the technician informs the surgeon, who considers the current procedure and may consult with the neurophysiologist. The chief artifact during surgery is electrocautery, although there is potential for extensive artifact from the surrounding equipment. With artifact rejection and proper grounding, the effects of this interference are reduced to acceptable levels.

37

□ □ □
□ □ □
□ □ □

Troubleshooting in Evoked Potentials

Noise

Most noise is due either to stray inductance or to stray capacitance. These electrical phenomena induce current to flow in electrode and amplifier wires, thereby obscuring the evoked potential (EP). Effects of stray capacitance and inductance are most pronounced if the electrode impedances are high or unequal. This is because unequal impedance destroys the noise-reducing benefits of the differential amplifier. See Part I for further details about the mechanisms of noise and general principles of noise reduction.

Averaging of EPs can lead to errors in waveform identification. The most consistent noise signal is 60-cycle interference. If the stimulus frequency is a harmonic of 60 Hz, the 60-cycle artifact can be averaged and can obscure the recording. The stimulus rate must be selected carefully so that 60-cycle interference is minimized.

EPs are typically very small in amplitude, but opportunities for noise interference with EPs are actually less than with most other neurodiagnostic techniques, due to the averaging required. Most sources of noise are not entrained to the stimulus so that artifact and random noise are averaged out. Potential error is possible if only one trial is performed. Even a single - large-amplitude artifact can appear to be important after many averages. Therefore, superimposing at least two averaged trials is key to correct identification of the waves.

Even with artifact rejection and careful selection of stimulation frequency, EP waveforms are frequently superimposed on lower frequency waves. In this instance, it is important to ensure that components of a sinusoid do not comprise a complex wave that could be confused with an EP.

Poor or Unusual Waveforms

Improper Electrode Position

As with most neurodiagnostic tests, the most common reason for poor results is poor technique. Improper electrode position will cause the wave to be absent or in the wrong configuration. The most dangerous result is the misidentification of waves, leading to an error in the final impression.

Improper electrode position is most common with the visual-evoked potential (VEP) and somatosensory-evoked potential (SEP). The landmarks for brain stem auditory-evoked potential (BAEP) electrode position are more obvious. For the VEP, the electrodes may be placed either too high or too low on the occiput. If too low, there may be excessive artifact from muscle, and the amplitude of the waveform may be reduced. If the electrodes are too high, the amplitude of the P100 may be reduced or the waveform may be changed.

Anatomic Variability

Anatomic variation is a common reason for absent or unusual waveforms on evoked responses. The most common of these affects the VEP. Some patients have a tilt in the normal orientation of the dipole, making the region of maximum positivity more anterior than normal. This is described in detail in the section on VEP waveform identification in Chapter 34.

Anatomic variation has very little effect on SEPs and BAEPs. In some patients, wave I of the BAEP cannot be identified. In this situation, it is important to use an electrode in the external auditory canal. This will aid in identification of wave I and distinction from the cochlear microphonic potential.

V

Polysomnography

38

Physiologic Basis of Sleep and Sleep Disorders

EEG during sleep is introduced in Part II. Sleep is used during routine EEG as an activation method to evoke epileptiform activity. Polysomnography (PSG) is the recording of EEG and other physiologic parameters during sleep. The most common sleep disorders evaluated by PSG are narcolepsy and sleep apnea. Insomnia is probably the most common sleep disorder, but PSG is more helpful for complaints of excessive daytime sleepiness. Part V covers the basic physiology of sleep and subsequently describes the methods and interpretation of PSG recordings.

Physiologic Basis of Sleep

The sleep-wake cycle is controlled by the reticular activating system. The reticular activating system consists of the brain stem reticular formation, posterior hypothalamus, and basal forebrain. These sites should be conceptualized as a continuous and indistinct structure rather than as separate nuclei.

The exact mechanisms of sleep and wake onset are not known. Activity in the pontine reticular formation, midbrain, and posterior hypothalamus are important for wakefulness. Activity in the medullary reticular formation is important for the generation of sleep. Sleep and wake may be integrated in the basal forebrain.

Wakefulness is probably a function of tonic activity in cells that project to the cortex. This activity increases neuronal excitability and may gate reactions to exogenous stimuli. Sleep develops as an active process that is generated by sleep-promoting neurons, such as the serotonergic raphe nuclei. This activation is probably promoted by a reduction in exogenous

Table 38.1   Sleep Stages

Stage	EEG Activity							EMG Activity
	α	β	θ	δ	V	K	S	
Awake	+	+	±	−	−	−	−	+
1A	±	−	+	±	−	−	−	±
1B	±	±	+	−	±	−	−	±
2	−	±	+	+	+	+	+	±
3	−	−	+	+	±	±	±	−
4	−	−	+	+	±	±	±	−
REM	−	+	+	+	−	−	−	−

α = alpha rhythm; β = beta rhythm; θ = theta rhythm; δ = delta rhythm; V = vertex waves; K = K complexes; S = sleep spindles; + = present; ± = may be present but not prominent; − = not present to a minor degree.

and endogenous stimuli that indicates a need for or an expectation of sleep. The tonic activating discharge and the response to exogenous stimuli are then suppressed, as are the patterned spontaneous activities normally seen while awake.

Years of sleep deprivation experiments have not explained the need for sleep. One proposed theory promotes the concept of sleep as a time for data management and reorganization. During the waking state, the brain receives a great deal of information on everything from music to tennis to physics. Much of this information is not ordered in a conceptual format, and the brain cannot access the information in a structured way. For example, there is a great difference between owning a tape of a lecture and understanding its content. Some data processing can occur in the waking state, but sleep may be required to organize the day's input, integrate it with existing data, and perhaps discard information that is seldom accessed or is judged by the brain to be useless or uninteresting.

Sleep Stages

Waking State

EEG in the waking stage is discussed in the Chapter 13 and summarized in Table 38.1. The adult waking EEG consists of predominantly fast frequencies. When the eyes are closed, a posterior dominant alpha rhythm predominates (Figure 38.1).

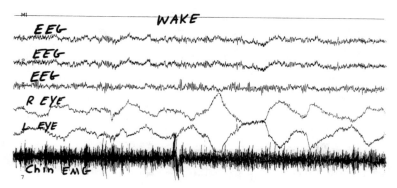

Figure 38.1 Waking state. There is a posterior predominant alpha rhythm with faster frequencies superimposed. Eye movements are conjugate.

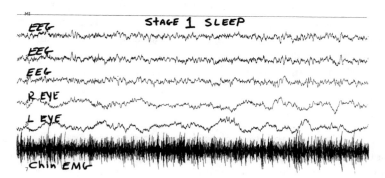

Figure 38.2 Stage 1 sleep. There is loss of the well-organized alpha rhythms and the appearance of some theta rhythms.

Sleep Stage 1

Stage 1 is usually separated into stages 1A (light drowsiness) and 1B (deep drowsiness). Stage 1A is characterized by desynchronization of the background, with loss of the posterior-dominant alpha rhythm. Theta activity is present but does not predominate (Figure 38.2).

Stage 1B is similar to stage 1A except that slow waves, mainly in the theta range, appear. Vertex waves may be seen during this stage. Positive occipital sharp transients of sleep are seen during this stage.

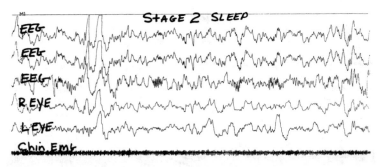

Figure 38.3 Stage 2 sleep. There are well-formed sleep spindles and vertex waves.

Sleep Stage 2

Stage 2 is light sleep. The background consists of a mixture of frequencies (Figure 38.3). Delta activity is present although not as prominently as in deeper stages of sleep. Theta and faster frequencies are superimposed. Differentiation from Stage 1B is made by the appearance of sleep spindles. Fusion of sleep spindles with vertex waves results in the K complex. Vertex waves and K complexes are frequent.

Sleep Stage 3

Stages 3 and 4 are slow-wave sleep. Stage 3 is characterized by delta activity with a frontal predominance. Sleep spindles, vertex waves, and K complexes persist but are not as prominent as during stage 2. Mittens are seen during this stage and are composed of a vertex wave fused to the end wave of a spindle. The small spindle wave is the thumb of the mitten and the slow vertex wave is the hand.

Sleep Stage 4

Stage 4 sleep is characterized by a predominance of slow activity in the delta range (Figure 38.4). The delta has a frontal predominance. Although some faster frequencies may be superimposed, sleep spindles and vertex waves are seldom seen and, if present, are poorly formed.

Rapid Eye Movement Sleep

Rapid eye movement (REM) sleep is characterized by the predominance of low-voltage fast activity (Figure 38.5). Electro-oculography and

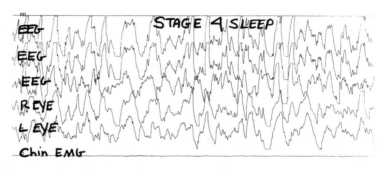

Figure 38.4 Stage 4 sleep. Delta activity predominates with very little EMG activity.

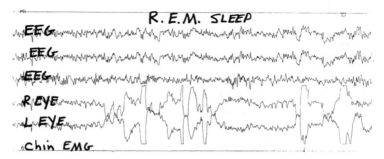

Figure 38.5 Rapid eye movement sleep. Eye movements are predominant, along with a mixed frequency EEG pattern. There is little EMG activity.

electromyography recordings are especially helpful in differentiating this stage from a normal drowsy pattern.

Rapid eye movement sleep usually does not occur within 60 minutes of sleep onset. Sleep-onset REM is seen in patients with narcolepsy, however. Early-onset REM may also be seen in some patients with sleep-deprivation, delirium tremens, and brain stem lesions.

Clinical Indications for Polysomnography

PSG includes not only nocturnal sleep testing, but also multiple sleep latency testing and ambulatory PSG. Detailed indications for sleep testing, recommended in the guidelines of the American Electroencephalographic Society (1994) (referred to as the *Guidelines* here), are presented below.

Briefly, the following are general clinical recommendations that are open to personal bias.

- Nocturnal PSG is indicated in patients who have clinical evidence of sleep apnea or who have excessive daytime sleepiness. These conditions suggest a nocturnal sleep disorder.
- Multiple sleep latency testing is indicated when narcolepsy is suspected. Multiple sleep latency testing cannot be used to support the diagnosis of narcolepsy if the clinical history is not consistent. Excessive daytime sleepiness, alone, is probably not an indication for multiple sleep latency testing.

The *Guidelines'* official recommendations list the following indications for sleep monitoring:

- Episodes of sleep at inappropriate times
- Insomnia
- Hypersomnia
- Atypical behavioral events during sleep (e.g., somnambulism, seizures, respiratory abnormalities, excessive movements)
- Assessment of effectiveness of treatment for sleep disorders

Long-duration EEG monitoring of patients with suspected seizures usually does not require all of the physiologic monitoring commonly performed during PSG studies. Measurement of some physiologic parameters may be helpful, however, particularly in patients who may have autonomic components to the seizures.

39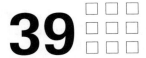

Technical Aspects of Polysomnography

The technical recommendations for polysomnography (PSG) are taken largely from the Guidelines in EEG, Evoked Potentials, and Polysomnography (American Electroencephalographic Society, 1994). For the duration of this chapter, these recommendations are referred to as the *Guidelines*.

Nocturnal Polysomnography

Measured Physiologic Parameters

The *Guidelines* recommends that the following physiologic parameters be measured:

- EEG
- Electro-oculogram (EOG)
- Submental EMG
- ECG
- Respiration
- Blood oxygenation
- Expired carbon dioxide
- Body and limb movement
- Audiovisual monitoring and behavioral observation
- Linear and elapsed time

These parameters are discussed individually. Not all laboratories record all of these parameters; however, this is recommended for accurate interpretation of the recordings.

Electroencephalogram

The *Guidelines* recommends that at least six channels of EEG be recorded. The following electrode positions should be used as a minimum:

- Fp1 and Fp2
- C3 and C4
- O1 and O2
- T3 and T4

Electrodes are attached using the same techniques described for routine EEG. Collodion is more dependable for long-term recording than the use of electrode gel alone and is therefore preferable for PSG.

Montages are determined by the examiner, but he or she should follow guidelines for routine EEG montages as described by the American Electroencephalographic Society (1994). Only one montage should be used to facilitate rapid sleep scoring. Paper speed for PSG is routinely set at 10 mm/sec, although faster speeds are occasionally helpful. When data are displayed on a screen, the display should conform to this standard format.

Electro-Oculogram

Two channels are used for routine EOG recordings. Electrodes are placed in the following positions:

- 1 cm above and 1 cm lateral to the left eye
- 1 cm below and 1 cm lateral to the right eye
- Left ear or mastoid
- Right ear or mastoid

The two channels are each eye lead in reference to the ipsilateral ear. Using this montage, eye movements can be clearly differentiated from frontal slow activity. Eye movements will produce potentials of opposite polarity in the two eye leads. Frontal slow activity will produce either slow waves of the same polarity or independent slow waves in the two channels.

Submental Electromyogram

Submental EMG is recorded using standard cup electrodes placed underneath the chin. The electrodes are connected to a standard EEG amplifier with the low-frequency filter set at 10 Hz and the high-frequency filter set at 70 Hz. Gain is adjusted for each individual but is in the same range as for EEG, or about 7 μV/mm.

Submental EMG is reduced in deep stages of sleep and virtually abolished in rapid eye movement (REM) sleep. The absence of EMG activity aids in identification of REM sleep.

Electrocardiogram

The ECG is recorded using two electrodes on the chest, usually on the rostral sternum and lateral chest. Standard self-stick ECG electrodes are satisfactory. The low-frequency filter is set at 5 Hz and the high frequency filter at 70 Hz. Gain is adjusted for each individual but is usually set at approximately 75 µV/mm. Available settings differ between machines.

Recording of ECG serves two basic purposes. First, heart rate can change with respiratory distress, so that patients with sleep apnea and resultant hypercarbia and hypoxia may have initial tachycardia followed by profound bradycardia. In this situation, ECG gives an estimate of the severity of the apnea. The second purpose of ECG monitoring is to identify cardiac artifact in EEG channels. This is seldom a problem with PSG because the technician should have minimized artifact before beginning the study. Also, bipolar montages greatly reduce ECG contamination.

Respiration

Diagnosis of sleep apnea requires knowledge of both respiratory effort and airflow. Respiratory effort is recorded using thoracic and abdominal strain gauge transducers, intercostal EMG, or thoracic and abdominal impedance. Airflow is usually monitored using thermal sensors near the nares and mouth. Alternating current recordings can be made if the time constant is sufficiently long (i.e., ≥1 second); however, direct current recordings are preferable.

Absence of airflow with preserved and even enhanced respiratory efforts indicates obstructive sleep apnea. Absence of airflow with depression in respiratory effort indicates central sleep apnea. Changes in respiration have to be correlated with blood oxygenation and expired carbon dioxide.

Blood Oxygenation

The pulse oximeter is most commonly used for measurement of oxygen saturation. Output of the oximeter is fed to the recorder by a direct current–coupled amplifier, since absolute measurements require steady-state direct current recordings. The oximeter is fastened to an earlobe or finger. The oximeter is fairly accurate but may give a falsely high reading in patients with carbon monoxide in their blood (i.e., smokers). Oximeters may give falsely low results in patients with cool extremities or poor peripheral circulation.

Expired Carbon Dioxide

Small tubes are placed below each nostril and near the mouth for sampling expired air. The air at end-expiration is largely alveolar, so that determination of carbon dioxide content is a fairly good indication of gas exchange. Patients with obstructive disorders will have a fall-off in expired carbon dioxide content during the obstruction and may have higher carbon dioxide content after clearing of the obstruction.

Body Movement

A surface electrode is placed over the tibialis anterior on one side for recording EMG. This can reveal the presence of myoclonus and may aid in the diagnosis of restless legs syndrome. Alternatively, accelerometers, which are small devices taped to the limb, can be used. Accelerometers produce a signal with a very small amount of movement. They are not used as much as surface EMG because of their expense and the different type of connection to the input amplifiers that they require. Because submental EMG is already recorded, placing additional EMG leads is conceptually and technically easier.

Video for Behavioral Observation

Monitoring of patient behavior using a closed-circuit camera is essential. The other physiologic parameters can often be recorded by the same video tape recorder, after analog-to-digital conversion. Split-screen viewing of the video image, EEG, and physiologic signals is desirable, although there is the potential for error if the resolution is not satisfactory.

The camera is positioned so that it can easily view the patient in bed. The camera should be able to provide a good image even in low light that is conducive to sleep. Additional light can be provided by an infrared source. These light sources will activate the detectors in the cameras but will not alert the patients. Audio monitoring is provided by a sensitive microphone placed such that it can detect vocalizations and respiratory effort. The recording equipment should be located outside of the patient's room so that machine noises and adjustments by the technician do not interfere with the patient's sleep. The most important aspects of behavior to observe are muscle twitches, signs of arousal, axial and limb movements, respiratory effort, and seizures.

Time

Time of onset and cessation of recording should be noted on the record. If a paper record is made, time can be calculated from the number of pages between onset time and an event. If a video recording is made, most video equipment provides for a digital time marker on the screen. Some laboratories record data on both videotape and paper. This is, in general, discouraged, because of the difficulty in precisely comparing events at identical times. Accurate time markers can minimize this error.

Recording Protocol for the Standard Nocturnal Study

The following guidelines summarize the requirements for a standard nocturnal study:

- Make the room comfortable and quiet. Place the recording equipment in a separate room.
- Begin as close to normal sleep time as possible.
- Minimize interruptions. Extra electrodes and sensors facilitate maintaining adequate recording if the patient dislodges primary electrodes and sensors.
- Duration of recording should ideally be 8 hours, with 6.5 hours as a minimum.

Multiple Sleep Latency Test

The multiple sleep latency test (MSLT) is performed in the daytime and can be performed in standard EEG laboratories without special equipment. Patient preparation is minimal, although it is important to ensure that no sedatives are taken within 1 week of the test, since the results will be influenced by sedative drug effect or sedative withdrawal. The *Guidelines* recommends performing the MSLT during the day following a nocturnal sleep study, so that the quality of sleep is known.

Conventional EEG electrodes are placed, and a waking recording is made. The patient is asked to go to sleep. The technician marks the time on the record.

The MSLT is performed as follows:

1. Patient has a normal night's sleep prior to the recording. Some neurophysiologists believe that it is important to have the patient under PSG study to evaluate the quality of the night's sleep. This helps to determine whether a positive MSLT might be caused by a disorder of nocturnal sleep, rather than being primary. A PSG recording is probably not necessary in all patients.

Table 39.1   Montages Used in Polysomnography[a, b]

Recording	Leads
EEG	C3-A2
	C4-A1
	O1-A2
	O2-A1
Electro-oculogram	OS-A1
	OD-A2
EMG	Submentalis

OS = left eye; OD = right eye.
[a]There are no official recommendations; however, these are adequate for staging routine records.
[b]Only EEG, electro-oculogram, and EMG channels are shown here. Other physiologic parameters are described in the text.

2. Electrodes are placed according to the 10–20 Electrode Placement System. The entire array is probably not necessary; however, it is easily placed in most EEG laboratories. If a limited array is placed, central and occipital leads are essential for identification of central vertex activity and the posterior dominant rhythm. (Samples of montages for EEG and noncerebral electrodes are shown in Table 39.1.) In addition to EEG leads, electrodes should be placed for monitoring the following physiologic parameters:
    a. EOG
    b. Submental EMG
    c. ECG
3. At least four naps are begun at scheduled intervals. The technician lowers the lights and asks the patient to go to sleep. Approximately 15 minutes are recorded before the first nap. After the "goodnight" command, recordings are made until the following criteria are met.
    a. 20 minutes without sleep
    b. 15 minutes of continuous sleep
    c. 20 minutes of interrupted sleep, even if less than 15 minutes of sleep occurred

40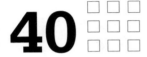

Interpretation of Polysomnographic Recordings

Interpretation of Nocturnal Polysomnogram

Sleep Staging and Interpretation of Nocturnal Polysomnography

Grading of sleep records is typically done in 20- to 40-second epochs. The 40-second epoch is convenient because this is the time for two pages of recordings at a paper speed of 15 mm/sec. An epoch is classified according to the predominant pattern during the epoch. For example, an epoch characterized mainly by a desynchronized background may be classified as stage 1 even though there is occasionally some posterior alpha activity.

Sleep onset is defined as either the first of three contiguous epochs of stage 1 sleep or the first epoch of any stage 2, 3, or 4 sleep. Three consecutive epochs of stage 2, 3, or 4 sleep are not required. With simultaneous monitoring of many physiologic variables, the amount of generated data can be overwhelming. The *Guidelines* (American Electroencephalographic Society, 1994) recommends the following sleep measurements:

- Total time in bed
- Duration of interspersed wakefulness
- Total sleep time
- Sleep latency
- Rapid eye movement (REM) latency
- Number of awakenings
- Time in each sleep stage (actual and percentage)

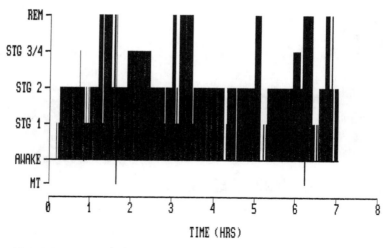

Figure 40.1 Histogram of sleep stages during a night of polysomnographic recording in a normal patient.

Sleep efficiency is the percent of total time in bed spent asleep. In addition, graphs of sleep stage progression are drawn (Figure 40.1). These are usually done using simple computer programs.

The following respiratory measurements and determinations are made:

- Respiratory rate in the wake and sleep states
- Presence of snoring
- Presence of paradoxical respiratory patterns
- Number and type of apneic episodes
- Frequency and degree of oxygen desaturation

ECG data are analyzed for the following:

- Mean and range of heart rate during wake and sleep states
- Arrhythmias, if present
- Cardiac response to respiratory changes (e.g., apnea)

EMG data are analyzed for myoclonus, and differentiation is made between myoclonus associated with arousal, myoclonus associated with epileptiform activity on EEG, and myoclonus not associated with other physiologic changes.

Table 40.1 Polysomnography Findings in Common Sleep Disorders*

Disorder	Findings
Narcolepsy	Rapid eye movement–onset sleep
Obstructive sleep apnea	Respiratory effort without air movement Eventual arousal
Central sleep apnea	Loss of respiratory effort during drowsiness or deep sleep Eventual arousal
Drug-related insomnia	Fragmented rapid eye movement sleep periods

*This table presents the most common distinguishing findings.

Polysomnographic Findings in Common Sleep Disorders

Sleep disorders can be classified into the following categories:

- Hypersomnias
- Insomnias
- Disorders of the sleep-wake cycle
- Arousal and paroxysmal disorders in sleep
- Excessive daytime sleepiness

Some investigators include seizures induced by sleep as a sleep disorder. This is really an underlying seizure disorder with sleep as an activating method, however. The neurophysiologic findings in specific sleep disorders are summarized in Table 40.1.

Narcolepsy

Narcolepsy is characterized by daytime sleep attacks. There are two types of narcolepsy: (1) non-REM, or isolated, narcolepsy and (2) REM, or compound, narcolepsy. Non-REM narcolepsy is characterized by non-REM sleep during attacks. Night sleep is normal. Patients with REM narcolepsy have REM sleep during their daytime attacks. At night, there is sleep fragmentation and shortened REM latency. The multiple sleep latency test (MSLT) may detect short REM latency or sleep-onset REM. The MSLT tests naps but may catch a narcoleptic sleep attack.

Sleep Apnea

Sleep apnea is probably the most common clinical reason for ordering polysomnography. There are three basic types of sleep apnea: (1) obstructive, or peripheral, apnea; (2) nonobstructive, or central, apnea; and (3) mixed apnea.

All types are characterized by loss of air flow for 10 seconds or more. Patients with obstructive sleep apnea continue to have respiratory effort that gradually increases because the movements are ineffectual (Figure 40.2). Eventually, partial arousal results in opening of upper airway passages and restoration of ventilation. Patients with central sleep apnea lose air movement because of loss of respiratory drive. With subsequent hypoxia and hypercarbia, there is partial arousal and restoration of normal ventilatory effort.

Interpretation of the Multiple Sleep Latency Test

Measurements

The following physiologic measurements are made during the multiple sleep latency test: (1) latency from "goodnight" to sleep onset, and (2) latency from sleep onset to REM sleep. Forty-second epochs are scored according to the predominant background. If an epoch is mainly desynchronized with slow roving eye movements but contains a small amount of posterior dominant alpha, the epoch is still scored as stage 1. Sleep onset is identified as the first of three consecutive stage 1 epochs, or any epoch of stage 2, 3, 4, or REM.

Mean sleep latency is the average of the sleep latencies determined for each nap. Some neurophysiologists do not consider a test to be interpretable unless the patient falls asleep with two or three of the naps.

Interpretation

The most characteristic abnormality found with multiple sleep latency tests is short sleep latency. A mean sleep latency of less than 5 minutes is virtually diagnostic of hypersomnolence. Latency of 10 minutes or more is normal. A mean sleep latency between 5 and 10 minutes is borderline. The report may indicate that consistent mean sleep latency of less than 10 minutes is suggestive of a sleep disorder but is not diagnostic.

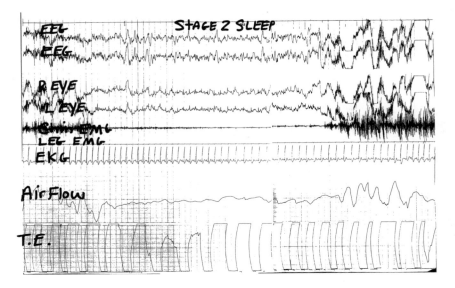

Figure 40.2 Obstructive sleep apnea. There is attenuation of airflow with continuation of thoracic effort. Eventually, arousal is accompanied by an increased effort and movement of air (see the airflow tracing and compare with the thoracic effort [TE] at the bottom of the figure).

Mean sleep latency is altered by the following conditions:

- Sleep deprivation
- Certain medications, especially sedatives, antihistamines, and stimulants
- Withdrawal of some medications
- Age

Withdrawal of medications such as benzodiazepines and barbiturates can have sustained effects; therefore, the medications should be stopped at least 2 weeks before the study.

Many patients with excessive daytime sleepiness will have shorter sleep latencies. Patients with narcolepsy will often have sleep-onset REM periods. The interpreter should be sure that the patient is not sleep-deprived before making the conclusion of sleep-onset or short-latency REM periods.

Glossary

Aliasing   Alteration in waveform due to digital sampling at too slow a rate. Some frequencies may be mistaken for slower frequencies.

Alpha   EMG activity in the 8- to 12-Hz range. This term usually is applied to the posterior activity seen in the waking state with the eyes closed (*alpha rhythm*) or the frontal activity seen in some patients with severe brain damage (*alpha coma*).

Alpha coma   Coma due to severe brain damage, characterized by a relative loss of normal activity and the presence of activity in the alpha range, most prominent in the frontal regions. This activity signifies a poor prognosis for functional recovery.

Ampere   A unit of current. One coulomb of charge flowing past a point in a conductor each second is a current of one ampere (1 amp) (from André Ampere, an eighteenth-century French physicist).

Amplifiers   Devices that magnify a signal so that it is large enough to drive a display unit. Ideally, they produce no change in the waveform of the signal.

Analog data   Data represented by continuous fluctuations in voltage. Compare with Digital data.

Analog-to-digital (A/D) converter   Electronic device that converts an analog signal into a digital signal using a defined sampling rate and voltage resolution.

Anode   The positive terminal of a power supply.

Antidromic   Stimulation of a nerve so that the action potential is conducted in the opposite direction to normal nerve impulse flow. Antonym: orthodromic.

Axonotmesis   In nerve trauma, breakage of the axons with the connective tissue sheath remaining intact.

Beta   EEG activity above 12 Hz. Beta is most commonly seen in the frontal regions after sedation and with skull defects. This activity is normal.

Blink reflex   EMG procedure. Brain stem reflex with stimulation of the trigeminal nerve and activation of facial muscles.

Breach rhythm   EEG pattern characterized by a localized region of prominent beta activity. This rhythm is due to a skull defect, giving less attenuation of cortical potentials.

Brief small-amplitude polyphasic motor unit potential (BSAP or BSAPP)
Descriptive term for myopathic motor unit.

Capacitor   A circuit element with the capacity to store energy in the form of an electric charge across two separated conducting plates.

Cathode   The negative terminal of a power supply.

Charge   A quantity of negatively charged electrons or positively charged holes. The unit of charge is the coulomb.

Circuit   A closed loop of circuit elements (such as resistors or capacitors) through which current flows.

Complex repetitive discharge   Repetitive discharge of several muscle fibers. This EMG pattern is usually considered abnormal.

Conduction block   Segment slowing or block of nerve conduction velocity.

Conductor   A substance that is conducive to the flow of electrons. This type of material typically has unpaired electrons in orbitals that can fairly easily be encouraged to move within the material.

Coulomb   A unit of measure of charge. One coulomb is the charge carried by 6.24×10^{18} electrons (or holes) (from Charles de Coulomb, an eighteenth century French physicist).

Current   The flow of charge. Current can be described as either the flow of negatively charged electrons in one direction or the flow of positively charged holes in the opposite direction.

Decibel (dB)   A unit of measure of electrical signal intensity or sound intensity. For electrical signals, the number of decibels difference between two signals is equal to 20 times the log of the ratio of the amplitudes of the signals. For example, a 1,000-fold difference in signal intensity is a 60-dB difference.

Delta   EEG activity in the frequency range below 4 Hz. Delta waves may be single or multiple. Interpretation depends on the clinical situation. Delta activity is a normal component of sleep; however, delta in awake adult patients is always abnormal. The implications of delta activity differ depending on conformation and distribution. Compare with Frontal intermittent rhythmic delta activity (FIRDA) and Polymorphic delta activity.

Digital data   Data represented by discrete data points over time. Compare with Analog data.

Displays   Devices that show the change in signal with time and/or topography. Types include cathode x-ray tube and chart (paper) display.

Dwell time   Sampling time of an analog-to-digital converter. This is the interval between samples. Preferred terms are *sampling rate* or *sampling interval*.

Early recruitment   Abnormal EMG pattern. With increased muscular effort, excessive numbers of units are recruited because the contraction with each is inefficient.

Electron   A negatively charged atomic particle. It is the smallest unit of charge.

F wave   A motor nerve is stimulated and the response recorded from the muscle. The first potentials are the M response. At 30–55 ms, the secondary response is the F wave.

Fasciculation Spontaneous discharge of a motor axon and its muscle fibers. It may be normal, although it is seen in axonal neuropathies, especially motoneuron disease.

Fibrillation potentials Spontaneous EMG activity due to single muscle fiber action potentials. It is common in denervation and myopathies.

Filters Simple electric circuits that de-emphasize unwanted electrical signals. Common types are high-frequency filter, low-frequency filter, and 60-Hz filter. Filters may be active or passive.

14-Hz and 6-Hz positive spikes Normal variant EEG patterns.

Frontal intermittent rhythmic delta activity (FIRDA) Episodic slow activity from the frontal regions, suggestive of a disconnection between deep nuclei and the cerebral cortex. This EEG pattern is considered abnormal.

Frontal sharp transients Spontaneous EEG sharp waves. Normal in neonates.

Grid The signal inputs of amplifiers, for example, G1 and G2. The term is derived from grids in tube devices.

Ground A common reference for the patient and amplifiers. It may or may not be in continuity with the building ground.

H reflex Electrophysiologic equivalent of the tendon reflex, typically elicited by stimulation of the tibial nerve and recording from the soleus.

Hole The opposite of an electron. More accurately represented as the absence of an electron. It therefore has a positive charge.

Impedance Resistance of a circuit when dependent on frequency. Impedance is used especially when a circuit involves capacitive elements.

Inductor A circuit element that can store energy in a magnetic field created by moving charge.

Kirchhoff laws Basic laws governing circuit theory (from Gustav Kirchoff, a nineteenth-century German physicist).

Lambda waves Occipital waves thought to be related to visual exploration.

Leak current The usually small amount of current that flows from a circuit to ground. If a patient and equipment are not properly grounded, the leak current may be sufficient to affect electrically sensitive organs, such as the heart.

M response The response caused when a motor nerve is stimulated during nerve-conduction studies, the muscle is excited, and the electrical activity is recorded by surface electrodes.

Mu rhythm Central 10- to 12-Hz rhythm, characteristically abolished by movement of the contralateral hand. This is a normal EEG rhythm.

Myopathic motor unit Low-amplitude potential with multiple phases. This is an abnormal EMG pattern.

Myotonia Repetitive muscle fiber action potentials seen on EMG in myotonic dystrophy, myotonia congenita, paramyotonia congenita, and hyperkalemic periodic paralysis.

Neurapraxia In nerve trauma, disruption of nerve fiber function without transection of the axons.

Neuropathic motor unit High-amplitude, long-duration polyphasic motor unit potential. This is an abnormal EMG pattern.

Neurotmesis In nerve trauma, complete transection of the nerve.

Noise Loosely, recorded electrical activity that is unwanted for analysis.

Strictly, electrical activity recorded that does not originate in the patient but rather in the electrodes, wires, equipment, or any combination thereof. The latter definition does not include muscle artifact.

Ohm   The unit of resistance. A 1-ohm resistance allows 1 amp of current to flow from a 1-V battery (from Georg Ohm, a nineteenth-century German physicist).

OIRDA   *See* Posterior intermittent rhythmic delta activity.

Orthodromic   Stimulation of a nerve so that conduction of the action potential is in the same direction as normal nerve impulses. Antonym: antidromic.

Polymorphic delta activity (PDA)   Irregular delta waves with theta superimposed. Implies a focal structural lesion.

Positive occipital sharp transients of sleep (POSTS)   Occipital sharp waves seen in sleep. This is a normal EEG pattern.

Positive sharp wave   Muscle fiber action potential seen in EMG recordings. Seen in denervating diseases and myopathies and similar to fibrillation potentials. This is an abnormal EMG pattern.

Posterior intermittent rhythmic delta activity (PIRDA)   Similar to FIRDA and has the same implications as FIRDA, except with posterior predominance. It is seen in children and is an abnormal EEG pattern. Also called OIRDA.

Posterior slow waves of youth   Slow waves superimposed on the waking background. It is a normal EEG pattern.

Potential difference   The amount of energy required to separate a given quantity of charge. This is a measure of the ability to do work. It is measured in volts.

Power   The rate at which energy can be transferred from a power supply to electrons. Also, the square of the amplitude of a specific frequency found after frequency analysis of a waveform.

Power supply   A circuit element that imparts energy to electrons, which subsequently descend the electrical gradient toward the ground or opposite pole of the power supply. It may be a battery (direct current), alternating current line power, or output of a transformer.

Pseudomyotonic discharge   Archaic term for complex repetitive discharge.

Reduced recruitment   Abnormal EMG pattern characterized by a reduced number of motor units activated by voluntary contraction. It is characteristic of denervating diseases.

Resistor   A circuit element that opposes the flow of electrons by dissipating voltage imparted to the electrons.

Sampling interval   Interval between samples measured by an analog-to-digital converter.

Sampling rate   Rate of sampling of an analog-to-digital converter. Sampling rate is the inverse of Sampling interval.

Secondary demyelination   Peripheral neuropathy caused by damage primarily to the axon or neuron that results in some damage to the myelin. This secondary demyelination causes a slowing of nerve conductions but to a much lesser extent than would be expected with primary demyelinating neuropathies.

Semiconductor   A material that is by nature a nonconductor but has been doped with a material to slightly increase its conductivity.

Slow waves of youth   *See* Posterior slow waves of youth.

Stimulators   Devices that activate sensory nerve fibers to produce an evoked response from a biological system. Types include not only direct electrical stimulators but also visual and auditory stimulators.

Theta   EEG activity in the frequency band from 4 Hz to 7 Hz. Theta activity is normal in young children in the waking state and in sleep in patients of all ages. Theta activity in the waking state of adults is abnormal.

Time constant   For filters, the time taken for the response to a step change in signal voltage to return to 37% $(1/e)$ of baseline. Measured in seconds.

Transducers   Devices that transform biological energy into electrical energy. EEGs and EMGs are already electrical and do not need transduction. Muscle tension and limb movements require transduction.

Transistor   A circuit element that uses one input to gate the flow through two other terminals. It is therefore a key element in amplifiers.

Volt   A measure of electrical potential difference between two points. This is the driving force for movement of electrons. One volt of potential difference can drive 1 coulomb of charge per second through a resistance of 1 ohm (from Count Alessandro Volta, a nineteenth-century Italian physicist).

Voltage resolution   A measure of the ability of an analog-to-digital converter to discern voltage differences. Determined by the number of bits of the converter. For example, a 12-bit converter can define 4,096 (2^{12}) voltage levels. If the converter is set to have an analog input range of –10 V to +10 V, the voltage resolution is 20/4,096 = 0.0049 V.

□ □ □
□ □ □
□ □ □

Annotated Bibliography

American Electroencephalographic Society. Guidelines in EEG, evoked potentials, and polysomnography. J Clin Neurophysiol 1994;11:2–127. *Required reading for everyone who performs or interprets EEGs and evoked potentials.*

Aminoff MJ. Electrodiagnosis in Clinical Neurology (3rd ed). New York: Churchill Livingstone, 1992. *Covers clinical neurophysiology with a moderately comprehensive approach. Well written and well edited.*

Chiappa KH. Evoked Potentials in Clinical Medicine (3rd ed). New York: Raven, 1997. *This latest edition was announced in 1996. Previous editions are excellent comprehensive texts of evoked potentials.*

Culebras A. Clinical Handbook of Sleep Disorders. Boston: Butterworth–Heinemann, 1996. *Comprehensive textbook of sleep disorders with essentials of diagnosis and treatment. Includes discussion of how to set up a sleep lab, self-help suggestions for patients, and an overview of pediatric sleep disorders.*

Daly DD, Pedley TA (eds). Current Practice of Clinical Electroencephalography. New York: Raven, 1990. *An excellent text. Especially good figures. A good reference to use while reading confusing EEGs.*

Dimitrijevic MR, Halter JA. Atlas of Human Spinal Cord Evoked Potentials. Boston: Butterworth–Heinemann, 1995. *Excellent explanations and diagrams of intraoperative evoked potentials. Intended for those already well versed in evoked potentials.*

Dyck PJ, Thomas PK, Griffen JW, et al. (eds). Peripheral Neuropathy (3rd ed). Philadelphia: Saunders, 1993. *Comprehensive text on peripheral neuropathy. Excellent reference.*

Ekstedt J, Nilsson C, Stalberg E. Calculations of the electromyographic jitter. J Neurosurg Psychiatry 1974;37:526.

Hughes JR. Two forms of the 6/sec spike and wave complex. EEG Clin Neurophysiol 1980;48:535.

Kimura J. Electrodiagnosis in Diseases of Nerve and Muscle: Principles and Practice (2nd ed). Philadelphia: FA Davis, 1989. *A solid text for nerve conduction velocities and EMG. Not only covers the details of the individual tests but also discusses some clinical aspects of neuromuscular disorders.*

Kryger MH, Roth T, Dement WC. Principles and Practice of Sleep Medicine. Philadelphia: Saunders, 1989. *Comprehensive text on polysomnography. Considered a bible by many sleep-disorder physiologists.*

Liveson JA. Peripheral Neurology: Case Studies in Electrodiagnosis. Philadelphia: FA Davis, 1991. *Good annotated case presentations. Discusses not only the implications of nerve conduction velocities and EMG findings but also what studies are indicated.*

Medical Consultants on the Diagnosis of Death to the President's Commission for the Study of Ethical Problems in Medicine and Biomedical and Behavioral Research. Guidelines for the determination of death. JAMA 1981;246:218.

Miller CR, Westmoreland BF, Kiass DW. Subclinical rhythmic EEC discharge of adults (SREDA): further observations. Am J EEG Technol 1985; 25:217.

Misulis KE. Basic electronics for clinical neurophysiology. J Clin Neurophysiol 1989;6:41.

Misulis KE. Spehlmann's Evoked Potential Primer (2nd ed). Boston: Butterworth–Heinemann, 1994. *Update of a solid evoked potential text. Intended for those new to the field.*

Misulis KE, Fenichel GM. Genetic forms of myasthenia gravis. Pediatr Neurol 1989;5:205.

Perotto A. Anatomical Guide for the Electromyographer: Limbs and Trunk (3rd ed). Springfield, IL: Thomas, 1994.

Russell GB, Ridichok LD. Primer of Intraoperative Neurophysiologic Monitoring. Boston: Butterworth–Heinemann, 1995. *Discussion of a broad range of intraoperative techniques from electrocorticography to evoked potential monitoring, transcranial Doppler, and basic physiology.*

Schaumburg HH, Berger AR, Thomas PK. Disorders of Peripheral Nerves. Philadelphia: FA Davis, 1992. *Discusses the essentials of peripheral nerve diseases, including mononeuropathies.*

Task Force for the Determination of Brain Death in Children. Guidelines for the determination of brain death in children. Arch Neurol 1987;44:587.

Index

Abductor pollicis brevis, EMG studies of, 227
Absence seizures, 84, 137
  three-per-second spike-wave complex in, 138–140
Acetylcholine receptors, 189
  in myasthenia gravis, 229, 271
Acetylcholinesterase deficiency, 273
Acoustic neuromas, brain stem auditory-evoked potentials in, 293, 301
Action potentials, 8–10
  compound motor, 195. *See also* Compound motor action potentials (CMAPs)
  conductance changes in, 9
  from muscle fibers, 189–190
  propagation of, and nerve conduction, 10
  sensory nerve, 198–199
    low-amplitude, 200
    medial-radial comparisons, 252
    unstable waveform of, 275
Activation methods for EEG, 97, 129–134
  hyperventilation, 129–130
  photic stimulation, 130–132
  sleep, 132–134
  withdrawal of anticonvulsants, 134
Active filters, 34
Active sleep, neonatal, 161–162
Aging
  alpha rhythm in, 104
  effect on nerve conduction, 199
  and EPs, 289
  and maturation of EEG, 162–164
  and maturation of posterior dominant rhythm, 112–113
  and recording sensitivity of EEG, 96

  sleep stages in, 118
  theta rhythm in, 106
Aliasing, 50, 353
Alpha rhythm, 104–105, 111, 353
  in children, 104, 112–113
  in coma, 105, 353
  posterior dominant, 111
    maturation of, 112–113
    sedation affecting, 176
    slowing of, 151
  sharp waves in, 135
  slow variant of, 127
Ambulatory EEG monitoring, 174–175
Ampere, 5, 353
Amplifiers, 37, 41–45, 353
  in active filters, 34
  balanced, 43
  differential, 43–45, 123–124
  driver, 42
  interface with electrodes, 66–68
  and preamplification, 42
Amplitude
  absolute, 50
  digital analysis of measurements, 47, 50
  of EPs, 289
  integrated, 50
Amyotrophic lateral sclerosis, 259
  EMG and nerve conduction velocity findings in, 247
Amyotrophy, diabetic, 261
Analog data, 353
Analog signal, 48
Analog-to-digital (A/D) conversion, 48–50, 169–170, 185, 353
Anatomic anomalies
  affecting EPs, 332
  in innervation, 279–280

Anesthesia
  affecting EEG patterns, 176
  affecting EPs, 327, 328, 329
Anions, 6
Anode, 353
Anoxic encephalopathy, 137, 148
Anterior interosseous syndrome, 253
Anticonvulsants, withdrawal of, in acti-
    vation of epileptiform activity,
    134
Antidromic stimulation, 197–198, 353
Apnea in sleep, polysomnography in,
    340, 349, 350
Arbovirus encephalitis, 137
Artifacts
  in ambulatory EEG, 174
  from electrocardiography, 121
  from electromyography, 120–121, 217
  in EPs, 331
    in monitoring, 329
    rejection of, 287
    VEPs, 312
  eye movement, 109, 118–120
  glossokinetic, 122
  high-voltage, in electromyography,
    217
  machine, 124
  movement, 71–72
    from electrode-gel interface,
      122–123
    from electrode leads, 123–124
  rejection of, 52–53
    in EP studies, 287
  removal with 60-Hz filters, 35, 97
  respiratory movement, 85
  shock, in sensory nerve conduction
    studies, 197, 206
  and signal-to-noise ratio, 69–70
  sources of, 97
  in telephone transmission EEG, 97
Ataxia, Friedreich's, 262
Atomic structure and charge, 3
Atrophy, spinal muscular, 260
Audiometry
  BAEP technique in, 303–304
  pure tones in, 294
Auditory-evoked potentials, brain stem,
    285, 293–304
Averaging of responses, 47, 51–52
  artifact rejection in, 52–53
  in EPs, 285, 286, 331

in sensory conduction studies, 187
and signal-to-noise ratio, 70
Axon hillock depolarization, 10, 80
Axonal neuropathies, 244, 259
Axonotmesis, 353

Balanced amplifier, 43
Band width, 29
Barbiturates
  coma from, burst-suppression pattern
    in, 148
  for sedation, 134
Becker muscular dystrophy, 263, 264
Bell's palsy, blink reflex in, 212
Beta activity, 105, 106, 111, 353
  drugs affecting, 106, 111
  sedation affecting, 176
Biceps brachii, EMG studies of, 227
Biceps femoris short head, EMG studies
  of, 227
Biological calibration in EEG, 94
Biological tissues, electrical properties
  of, 6–15
Blindness
  congenital, occipital spikes in, 147
  cortical, VEPs in, 315
Blink reflex, 210–214, 353
Blocking
  of muscle fiber action potentials,
    234, 235, 236
  of nerve conduction velocity, 200,
    354
    myelin lesions affecting, 190
Botulism, 229, 231, 232, 233, 272, 274
Brachial plexus lesions, 245, 255, 256
Brain death
  BAEP tests in, 302
  in children, 156–157, 158
  determination with EEG, 96,
    157–158
  duration of EEG recording in, 96
  guidelines for determination of,
    155–158
  in newborn, 168
Brain electrical activity. *See* Electroen-
    cephalography
Brain mapping, 48, 171–172
Brain stem auditory-evoked potentials
    (BAEPs), 285, 293–304
  in acoustic neuromas, 293, 301
  anatomic variations affecting, 332

in audiometry, 303–304
in brain stem tumors and strokes, 301–302
in childhood, 300
in coma and brain death, 302
data analysis in, 297–300
in diabetes mellitus, 302
electrode placement in, 295
interpretation of, 295–300
in intraoperative monitoring, 293, 327–328
in meningitis, 302
montages in, 295
in multiple sclerosis, 302
neonatal, 300–301
recording parameters for, 295, 296
stimulus in, 293–295
    intensity of, 294–295, 296
    rate of, 294, 296
    type of, 293–294
    waveform identification and origin in, 295–297
Brain stem lesions
    blink reflex in, 212–213
    myokymia in, 223
Breach rhythm, 106, 353
Brief small-amplitude polyphasic motor unit potentials, 220, 221, 354
Burst-suppression EEG pattern, 139, 142, 148
    differentiation of, 149, 162

Calcium
    conductance of, 6–8
    role in neuromuscular function, 189
Calibration in EEG, 93–94
    biological, 94
    square wave, 93–94
Capacitance, 25–26
    of skin-gel-electrode interface, 65
    stray, 69, 70, 73, 123, 331
Capacitative current, 25–26
Capacitors, 18, 24–26, 354
    in resistor-capacitor circuits, 29–34
Carbon dioxide expiration, measurements of, 344
Carnitine palmityl transferase deficiency, 266
Carotid endarterectomy, intraoperative monitoring in, 175–177, 320, 329

Carpal tunnel syndrome, 201, 245, 247, 251–252
Cathode, 354
    cathode ray tube displays, 55–58
    in color, 58
    compared to oscilloscopes, 58
    flicker-fusion frequency in, 57
    line triggering in, 56
    stimulus triggering in, 56
    takeoff, 56
Cations, 6
Cerebral cortical potentials, 79–81
Cerebrovascular disease, quantitative EEG in, 172
Cervical radiculopathy, 245
Charcot-Marie-Tooth disease, 261–262
Charge, 3, 6, 354
Children
    absence seizures, 138–139
    alpha rhythms, 104, 112–113
    BAEPs, 300
    behavioral disorders, 146
    benign focal epilepsies, 145–146
    beta rhythm, 106, 112
    brain death, 156–157, 158
    EEG recording sensitivity, 96
    intermittent rhythmic delta activity, 153
    maturation of posterior dominant rhythm, 112–113
    montages for, 91
    muscle fiber density, 237
    occipital epilepsy, 145–146
    posterior slow waves of youth, 106, 113, 151, 357
    rolandic epilepsy, 145
    sleep patterns, 118
    theta rhythm, 112
    vertex waves, 114
Chloral hydrate sedation, 133
Chloride
    conductance of, 6–8
        abnormalities in, 223
    role in neuromuscular function, 189
Chloriding of electrodes, 64, 86
Circuits, 17–27, 354
    elements of, 17–18
    laws of, 18–21
Collision technique in diagnosis of Martin-Gruber anomaly, 279
Collodion for electrode application, 87

Collodion for electrode application—
  continued
  in ambulatory monitoring, 174
  in intensive care unit monitoring,
    175
  in intraoperative monitoring, 176
Coma
  alpha, 105, 353
  barbiturate, burst-suppression pattern
    in, 148
  and brain death studies, 155–158
  BAEP tests in, 302
Common mode rejection, 43, 71
Complex partial seizures, 138, 144
Complex repetitive discharge, 224, 354
Complex waveforms, 29
Compound motor action potentials
    (CMAPs), 195
  decremental response in, 229
  early positive component to, 275
  low-amplitude, 200
  measurements of, 196
  in repetitive stimulation studies, 230
  unstable waveform of, 275
Computer use
  analog-to-digital conversion, 48–50,
    169–170, 185, 353
  in digital filtering, 34–35, 170, 186
  displays with, 55–62
    on paper, 59–62
    on screen, 55–59
Computerized equipment
  in electroencephalography, 169–172
  in electromyography, 185, 239–241
Condensation in brain stem auditory-
    evoked potentials, 294
Conductance, 7
  changes in action potentials, 9
  compared to resistance, 24
  doping affecting, 37
Conduction. *See* Nerve conduction
Conduction block, 200, 354
  from myelin lesions, 190
Conductors, 3–4, 354
Cortical blindness, visual-evoked poten-
    tials in, 315
Cortical fields of dipole, 82
Cortical organization, 79–80
Cortical potentials, cerebral, 79–81
Coulomb, 5–6, 354
Cranial nerves, evaluation with blink

  reflex, 210–213
Creutzfeldt-Jakob disease, 137, 149
Cubital tunnel, ulnar nerve entrapment
    in, 247, 254
Current, 5, 354
  capacitative, 25–26
  in ground loops, 74
  Kirchhoff's law, 20
  leakage, 73–75, 181–182, 355
  relation to resistance and voltage,
    18–19
Cushing's syndrome, 266

Damping, for overshoot of EEG record-
    ing pens, 60, 95
Death, cerebral. *See* Brain death
Decibels, 354
  in BAEP tests, 294
  and turnover frequency, 34
Dejerine-Sottas disease, 262
Delta activity, 105, 106–107, 111, 117,
    354
  intermittent rhythmic, 107, 153, 355
  in newborn, 167–168
  polymorphic, 152–153
    intraoperative, 176
  posterior intermittent rhythmic, 153,
    156
  in waking records, 151
Delta brushes, neonatal, 163
Deltoid muscle, EMG studies of, 227
Dementia, brain mapping in, 171
Demyelination
  distal motor latency in, 200
  F-wave response in, 207, 209
  neuropathies in, 244, 258–259
  secondary, 356–357
Dendrites, depolarization of, 80
Depolarization
  action potentials in, 8–10
  of axon hillock, 10, 80
  of dendrites, 80
  and nerve conduction, 10
  paroxysmal shifts in, 82–84
  in postsynaptic muscle membrane,
    189
  and transmitter release, 11
Depth electrodes, 88
Dermatomyositis, 266
Diabetes mellitus
  BAEP tests in, 302

neuropathy in, 260–261
Differential amplifiers, 43–45, 123–124
Digital data, 354
Digital filters, 34–35, 170, 186
Digital signal analysis, 47–53
  analog-to-digital conversion in,
    48–50, 169–170, 185, 353
  in electroencephalography, 169–172
  in electromyography, 47, 239–241
  quantitative, 50–53
Digitorum brevis, extensor, EMG studies of, 227
Digitorum communis, extensor, EMG
    studies of, 227, 237
Diode function
  of gel-electrode junction, 64
  semiconductor, 39
Dipole
  cortical fields of, 82
  epileptiform, 82
  positive-negative, 80, 81
  of spikes and sharp waves, 135
  tongue as, 122
Dispersed waveform in nerve conduction studies, 200–201
Displays, 55–62, 354
  digital versus paper, for EEG, 86
  paper, 59–62
    dot matrix printers in, 60–61
    pens in, for EEG, 55, 59–60
  screen, 55–59
    cathode ray tubes in, 55–58
    digital, for EEG, 58–59
    liquid crystals in, 59
Doped materials
  in semiconductors, 37
  in transistors, 40
Doppler studies, transcranial, for brain
    death, 156
Dot matrix displays, 60–61
Driving response, photic, 130–131
Drowsiness, rhythmic temporal theta of,
    127
Drugs
  affecting beta rhythm, 106, 111
  anticonvulsant, withdrawal of, 134
  insomnia from, polysomnography in,
    349
  for sedated sleep, 133–134
Duchenne-type muscular dystrophy,
    263, 264

Dwell time in analog-to-digital conversion, 48, 354
Dystrophies, muscular, 263–265

Early recruitment, 225, 354
Eaton-Lambert syndrome, 274
EEG. *See* Electroencephalography
Electrical safety, 73–75, 181–182
Electricity, physics and biology of, 3–15
Electrocardiography
  artifacts from, 121
  grounds causing leak current,
    181–182
  monitor causing noise, 180
  and neonatal EEG, 159
  in polysomnography, 343, 348
Electrochemical gradient, 7
Electrode pops, 72, 179
Electrodes, 63–68
  application with collodion, 87
    in ambulatory monitoring, 174
    in intensive care unit monitoring,
      175
    in intraoperative monitoring, 176
  chloriding process, 64, 86
  depth, 88
  for electroencephalography, 63–66,
    86–90
  for electromyography, 66, 188, 215
    coaxial, 215
    monopolar, 215
    single-fiber, 215
  for EPs, 63–66
    improper placement of, 332
  eye lead placement, 119–120
  gel placement, 87
  gel smear detection, 71
  interface with amplifiers, 66–68
  leads causing movement artifacts,
    123–124
  needle, 66, 87, 188
  for nerve conduction studies,
    187–188
  nonreversible, 64
  placement of
    for BAEP tests, 295
    for electroencephalography, 88–90
    errors in, 181
    for VEPs, 309
  reversible, 64
  ring, 187–188

Electrodes—*continued*
skin-gel-electrode interfaces, 65–66
movement artifacts from, 123
sphenoidal, 88
subdural strip, 88
surface, 86–87
Electroencephalography
activation methods in, 97, 129–134
alpha rhythms, 104–105, 111, 353
slow variant of, 127
amplifiers in, 44–45
benign epileptiform transients of
sleep, 127
beta rhythms, 105, 106
for brain death, 96, 157–158
breach rhythm, 106, 353
calibration in, 93–94
cortical potentials in, 79–81
delta rhythms, 105, 106–107, 111,
117, 354
digital displays for, 58–59
digital signal analysis in, 47–48,
169–172
duration of recording, 96
electrodes in, 63–66, 86–90
epileptiform activity in, 81–84
and EPs, 285, 286, 305
equipment in, 85–86
filters in, 96–97
14- and 6-Hz positive spikes,
126–127, 142, 355
indications for, 103
interpretation of, 101, 103–104
laboratory studies, 98–99
lambda waves, 116, 125, 355
localization of activity in, 107–109
maturation of posterior dominant
rhythm, 112–113
mitten waveforms, 127–128, 338
monitoring with, 173–177
montages in, 90–91
mu rhythm, 124–125
in multiple sleep latency test,
345–346
neonatal, 159–168
noncerebral potentials in, 118–124
normal patterns, 111–128
variants of, 124–128
pen display in, 55, 59–60
pen pressure and damping in, 60,
94–95

physiologic basis of, 79–84
in polysomnography, 335, 342
potentials recorded in, 13–15
quantitative analysis, 169–172
recording sensitivity, 95–96
reports and record keeping, 99–102
rhythmic temporal theta of drowsiness, 127
rhythms in, 104–107
generation of, 79–81
normal patterns of, 111–128
routine recordings, 93–97
sawtooth waves in, 117
scalp potentials in, 81
in sleep disorders, 335, 342
sleep patterns, 113–118. *See also*
Polysomnography, nocturnal;
Sleep
slow activity, 107, 151–154
spikes and sharp waves, 81, 105, 107,
135–149
technical requirements for, 85–102
telephone transmission of, 97–98
theta rhythms, 105, 106, 111, 117,
357
troubleshooting in, 179–182
variant patterns, normal, 124–128
waking rhythms, 111–113
wicket spikes, 125, 142
Electromyography, 215–227. *See also*
Muscle
abnormal activity in, 219–226
cathode ray tubes in, 55–58
common errors in, 277–278
digital signal analysis in, 47, 239–241
electrodes in, 66, 188, 215
equipment for, 185–188
fasciculations in, 220, 221, 222
fibrillations in, 220, 221
findings in common neuromuscular
problems, 243–249
insertional activity in, 217–218
abnormal, 219
in intraoperative monitoring,
240–241
machine settings in, 215–216
motor unit potentials in, 192–194,
218, 219
abnormal, 224–225, 227
digital analysis of, 239–240
and muscle artifacts in EEG, 120–121

muscles studied in, 227
myokymia in, 222–223
myotonic discharges in, 220, 223–224
neuromuscular transmission tests,
    229–237
no recordable potentials in, 277
normal activity in, 217–219
paired stimulation test, 232–233
phasic activation and polyphasic
    potentials compared, 278
in polysomnography, 344, 348
    submental recordings in, 342–343
poor motor unit potential waveform
    in, 277
    fibrillation potentials with,
        277–278
positive sharp waves in, 220, 221–222
potentials recorded in, 13–15
quantitative analysis, 239–241
recruitment in, 218, 220
    abnormal, 225–226
    digital analysis of, 240
repetitive stimulation test, 229–232
single-fiber, 233–237
    blocking in, 234
    fiber density determination in,
        236–237
    jitter analysis in, 233–236
in sleep, 118
spontaneous activity in, 218
techniques, 216–217
ultra-short duration spontaneous
    potentials in, 278
voluntary and spontaneous activities
    compared, 278
Electrons, 3, 354
Electro-oculogram in polysomnography,
    342
Electrotonic conduction, 10
Emery-Dreifuss muscular dystrophy, 264
EMG. *See* Electromyography
Encephalitis
    arbovirus, 137
    herpes simplex, 137, 148
Encephalopathy, anoxic, 137, 148
Endocrine myopathies, 265–267
EP. *See* Evoked potentials (EPs)
Epileptiform activity, 81–84
    in absence seizures, 84
    activation methods, 129–134
    and benign transients of sleep, 127

brain mapping in, 171
compared to rhythmic temporal
    theta of drowsiness, 127
focal spikes in, 143–146
generalized, 84
in neonates, 165–167
paroxysmal depolarization shifts in,
    82–84
periodic lateralized discharges in,
    144, 147–148
rhythmic slow waves in, 153–154
spikes and sharp waves in, 82, 105,
    107
and telemetric monitoring for
    seizures, 173–174
Equilibrium potential, 7–8
Equipment
    for electroencephalography, 85–86
    for EPs, 288–289
    for nerve conduction studies and
        EMG, 185–188
Erb's palsy, 255
Erb's point stimulation for somatosenso-
    ry-evoked potentials, 318, 320
Evoked potentials (EPs), 285–290
    anatomic variations affecting, 332
    artifact rejection and analysis time,
        287
    averaging for, 285, 286
    brain stem auditory, 285, 293–304
    cathode ray tubes in, 55, 57
    digital signal analysis, 47
    electrodes in, 63–66
        improper placement of, 332
    equipment for, 288–289
    interpretation of, 290
    interside differences in, 289
    in intraoperative monitoring,
        327–329
        artifacts in, 329
    motor, 285
    neural generators of, 285–286
        in nerve fiber bundles, 286
        in nuclei, 286
    noise in, 331
    normative data, 289
    photic, 130–131
    poor or unusual waveforms in, 332
    replication of waveforms, 289
    sensory, 285
    somatosensory, 285

Evoked potentials (EPs)—*continued*
   troubleshooting in, 331–332
   visual, 285, 305–316
Excitatory postsynaptic potentials, 11,
      79, 80
Eye leads, placement of, 119–120
Eye movements, 118–120
   compared to frontal slow-wave activ-
      ity, 85, 109
   in neonatal EEG, 159
   rapid, in sleep, 117, 118
      in childhood, 118

F wave, 354
   conduction study, 206–209
   mistaken for H reflex, 276–277
Facial nerve lesions, blink reflex in,
      212–213
Facioscapulohumeral dystrophy, 264, 265
Far-field potentials, 13, 81
   recording of, 13, 15
Farad, 25
Fasciculations, 220, 221, 222, 355
Fast spike-wave complex, 141–142
Fatigue or weakness, 245
Fibrillation potentials, 193, 355
   in electromyography, 220, 221
   with poor motor unit potential wave-
      form, 277–278
Field-effect transistor, 40, 41
Field potentials, 13–15, 135
Filters, 29–35, 355
   active, 34
   digital, 34–35, 170, 186
   in electroencephalography, 96–97
   in electromyography, 186
   high-frequency, 32
   low-frequency, 32
   notch, 35
   passive, 29–34
   60-Hz, 35, 97
   for SEPs, 320
   in square wave calibration, 93
Flicker-fusion frequency, 57
Focal activity
   slowing, 152–153
   spikes, 142–147
Focal loss of EEG patterns, 154
Footdrop, 245
14- and 6-Hz positive spikes, 126–127,
      142, 355

Frequencies, filtering of, 29–35
Frequency dependence
   of capacitative current, 26
   of circuits, 18
Friedreich's ataxia, 262
Frontal activity
   delta, intermittent rhythmic, 107,
      153, 355
      sedation affecting, 176
   sharp transient, 355
   slow wave compared to eye move-
      ments, 85, 109

Gastrocnemius muscle, medial, EMG
      studies of, 227
Gaze, and eye movement detection,
      120
Gel, electrode, 63–64, 87
   in nerve conduction studies, 187
   smear detection, 71
Generalized activity
   slowing, 151–152
   spike-wave discharge, 136–142
Glaucoma, visual-evoked potentials in,
      315
Glossokinetic artifact, 122
Gluteus medius, EMG studies of, 227
Gold neuropathy, myokymia in, 223
Goldman constant field equation, 8
Grid, 355
Ground, 355
   faulty connections in, 73–74, 99
Ground loops, current in, 74
Guillain-Barré syndrome, 208, 223, 247,
      258
Guyon's canal, ulnar nerve entrapment
      in, 247, 253–254

H reflex, 209, 210, 355
   compared to F wave, 276–277
Hand
   pain or weakness in, 245
   variations in innervation of muscles,
      279–280
Harrington rod instrumentation, soma-
      tosensory-evoked potentials in,
      317, 329
Hearing loss, audiometry in, 294,
      303–304
Hereditary neuropathies, 261–262
Herpes simplex encephalitis, 137, 148

High-frequency filters, 32
Holes, 6, 355
Humeroperoneal dystrophy, 264
Hyperpolarization, 9, 83
Hyperthyroidism, beta rhythm in, 106
Hyperventilation as activation method
    in EEG, 97, 129–130, 138
Hypothyroidism, 266
Hypsarrhythmia, 139, 142

Impedance, 355
    in electrode-amplifier interface,
        67–68
Inclusion body myositis, 266
Inductance, stray, 70, 73, 123, 331
Inductors, 18, 26–27, 355
Inertia of EEG recording pens, 60,
    94–95
Inflammatory myopathies, 265, 266
Infraspinatus muscle, EMG studies of,
    227
Inhibitory postsynaptic potentials, 11,
    12, 79, 80
Ink-jet printers, 61–62
Insertional activity in electromyogra-
    phy, 217–218, 219
Insomnia, drug-related, polysomnogra-
    phy in, 349
Intensive care unit monitoring, 175
Intermittent rhythmic delta activity,
    107, 153, 355
Interosseous muscle, first dorsal, EMG
    studies of, 227, 237
Interpotential intervals for two muscle
    fibers, 234
    mean consecutive differences of, 235
Interpretation
    of BAEPs, 295–300
    of electroencephalograms, 101,
        103–104
        in neonatal EEG, 161–168
    of EPs, 290
    of multiple sleep latency test,
        350–351
    of nerve conduction abnormalities,
        200–213
    of nocturnal polysomnogram,
        347–350
    of SEPs
        median nerve, 320–322
        tibial nerve, 325

Intersample interval in analog-to-digital
    conversion, 48
Intraoperative monitoring
    electroencephalography in, 175–177
    EMGs in, 240–241
    EPs in, 327–329
        brain stem auditory, 285, 293,
            327–328
        somatosensory, 317, 320, 327,
            328–329
        visual, 316, 327
Ions
    fluxes of, 6–8
        and depolarization in muscle
            membrane, 189
    negative, 6
    positive, 6
Isaac's syndrome, 269

Jitter
    analysis in single-fiber EMG,
        233–236
    examination with line triggering, 56
Junction, neuromuscular, 189
Junction bipolar transistor, 40–41
Junction potentials
    discharge causing electrode pops, 72,
        179
    gel-electrode, 64
        movement affecting, 72, 123

K complexes in sleep, 114, 115, 116
Kirchhoff's laws, 355
    current, 20
    voltage, 21

Lambda waves, 116, 125, 355
Laser printers, 61
Latencies
    in EPs, 289
        in BAEP data, 297–300, 305
        in SEP data, 305, 317
        in VEP data, 305, 312
    multiple sleep latency tests, 340,
        345–346
Latency measurements
    digital analysis of, 47, 50
    H reflex, 209, 210
    motor nerve, 197
        distal, increased, 200
        F-wave studies in, 208

Latency measurements—*continued*
  sensory nerve, 198–199
    peak, 199
    takeoff, 199
Lateralized epileptiform discharges,
    periodic, 144, 147–148
Leakage current, 73–75, 181–182, 355
Lennox-Gastaut syndrome, 137,
    140–141
Leprosy, 258
Ligament of Struthers compressing
    median nerve, 253
Limb-girdle muscular dystrophy, 263,
    264
Liquid crystal displays, 58
Localization of EEG activity, 107–109
Low-frequency filters, 32
Lumbar region
  plexopathy, 245
  radiculopathy, 245

M response, 195, 355
Machines, artifacts from, 124
Magnetic fields
  changes affecting electron flow,
    26–27
  and ground loops, 74
  and stray inductance, 70, 123
Mapping of brain, 171–172
Martin-Gruber anomaly, 201, 279, 280
Masking, in brain stem auditory-evoked
    potentials, 294
Median nerve, 251–253
  in anterior interosseous syndrome,
    253
  in carpal tunnel syndrome, 251–252
  compression by ligament of
    Struthers, 253
  conduction velocity studies, 201
  F-wave study, 208, 209
  in Martin-Gruber anomaly, 279, 280
  in pronator teres syndrome, 252–253
  SEPs, 318–322
Membrane potentials, 6–8
  resting, 6–7
    in neural tissue, 38
  rhythmic oscillation of, 81
Meningitis, brain stem auditory-evoked
    potential tests in, 302
Meralgia paresthetica, 245
Metabolic myopathies, 265–267

Mitochondrial myopathies, 265, 267
Mitten waveforms, 127–128, 338
Monitoring
  ambulatory, 174–175
  with electroencephalography,
    173–177
    telemetric, for seizures, 173–174
  in intensive care unit, 175
  intraoperative. *See* Intraoperative
    monitoring
Mononeuropathies, 251–258
  multiple, 257–258
  polyneuropathies with, 281
Montages, 90–91
  bipolar, 90, 108
  in BAEP tests, 295
  in digital EEG, 170
  and localization of activity, 107–108
  in neonatal EEG, 160–161
  in polysomnography, 346
  referential, 90
Motor evoked potentials, 285
Motor function, mechanisms in,
    189–190
Motor nerves
  activation of, 189–190
  compound action potentials, 195–197
  conduction studies, 195–197
  degeneration of, 240
  disorders of, 190–191, 245
  F-wave study, 206–209
  multifocal neuropathy, 259
Motor-sensory neuropathies, hereditary,
    261–262
Motor system components, 188–189
Motor unit potentials in EMG, 192–194,
    217, 218, 219, 220
  abnormal, 224–225
  digital analysis of, 239–240
  evaluation of, 217, 218, 219, 220
  myopathic, 225
  neuropathic, 224–225
  polyphasic, 221, 278
    brief small-amplitude, 220, 221, 354
  poor waveforms of, 277
    fibrillation potentials with,
      277–278
Movements
  artifacts from, 71–72, 122–124
  recordings in sleep, 344
Mu rhythm, 124–125, 355

Multiple sclerosis, 231
  BAEP tests in, 302
  myokymia in, 223
  SEPs in, 314, 317
  VEPs in, 314
Multiple sleep latency test, 340,
    345–346, 350–351
Multiplexed signal in telephone trans-
    mission EEG, 97–98
Muscle. *See also* Electromyography
  artifacts, 120–121
  disorders, 263–269
    continuous fiber activity,
      267–268, 269
    dystrophies, 247, 263–265
    inflammatory, 265, 266
    metabolic, 265–267
  extrafusal and intrafusal fibers,
    189–190
  physiology, 188–191
  postsynaptic membrane depolariza-
    tion, 189
  summed potentials of multiple
    fibers, 193, 195
Myasthenia gravis, 229, 230, 232, 233,
    236, 247, 271–272
Myasthenic syndromes, 229, 231, 232,
    233, 272, 274
  neonatal, 272–273
Myelin
  affecting nerve conduction, 10
  disorders of, 190, 191. *See also*
    Demyelination
Myelopathy, somatosensory-evoked
    potentials in, 317, 320
Myoclonic epilepsy, juvenile, 137
Myoclonus detection in sleep, 344,
    348
Myokymia in electromyography,
    222–223
Myopathic motor unit potentials, 225,
    355
Myopathy, 244, 248
Myositis, 265, 266
Myotonia
  compared to complex repetitive dis-
    charge, 278
  congenita, 267, 268
  in electromyography, 220, 355
Myotonic discharges in electromyogra-
    phy, 220, 223–224, 265

Myotonic dystrophy, 264, 265

N-doped materials
  in semiconductors, 37
    and NP junctions, 38
  in transistors, 40
Narcolepsy
  polysomnography in, 340, 349
  REM-onset sleep in, 117
Near-field potentials, 13
  bipolar, 13–15
  unipolar, 13
Needle electrodes, 66, 87, 188
Nernst equation, 7
Nerve conduction, 10, 195–214
  action potential propagation in, 10
  age affecting, 199
  blink reflex study, 210–213
  common errors in, 275–277
  dispersed waveform in, 200–201
  early positive potential in, 275
  electrotonic, 10
  equipment for, 185–188
  excessive 60-Hz interference in, 276
  F wave in, 206–209
    mistaken for H reflex, 276–277
  findings in common neuromuscular
    problems, 243–249
  guidelines for, 214
  H reflex in, 209, 210
    F wave mistaken for, 276–277
  high-voltage long-duration stimulus
    in, 277
  increased distal motor latency, 200
  interpretation of abnormalities,
    200–214
  low-amplitude potentials, 200
  median nerve, 201
  motor nerve studies, 195–197
  no recordable potentials in, 276
  normal data for, 193
  peroneal nerve, 204
  radial nerve, 204
  reduced velocity, 200
  routine studies, 195–199
  saltatory, 10, 189
  sensory nerve studies, 197–199
  sural nerve, 205–206
  and sympathetic skin response, 213
  temperature affecting, 199
  tibial nerve, 204–205

Nerve conduction—*continued*
ulnar nerve, 202–203
unstable waveforms in, 275
velocities of, 191–192
Nerve physiology, 188–191
Neurapraxia, 355
Neuromuscular function
abnormal, 190–191
evaluation of common problems in,
243–249
motor, 189–190
normal, 189–190
sensory, 190
transmission disorders, 244, 271–274
transmission tests, 229–237
paired stimulation, 232–233
repetitive stimulation, 229–232
single-fiber EMG, 233–237
Neuromuscular junction, 189
Neuromyotonia, 268, 269
Neuronal degenerations, 259–260
motor, 244
sensory, 244
Neuropathic motor unit potentials,
224–225, 355
Neuropathies
axonal, 244
demyelinating, 244
peripheral, 243–244, 245
Neurotmesis, 355
Neutrons, 3
Newborn
BAEPs, 300–301
electroencephalography in, 159–168
abnormal, 164–168
background abnormalities in,
167–168
burst-suppression pattern in, 148
duration of recording in, 96
dysmaturity in, 164–165
maturation of, 162–164
montages in, 91–92, 160–161
normal, 161–164
recording procedures, 159
spikes and sharp waves in, 107
epileptiform activity in, 165–167
intraventricular hemorrhage of, 82
myasthenic syndromes, 272–273
wake and sleep cycle in, 161–162
Nodes in circuits, 20
Noise, 355

from capacitance, 26
in EPs, 331
from induction, 18, 27
signal-to-noise ratio, 52, 69–70
60-Hz, 70–71. *See also* 60-Hz interference
sources of, 179–181
Nonconductors, 4
Normal EEG patterns, 111–128
Notch filters, 35
NP junctions, 38

Occipital activity
delta, intermittent rhythmic, 107,
153
in epilepsy, 137, 144, 145–146
sharp transients of sleep, positive, 82,
115–116, 356
spikes in congenital blindness, 147
Ohms, 17, 356
Ohm's law, 18–19
Optic neuritis, visual-evoked potentials
in, 312–313
Orthodromic stimulation, 197–198, 356
Oscilloscope displays compared to cathode ray tube, 58
Overshoot of EEG recording pens, 60, 95
Oximeters, pulse, 343

P-doped materials
in semiconductors, 37
and NP junctions, 38
in transistors, 40
Paired stimulation test, 232–233
Palmar branch of ulnar nerve, lesion in,
254
Palmar stimulation test in carpal tunnel
syndrome, 252
Palsy
Bell's, blink reflex in, 212
Erb's, 255
peroneal, 246, 247, 256
Panencephalitis, subacute sclerosing,
137, 149
Paper displays, 59–62
Parallel resistance, 23–24
Paralysis, periodic, 269
hyperkalemic, 267
hypokalemic, 267
Paramyotonia congenita, 268
Parietal sharp waves, 144

Paroxysmal depolarization shifts, 82–84
Partial seizures
    complex, 138, 144
    simple, 138, 143–144
Passive filters, 29–34
Pen EEG display, 55, 59–60
Periodic EEG patterns, 144, 147–149
    lateralized epileptiform discharges,
        144, 147–148
Periodic paralysis, 269
    hyperkalemic, 267
    hypokalemic, 267
Peripheral nerve disorders, 251–262
    diabetic neuropathy, 260–261
    hereditary, 261–262
    mononeuropathies, 251–258
    polyneuropathies, 258–260
Peroneal nerve
    accessory, 280–281
    conduction velocity studies, 204
    F-wave study, 209
    neuropathy, 256
    palsy, 246, 247, 256
    SEPs, 322
Peroneus longus, EMG studies of, 227
Petit mal variant, 140
Phantom spike-wave pattern, six-per-
    second, 139, 142
Phasic muscle activation, 278
Photic stimulation
    as activation method in EEG, 97,
        130–132
    driving response in, 130, 131
    EP in, 130, 131, 285, 305–309
    normal response in, 130–131
    photoconvulsive response in, 132,
        133
    photomyoclonic response in, 132
Photoconvulsive response to photic
    stimulation, 132, 133
Photomyoclonic response to photic
    stimulation, 132
Poliomyelitis, 260
Polyarteritis nodosa, 258
Polymorphic delta activity, 152–153
Polymyositis, 247, 265, 266
Polyneuropathies, 258–260
    demyelinating, 258–259
    mononeuropathies with, 281
Polyphasic motor unit potentials, 221,
    278

Polysomnography, nocturnal, 340,
    341–351
    indications for, 339–340
    interpretation of, 347–350
    physiologic parameters measured in,
        341–345
    requirements for standard studies, 345
Pops, electrode, 72, 179
Positive charge, flow of, 6
Positive occipital sharp transients of
    sleep, 82, 115–116, 356
Positive sharp waves in EMG, 220,
    221–222, 356
Postpolio syndrome, 260
Posterior dominant rhythm. *See* Alpha
    rhythm
Posterior intermittent rhythmic delta
    activity, 153, 356
Posterior interosseous syndrome, 255
Posterior slow waves of youth, 106, 113,
    151, 356
Postsynaptic potentials, 11–12
    excitatory, 11, 79, 80
    inhibitory, 11, 12, 79, 80
Potassium
    conductance of, 6–8
        in action potential, 9
    hyperkalemic periodic paralysis, 267
    hypokalemic periodic paralysis, 267
    role in neuromuscular function, 189
Potential(s)
    action, 8–10
    brief small-amplitude polyphasic,
        221, 225
    cortical, cerebral, 79–81
    equilibrium, 7–8
    evoked, 285–290
    extracellular, 13
    field, 13–15, 135
    membrane, 6–8
    motor unit, 192–194
    noncerebral, 118–124
    postsynaptic, 11–12
    resting, 6–7
    scalp, 81
Potential difference, 4–5, 356
    capacitor, 26
    in power supply, 17
Power, 356
Power spectral analysis of signals, 30,
    48, 53, 170–171

Power spectral analysis of signals—
  continued
  in intensive care unit monitoring, 175
Power spectrum, 29
Power supply, 17, 356
Preamplifiers, 42
  in electrode junction box, 69
Preterm infants, abnormal EEG patterns
    in, 166
Printers for paper displays, 60–62
  dot matrix, 60–61
  ink-jet, 61–62
  laser, 61
  thermal transfer, 62
Pronator teres
  EMG studies, 227
  syndrome, 247, 252–253
Protein, conductance of, 6–8
Protons, 3
Pseudo-beta-alpha-theta-delta rhythm in
    newborn, 167
Pseudomyotonic discharge, 356
Pseudotumor cerebri, visual-evoked
    potentials in, 314–315
Psychomotor variant EEG rhythm, 127
Pulse oximeters, 343
Pure tones in brain stem auditory-
    evoked potential tests, 294

Quantitative analysis, 50–53
  in electroencephalography, 169–172
    brain mapping in, 171–172
    digitized data in, 169–170
    monitoring with, 173–177
    and power spectral analysis,
      170–171
    spike detection in, 170
  in electromyography, 239–241
Quiet sleep, neonatal, 161–162

Radial nerve
  compression at spiral groove,
    254–255
  conduction velocity studies, 204
  neuropathy, 246
  in posterior interosseous syndrome,
    255
Radiation plexopathy
  compared to neoplastic infiltrations,
    255
  myokymia in, 223

Radiculopathy, 247
  diabetic, 251
Rapid eye movement (REM) sleep, 117,
    118
  in childhood, 118
  equivalence in newborn, 161
  in narcolepsy, 349
  in newborn, 164
Rarefaction in brain stem auditory-
    evoked potentials, 294
Record keeping in EEG, 102
Recruitment patterns in EMG, 218, 220
  abnormal, 225–226
  digital analysis of, 240
  early, 225, 263, 354
  reduced, 225, 356
Rectus femoris, EMG studies of, 227
Reduced recruitment, 225, 356
Refsum's disease, 262
Repetitive discharge of muscle fibers,
    220, 223–224
  complex, 224, 354
    mistaken for myotonia, 278
Repetitive stimulation test, 229–232
  common errors in, 278–279
  at fast rates, 231–232
  at slow rates, 230–231
Repolarization
  after prolonged depolarization, 82–83
  mechanisms in, 9
Reports
  for electroencephalography, 99–102
  for EPs, 290, 291
Resistance
  compared to conductance, 24
  in electrodes and amplifier input,
    66–67
  relation to current and voltage, 18–19
Resistor-capacitor circuits, 29–34
Resistors, 17–18, 21–24, 356
  in parallel, 23–24
  in series, 22–23
Respiration
  movements in
    artifacts from, 85
    in neonatal EEG, 159
  recordings in polysomnography, 343,
    348
Resting activity in electromyography,
    217, 218, 220
Resting potential, 6–7, 38

Restless legs syndrome, body movements recorded in, 344
Rhythm generation in EEG, 79–81
Rhythmic activity
  oscillations of membrane potentials, 81
  spikes in epilepsy, 82, 83
Ring electrodes, 187–188, 197
Rolandic epilepsy, 137, 144, 145
Roll-off, in frequency response, 34

Safety, electrical, 73–75, 181–182
Saltatory conduction, 10
  myelin lesions affecting, 190
  and neuromuscular function, 189
Sampling interval, 48, 356
Sampling rate in analog-to-digital conversion, 48–50, 287, 356
Sawtooth waves, 117
Scalp potentials, 81
Scapuloperoneal dystrophy, 264, 265
Schwartz-Jampel syndrome, 268, 269
Sciatic nerve lesions, 246, 257
  compared to peroneal palsy, 256
  piriformis syndrome, 257
  stretching, 257
Scoliosis surgery, somatosensory-evoked potentials in, 317, 329
Sedation, EEG patterns in, 176
Seizure activity. *See* Epileptiform activity
Semiconductors, 4, 18, 37–39, 357
Sensitivity of EEG recording, 95–96
Sensory evoked potentials, 285
Sensory function, mechanisms in, 190
Sensory nerve(s)
  action potential (SNAP), 198–199
    low-amplitude, 200
    medial-radial comparisons, 252
    unstable waveform of, 275
  conduction studies, 195–197
  degeneration, 244
Series resistance, 22–23
Serratus anterior, EMG studies of, 227
Sharp waves, 105, 107, 135–149
Shock
  artifact in sensory nerve conduction studies, 197, 206
  voltage recommended for nerve conduction studies, 214
Signal averaging. *See* Averaging of responses

Signal-to-noise ratio, 52, 69–70
Six-per-second spike-wave complex, 139, 142
60-Hz interference, 70–71, 123–124, 180–181
  excessive, 276
  filtering of, 35, 97
  rejection by differential amplifiers, 43, 124
Sleep
  as activation method in EEG, 97, 132–134
  alpha rhythm in, 116, 336–337
  apnea in, polysomnography in, 340, 349, 350
  benign epileptiform transients of, 127
  beta rhythm in, 106
  delta rhythm in, 106, 117, 338
  deprivation of, 134
  in EEG laboratory, 98–99
  electromyography in, 118
  generalized slowing in, 151–152
  indications for polysomnography, 339–340. *See also* Polysomnography, nocturnal
  K complexes in, 114, 115, 116, 337, 338
  multiple sleep latency test, 340, 345–346
  in newborn, 161–162
  normal EEG patterns in, 103, 113–118
    in childhood, 118
  physiologic basis of, 335–336
  positive occipital sharp transients in, 82, 115–116
  rapid eye movement (REM), 117, 118, 338–339
    in childhood, 118
  sedated, 133–134
  seizure activity in, 84
  slow waves in, 141, 338
  spindles in, 115, 117, 338
    in childhood, 118
  stages of, 114, 116–117, 336–339
    aging affecting, 118
  sequence of, 117–118
  theta rhythm in, 106, 114, 117, 337, 338
  vertex waves in, 114, 117, 337, 338
    in childhood, 118

Slow activity, 107, 151–154
  alpha variant, 127
  from eye movement, 119
  focal, 152–153
  and focal loss of EEG patterns, 154
  frontal activity compared to eye
      movement, 85, 109
  generalized, 151–152
  localization in montages, 109
  posterior, of youth, 106, 113, 151,
      357
  in posterior dominant rhythm, 151
  rhythmic waves in seizures, 153–154
  in sleep recordings, 151–152
  spike-wave complex in, 139, 140–141
  on waking background, 151
Slow-channel syndrome, 273
Slow-wave sleep in newborn, 162
Sodium
  channels for
    depolarization affecting, 8–10
    time dependent, 9
    voltage dependent, 9
  conductance of, 6–8
  role in neuromuscular function, 189
Somatosensory-evoked potentials (SEPs),
      285, 317–325
  in intraoperative monitoring, 317,
      327, 328–329
  of median nerve, 318–322
    interpretation of, 320–322
    stimulus and recording parame-
        ters in, 318–320
    waveform identification in, 320
  in multiple sclerosis, 314, 317
  in myelopathy, 317
  stimulus in, 317
  of tibial nerve, 322–325
    interpretation of, 324–325
    stimulus and recording parame-
        ters in, 322–323
    waveform identification in,
        323–324
  of ulnar nerve, 322
  waveform generation in, 317
Sphenoidal electrodes, 88
Spikes and sharp waves, 105, 107,
      135–149
  burst-suppression of, 139, 142
  compared to nonspike potentials,
      135–136

digital analysis of, 170
  in epileptiform activity, 82
  fast complex, 141–142
  focal, 142–147
    with epilepsy, 143–146
    without seizures, 146–147
  14- and 6-Hz positive, 126–127, 142
  frontal transients, 355
  generalized, 136–142
  hypsarrhythmia, 139, 142
  localization in montages, 108
  in newborn, 167
  normal, 136
  occipital, 144, 145–146, 147
  parietal sharp waves, 144
  periodic patterns, 144, 147–149
  positive, in electromyography, 220,
      221–222, 356
  rolandic, 144, 145
  six-per-second phantom pattern, 139,
      142
  slow complex, 139, 140–141
  temporal sharp waves, 144
  three-per-second complex, 138–140
  wicket, 125, 142
Spinal canal stenosis, 246
Spinal muscular atrophy, 260
Spinal surgery, somatosensory-evoked
      potentials in, 317, 328–329
Spindles, sleep, 115, 117
  in childhood, 118
Spontaneous activity in electromyogra-
      phy, 218
Square wave calibration in EEG, 93–94
Standard deviation in evoked potentials,
      289
Step voltage, 29
Steroid myopathy, 266
Stiff-man syndrome, 268, 269
Stimulators, 357
Stray capacitance, 69, 70, 73, 123
  in EPs, 331
Stray inductance, 70, 73, 123
  in EPs, 331
Strokes, brain stem auditory-evoked
      potential tests in, 301–302
Struthers ligament compressing median
      nerve, 253
Subdural strip electrodes, 88
Supraspinatus muscle, EMG studies of,
      227

Sural nerve, conduction velocity studies, 205–206
Surface electrodes, 86–87
Surgery, monitoring in. *See* Intraoperative monitoring
Sympathetic skin response, 213
Synaptic transmission, 11–12
and EPs, 286
Synchronous activation of neurons, and epileptiform activity, 81–82, 84

Tarsal tunnel syndrome, 246, 247, 256–257
Telemetric monitoring for seizures, 173–174
Telephone transmission of EEG, 97–98
Temperature affecting nerve conduction, 199
Temporal activity
sharp waves, 144
theta, 106
rhythmic, of drowsiness, 127
Tetanus, 267–268, 269
Thalamocortical afferents, activation of, 80
Thermal transfer printers, 62
Theta activity, 105, 106, 111, 117, 357
in newborn, 162
sharp waves in, 135
subclinical rhythmic discharge of adults, 146
temporal, 106
rhythmic, of drowsiness, 127
in waking records, 151
Thoracic outlet syndrome, 246, 247
SEPs in, 320
Three-per-second spike-wave complex, 138–140
Threshold in depolarization, 9
Tibial nerve
conduction velocity studies, 204–205
F-wave study, 209
neuropathy, 256–257
SEPs, 322–325
Tibialis anterior muscle, EMG studies of, 227, 237
Time
resolution of, and sampling rates, 48–49, 287
for sleep recordings, 344–345
Time constant, 357

in resistor-capacitor circuit, 32–33
and square-wave calibration, 93
Tongue movement, artifact from, 122
Tonic-clonic seizures, generalized, 138, 141, 142
Toxic axonal neuropathies, 259
Tracé alternant pattern in newborn, 162
Tracé discontinu pattern in newborn, 162
Transducers, 357
Transients
frontal sharp, 355
of sleep
benign epileptiform, 127
positive occipital, 82, 115–116, 356
spikes and sharp waves, 135
Transistors, 37, 39–41, 357
field-effect, 40, 41
unction bipolar, 40–41
Triceps muscle, EMG studies of, 227
Trigeminal nerve lesions, blink reflex in, 212–213
Troubleshooting
in electroencephalography, 179–182
electrical safety in, 181–182
electrode position in, 181
noise in, 179–181
in EP studies, 331–332
in nerve conduction studies and EMG, 277–279
Tumors
BAEP tests in, 301
VEPs in, 314
Turnover frequency, 34

Ulnar nerve
conduction velocity studies, 202–203
F-wave study, 209
in Martin-Gruber anomaly, 279, 280
neuropathies, 246, 253–254
cubital tunnel, 247, 253
Guyon's canal, 247, 253–254
palmar branch lesion, 254
SEPs, 322

Vastus medialis muscle, EMG studies of, 227
Velocities in nerve conduction, 191–192
motor, 195–197
reduced, 200

Velocities in nerve conduction—
  continued
  sensory, 197–199
Ventilator artifacts, 180
Vertex waves in sleep, 114, 117
  in childhood, 118
Video for behavioral observation in
    sleep, 344
Viral myositis, 266
Visual-evoked potentials (VEPs), 285,
    305–316
  anatomic variations affecting, 332
  artifacts in, 312
  in cortical blindness, 315
  electrode placement in, 309, 332
  in functional visual loss, 315
  interpretation of, 312–315, 316
  in intraoperative monitoring, 316,
    327
  in multiple sclerosis, 314
  in ocular and retinal disorders, 315
  in optic neuritis, 312–313
  in pseudotumor cerebri, 314–315
  recording parameters in, 308, 310
  stimulus in, 305–309
    flash, 305, 306

  half-field pattern-reversal,
    305–306, 309
  pattern-reversal, 305, 306–309
  in tumors, 314
  waveform identification in, 310–312
Volt, 17, 357
Voltage, 5
  drop across resistors, 17–18, 21
  Kirchhoff's law, 21
  levels in analog-to-digital conversion,
    48
  relation to current and resistance,
    18–19
  step, 29
Voltage resolution, 357
Volume conduction, 13

Waking state, 336–337
  EEG rhythms in, 111–113
  theta and delta activity in, 151
Warburg impedance, 65
White noise in brain stem auditory-
    evoked potential tests, 294
  Wicket spikes, 125, 142
  negative, in mu rhythm, 124–125